Contract Research and Development Organizations-Their History, Selection, and Utilization

Shayne C. Gad • Charles B. Spainhour
David G. Serota

Contract Research and Development Organizations-Their History, Selection, and Utilization

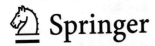 Springer

Shayne C. Gad
Gad Consulting LLC
Cary, NC, USA

David G. Serota
7th Inning Stretch Consulting LLC
Kalamazoo, MI, USA

Charles B. Spainhour
Scott Technology Park
Calvert Laboratories
Scott Township, PA, USA

ISBN 978-3-030-43075-7   ISBN 978-3-030-43073-3   (eBook)
https://doi.org/10.1007/978-3-030-43073-3

This Springer imprint is published by the registered company Springer Nature Switzerland AG
The registered company address is: Gewerbestrasse 11, 6330 Cham, Switzerland

Preface

Dr. Gad was privileged to start his career in toxicology more than 43 years ago in a testing laboratory that was a hybrid of a company lab and a contract testing lab (the Chemical Hygiene Fellowship of Carnegie Mellon Institute of Research, later known as Bushy Run Labs). This institution was a near-perfect environment to learn the practical aspects of regulatory toxicology testing while also being pushed to stay abreast of the then rapidly flowering science of toxicology. Though he has not been employed in the contract research environment full time since then, he has worked as a highly regarded safety and toxicology consultant for and utilizing such organizations on a daily basis since.

Alternatively, Dr. Spainhour started his career working for a small ethical pharmaceutical company by the name of Smith, Kline & French Ltd. During his 20-year tenure there, he managed to work in a variety of different disciplines in drug discovery and drug development, gaining knowledge and experience understanding the mechanics and the process of how drugs are discovered and developed. After taking leave to earn his V.M.D. and Ph.D., he started and ran his own veterinary practice, provided forensic consulting services, and performed research at Texas A&M University for 6 years. Eventually, he opted for an opportunity to work for a very small CRO, Pharmakon Research Laboratories, and learned firsthand what contract research is all about and over 26 years highly successfully grew and developed that business. The things that he learned along the way and the relationships that he established have been of critical importance in formulating his current views and strategies today.

Finally, Dr. Serota has spent his entire 40 plus years working in toxicology CROs. He, who was asked by the other authors to contribute to this new edition, spent 40+ years working entirely at three different CROs as both a senior scientist and a senior company leader. Having entered into the field of contract research toxicology at the exact same time that the GLPs were first being formulated and implemented, he has experienced many different and unusual situations over the years that make him well qualified to contribute to this publication. Combined, the three principal authors have more than approximately 110 years' experience working for and with CROs.

At least through the point of completion of initial studies in humans, virtually all pharmaceutical and medical device development is performed primarily by one form or another of contractor. It is only because of contract research organizations (CROs) that the recent advances in basic science have been translated to the medical wonders that have become available in the last quarter of a century, with the CROs providing the essential regulatory compliant underpinnings of science and technology. Success in pharmaceutical and medical device development requires many things, but the probability of a positive outcome is vastly improved if the individuals and companies seeking to develop these new products truly understand the armamentarium of technology available to them. The last 15 years has seen a shift in where both regulatory and investigative toxicology are performed in two senses. First, most such work is no longer performed in company laboratories but rather in specialized fee-for-service organizations, primarily guided by freestanding individuals who are paid for their expertise and experience. Second, while the contract CROs used to be almost entirely located in North America, Europe, and Japan, their locations are now ever increasingly global.

Raleigh, NC, USA
Clarks Summit, PA, USA
Kalamazoo, MI, USA

Shayne C. Gad
Charles B. Spainhour
David G. Serota

Selected Regulatory and Toxicological Acronyms

510(k)	Premarket notification for change in a device
AALAS	American Association for Laboratory Animal Science
AAMI	Association for the Advancement of Medical Instrumentation
ABT	American Board of Toxicology
ACGIH	American Conference of Governmental Industrial Hygienists
ACT	American College of Toxicology
ADE	Acceptable Daily Exposure
ADI	Allowable Daily Intake
AIDS	Acquired Immune Deficiency Syndrome
AIMD	Active Implantable Medical Device
ANSI	American National Standards Institute
APHIS	Animal and Plant Health Inspection Service
ASTM	American Society for Testing and Materials
AWA	Animal Welfare Act
CAS	Chemical Abstract Service
CBER	Center for Biologics Evaluation and Research (FDA)
CDER	Center for Drug Evaluation and Research (FDA)
CDRH	Center for Devices and Radiological Health (FDA)
CFAN	Center for Food Safety and Applied Nutrition (FDA)
CFR	Code of Federal Regulations
CIIT	Chemical Industry Institute of Toxicology
CPMP	Committee for Proprietary Medicinal Products (United Kingdom)
CPSC	Consumer Product Safety Commission
CSE	Control Standard Endotoxin
CSM	Committee on Safety of Medicines (United Kingdom)

CTC	Clinical Trial Certificate (United Kingdom)
CTX	Clinical Trial Certificate Exemption (United Kingdom)
CVM	Center for Veterinary Medicine (US Food and Drug Administration)
DART	Developmental and Reproductive Toxicology
DHHS	Department of Health and Human Services
DIA	Drug Information Association
DIC	Disseminated Intravascular Coagulation
DMF	Device (or Drug) Master File
DOE	Department of Energy
DOT	Department of Transportation
DSHEA	Dietary Supplement Health and Education Act
EEC	European Economic Community
EM	Electron Microscopy
EMA	European Medicines Agency
EPA	US Environmental Protection Agency
EU	European Union
FCA	Freund's Complete Adjuvant
FDA	US Food and Drug Administration
FDCA	Food, Drug, and Cosmetic Act
FDLI	Food and Drug Law Institute
FHSA	Federal Hazardous Substances Act
FIFRA	Federal Insecticide, Fungicide, and Rodenticide Act
GCP	Good Clinical Practices
GLP	Good Laboratory Practices
GMP	Good Manufacturing Practices
GPM	Guinea Pig Maximization Test
HEW	Department of Health, Education, and Welfare (no longer in existence)
HIMA	Health Industry Manufacturers Association
HSDB	Hazardous Substances Data Bank
IACUC	Institutional Animal Care and Use Committee
IARC	International Agency for Research on Cancer
ICH	International Conference on Harmonization
id	Intradermal
IDE	Investigational Device Exemption
IND(A)	Investigational New Drug Application
ip	Intraperitoneal
IRAG	Interagency Regulatory Alternatives Group
IRB	Institutional Review Board

IRLG	Interagency Regulatory Liaison Group
ISO	International Organization for Standardization
IUD	Intrauterine Device
iv	Intravenous
JECFA	Joint Expert Committee on Food Additives
JMAFF	Japanese Ministry of Agriculture, Forestry and Fisheries
LA	Licensing Authority (United Kingdom)
LAL	Limulus Amebocyte Lysate
LD_{50}	Lethal dose 50: the dose calculated to kill 50% of a subject population, median lethal dose
LOEL	Lowest Observed Effect Level
MAA	Marketing Authorization Application (EEC)
MD	Medical Device
MHW	Ministry of Health and Welfare (Japan)
MID	Maximum Implantable Dose
MOE	Margin of Exposure
MOU	Memorandum of Understanding
MRL	Maximum Residue Limits
MSDS	Material Safety Data Sheet
MTD	Maximum Tolerated Dose
NAS	National Academy of Science
NCTR	National Center for Toxicological Research
NDA	New Drug Application
NIH	National Institutes of Health
NIOSH	National Institute for Occupational Safety and Health
NK	Natural Killer
NLM	National Library of Medicine
NOEL	No-Observable-Effect Level
NTP	National Toxicology Program
ODE	Office of Device Evaluation
OECD	Organisation for Economic Co-operation and Development
OLAW	Office of Laboratory Animal Welfare
PDI	Primary Dermal Irritation
PDN	Product Development Notification
PEL	Permissible Exposure Limit
PhRMA	Pharmaceutical Research and Manufacturers Association
PL	Produce License (United Kingdom)
PLA	Produce License Application
PMA	Premarket Approval Application

PMN	Premanufacturing Notice
PMOA	Principal Mode of Action
po	Per os (orally)
PTC	Points to Consider
QAU	Quality Assurance Unit
RAC	Recombinant DNA Advisory Committee
RCRA	Resources Conservation and Recovery Act
RTECS	Registry of Toxic Effects of Chemical Substances
SARA	Superfund/Amendments and Reauthorization Act
sc	Subcutaneous
SCE	Sister chromatid exchange
SNUR	Significant New Use Regulations
SOP	Standard Operating Procedure
SOT	Society of Toxicology
SRM	Standard Reference Materials (Japan)
STEL	Short-Term Exposure Limit
TLV	Threshold Limit Value
TSCA	Toxic Substances Control Act
USAN	US Adopted Name Council
USDA	US Department of Agriculture
USEPA	US Environmental Protection Agency
USP	United States Pharmacopeia
WHO	World Health Organization

Contents

Contributors

Shayne C. Gad, PhD, DABT, Gad Consulting Services, Raleigh, NC, USA

Robin Guy, MS, DABT, RQAP-GLP, Robin Guy Consulting LLC, Toxicology, Safety Assessment & GLP Consulting, Lake Forest, IL, USA

Christopher Papagiannis, BS, Senior Director, Safety Evaluation/Principal Reserach Scientist, Charles River (CR-MWN), Mattawan, MI, USA

David Serota, PhD, DABT, 7th Inning Stretch LLC, Kalamazoo, MI, USA

Charles B. Spainhour, VDM, PhD, DABFS, DABT, DABFM, Spainhour Consulting, Chinchilla, PA, USA

Introduction

The research-driven components of the global healthcare industry represent an enormous economic and societal force in the world and even at the primary (new product developer) levels are composed of an incredibly diverse set of component organizations. These range from huge multinational corporations to "virtual" organizations, which have only a few part time employees, but are now truly global in scope. While primarily in the private sector, there are also those which are partially or fully funded by various government organizations. There is probably even room for a separate volume on funding models and means of funding for such organizations and the impact of such on development processes. There are "for pay" directories of these available services (e.g., Drug Information Association [DIA] 2018), but these are limited to those who pay for placement and are not at all comprehensive or objective. There are also lists maintained by organizations for their members, which are more comprehensive and less biased by pay-to-play, but never complete in content nor fully current.

For the purposes of this volume, the resulting products from all of the efforts of this sector of the global economy include drugs (pharmaceuticals, biologics, medical foods, nutraceuticals, vaccines, and so forth, intended for both humans and animals), medical devices, and diagnostics. All of these are highly regulated at both regional and a global level during their development and marketing. Though many of the service organizations referred to in this volume also do work for other industries, our focus will concentrate on their activities in the

© Springer Nature Switzerland AG 2020
S. C. Gad et al., *Contract Research and Development Organizations-Their History, Selection, and Utilization*, https://doi.org/10.1007/978-3-030-43073-3_1

more limited pharmaceutical and medical device industrial sectors. While there has always been an element of outsourcing of the research, development, and even manufacturing of these healthcare products, the twenty-first century has seen an almost complete shift to "virtual" approaches by companies developing and seeking to market the products. Currently it is estimated that more than 2000 CROs worldwide serve just the nonclinical and clinical development needs of these industries (more than 200 in just the "toxicology" space).

CROs (also called CSOs (contract service organizations) or PDOs (pharmaceutical development organizations)) span an amazing range of areas of operations and expertise. Though there are some organizations which present themselves as turnkey "we do it all," none of them meet that goal. Many present themselves as "full-service CROs," but most offer primarily distinct niche services and at best can readily subcontract other needed services. These services include:

Biological Pharmacology (in vitro screening, efficacy modeling, safety pharmacology, candidate in vivo screening for final selection), toxicology (genetic toxicology, animal toxicology, biocompatibility testing – with many subsets), pharmacokinetics, and metabolism.

Chemistry Synthesis, API manufacture, radiolabeled synthesis, analytical methods, bioanalytical methods, leachable, and extractable testing.

Clinical Phase I centers, CRA identification and training, statisticians, data and site management, report writing services and for-profit phase II/III sites. Centerwatch.com currently lists more than 54,000 ongoing clinical trials at US and foreign sites.

Dosage form Aspects Formulation developers, drug product manufacturers, CTM (clinical trial material) manufacturers (oral, topical, parenteral, and specifically delivery, labeling, patient kit preparation).

Regulatory IND, NDA, IDE, 510(K), PMA, CTD, DMF, and annual update writers and regulatory advisors.

Consultants Individuals or small groups which provide various scopes of expert guidance and services.

A more detailed breakdown of the scope and types of activities of CROs is provided in Chap. 4. Literally the services provided cover the entire range of activities involved in discovering, selecting leads, developing candidates, and securing market approval for the manufacture, distribution, and marketing of the products in the regulated healthcare industries. This volume will focus on those involved in taking an idea or molecule forward through candidate selection development to the point of getting regulatory approval to primarily market a product.

The authors must also state that most of our careers have been spent in the aspects involved in insuring the safety of products, and therefore we will tend to use the CROs ("toxicology labs") and activities in this area as examples. While such have been the subject of limited directories in the past (Freudenthal 1997; Jackson 1985 and Texas Research Institute 1986), these references have been limited to larger US toxicology facilities. More recently, there has been publication of annual directories by *Contract Pharma*, and DIA, which are actually compendiums of paid advertisements. The earlier edition of this book provided global directories of these facilities, which have been updated in this volume.

We should start by briefly considering the history of such commercial labs. The oldest in the United States is Food and Drug Research Laboratories or FDRL, which opened in the 1930s and then moved from its original site in suburban New Jersey to rural upstate New York. Subsequently, it went out of operation under the FDRL name in the late 1980s. However, the facilities are still in existence and operated under the name and ownership of Liberty Laboratories, which specializes in studies using domestic felines and dog disease model work. Many of the original FDRL employees continues to work at Liberty. However, Liberty has recently been bought, having been a special target of PETA in recent years. Similarly, the Chemical Hygiene Fellowship (CHF) of Carnegie Mellon Institute of Research (CMIR) started as the Union Carbide toxicology lab in 1937 but from its inception additionally performed testing under contract for other businesses.

Starting in the second half of the 1970s, a number of toxicology laboratories (Industrial Bio-Test (IBT), a University of Miami-operated lab; Cannon Laboratories; Bioassay Systems; Litton Biometrics; Tegaris Labs; Bushy Run, which in its earlier years was called the Chemical Hygiene Fellowship of Carnegie Mellon Institute and is perhaps the second oldest contract toxicology research laboratory; Borriston/Midatlantic Laboratories; Primate Research Institute (PRI); Utah Biomedical Test Laboratory (UBTL); HTI; and Oread

Laboratories), just to name a few of significant size, thrived initially but subsequently have gone out of existence. Additionally, just as in the industries they serve, there has been a continued series of acquisitions and mergers. For example, the current Charles River Laboratories includes what were once Sierra Biomedical, Bio-Research, Pathology Associates Incorporated, Argus Research, Redfield Laboratory (site now closed), Springborn Laboratories, MPI Research, WIL Research, and TSI Mason (also until site closed) among its parts. Hazleton become Corning which then evolved to Covance. These same trends and forces have been active in the other types of CROs. There have been noticeable trends where protracted periods of acquisition would be followed by fragmentation into separate laboratories. As has continued shifting generally, the expansion of services offered to expand market, revenues, and profitability. In extreme cases this has led to the evolution of some organizations (such as IQVIA – previously Quintiles, Covance, and MDS Pharma) which offer to "do it all" for the pharmaceutical industry. Periodic economic changes also have served to reshape the "population" of CROs. The history of CROs is the subject of Chap. 2 in this volume.

A vanishing number of companies seeking to develop a new regulated product have limited internal capability to perform the required technical and regulatory work needed to bring a product to market. Although the focus of this book is on drugs, devices, and diagnostics, the information contained herein is also applicable to dietary supplements, cosmetics, pesticides, and many other types of products. From this point on, such companies will be generally referred to as clients or sponsors. Previously, for various reasons, industry will need to contract work to external facilities, whether they are commercial contract laboratories, university laboratories, or even a member company's laboratory as in the case of a consortium study. This "virtual" approach has now become the norm even for the target drug and device companies. As with all contractual arrangements, careful planning and coordination coupled with thorough preparation are required in order to obtain the desired product or service, to avoid confusion and misunderstanding, and to produce a timely and cost-effective result. This volume primarily seeks to serve as a practical guide for those organizations that need to outsource some or all of their activities at external facilities.

The needs for and means of accessing CRO support services are different for each of the majority of client organizations. Such types of organizations can generally be broken down into two different categories. Smaller companies, which have no or only one marketed product and larger organizations, are referred to as "big pharma." The latter comprise traditionally fully integrated companies with multiple products on the market. Issues of timing, cash flow, and getting the product to a point where a "partner" will buy in or at least heavily support the continued development of a product versus taking a product all the way to market as well as what contract resources are needed and how they are to be managed as part of a development program tend to be very different. But the majority of the concerns and issues of individual contract research organization selection, monitoring, and management as presented in this book are common (FDA 1984).

Consultants

While consultants have existed and been active in the industrial hygiene, pharmaceutical, and medical fields for many years, the changes in how development is done, particularly the shift to a higher proportion of smaller and "virtual" companies and the virtual elimination of internal staff by established larger companies, have *transformed* consultants to inherent and critical parts of the process. This is now commonly referred to as the "gig" economy.

From the consultant side, this has meant a shift from consulting being either something done between jobs or late in a career while transitioning to retirement (e.g., "sun setting") to a legitimate long-term career option. For example, the lead author on this volume has been gainfully so employed for more than 26 continuous years.

Consultants may be either narrow or broad in focus in expertise and services offered. They may operate as individuals, with small support staff, or as members of a small group or as a group of employees working within a large consulting company. There are, as yet, few associations of such consultants. The premier version is the Roundtable of Toxicology Consultants (RTC; see www.toxconsultants.com), in which an international membership of more than 140 (currently) individuals has associated both to better market themselves and to be able to draw on mutual knowledge and experience in meeting client needs and supporting each other as "force multipliers while also ensuring adherence to a code of ethics and standards of practices."

Defining the Project

Development of the Study Record

The objective of a study or any research is to evaluate theories and hypotheses and to produce results supporting or disproving the theories. The written evidence of this work is called the study record and includes all records, documentation, and results of the development effort. Let us now consider the logical progression of such research activities and the development of the study record.

Research Plan

The development project begins with developing the study or project plan or simply thinking through what needs to be done and when. Whether the worker is performing internal research, concept evaluations, or work in support of regulatory requirements, this plan should be written down. When written, the research plan becomes the framework for the protocol or contract for the project and includes the hypothesis, the proposed methods, the observations to be made, and the expected results. Researchers should pay special attention to the level of detail in this plan. For example, in regulatory research environments, there are mandated requirements for inclusion of particular details in the protocol and a specified format. Optional experimental methods may be included in the protocol or amended into it as needed, but it needs to be emphasized that they must be recorded. Even if a written protocol or detailed contract is not specifically required for the project, it is useful to develop the habit of producing a protocol because it requires you and your colleagues to think clearly through the experimental design, resources required, and any potential issues. It also provides guidance for the actual conduct of the work and promotes consistency in performance (Fig. 1.1).

General Considerations

There are a number of general aspects to be considered in the operations of a CRO in the regulated environment with which we should be concerned. Most of these, of course, have to do with how things are documented. We will gener-

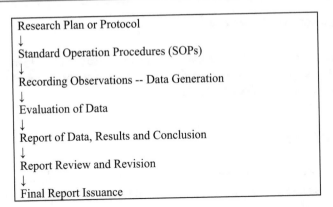

Fig. 1.1 Progression of a contracted study or project

ally use USFDA Good Laboratory Practices (first operative in July of 1979, currently FDA 2015) as our model in this volume, but the principles are the same internationally (Gad 2010, 2018) and for Good Manufacturing Practices and Good Clinical Practices.

Standard Operating Procedures

Some of the procedures performed during a study are routine for the laboratory. CROs formalize the documentation of these routine procedures into written standard operating procedures (SOPs). SOPs are detailed descriptions of such things as animal handling, equipment operation, methods for taking and recording data, and procedures for reagent receipt, storage, and preparation – the types of procedures that are common to all laboratory operations. SOPs should be written in sufficient detail as to promote consistency in performing the procedures, but not in such detail as to make implementation cumbersome from a quality assurance perspective. Having SOPs and insisting that they are followed provides the researcher with a measure of control over potential variables in the experiment.

Regulatory Performance

A good place to initiate an evaluation of any regulated facility is to examine its record of previous inspection results and responses to these. For FDA, these are easy to obtain (FDA 2002b; Gad 2018).

Data Recording

Once the study initiates, as each procedure is performed, it is essential to write down what one did, the date and time it was done, apply a signature, and record the observed results. The level of detail of any written record should enable someone else with equivalent technical training to repeat your experiment exactly as you did. Why? *Reproducibility*. That experimental results must be reproducible is a basic covenant of science. It is the process through which scientific conclusions and discoveries are confirmed. Reproducibility is promoted by the specific data-recording requirements for data that are submitted to FDA and equivalent non-US regulatory agencies. Reproducibility is also required in research performed to support a patent request.

For now, we wish to introduce you to the concept of "if you didn't write it down, you didn't do it." You, the researcher, have the burden of proof in regulated research, in protection of patent rights, and in defense of your work in professional circles. The issue is *completeness* of your records. The study record must be a complete documentation of all data and procedures performed. If you didn't write it down, you didn't do it as far as regulatory agencies and patent offices are concerned. In the experimental record, there are however some accepted shortcuts. Here, some of the hard preparatory work pays dividends. In the written record, one may include references to previously described methods and SOPs, state that they were followed exactly, or describe amendments to or deviations from them. Efficient ways of collecting data may be developed to encourage the complete recording of all required data. Later in this chapter, methods for recording procedures and observations will be discussed in detail.

The *accuracy* of recorded data is another important consideration because any observed result, if not recorded immediately, may not be recorded accurately. Don't lose data because of some rationalization about time, money, or one's ability to remember what happened. All data should be recorded directly into a notebook or onto a worksheet at the time of the observation. Keep in mind that transcribed data – data copied by hand or entered by a person into a computer – is often subject to error. If data are copies to a table or a spreadsheet, the entered data should be checked for complicity against the original data to ensure accuracy. In a regulated research work, all such work and data will also be audited and the accuracy and conformance to all procedures verified.

Analysis of the Data

When the laboratory work is done, the analysis of the data begins. Observed data are entered into formulae, calculations are made, and statistical analyses are performed. All these manipulations must be carefully recorded, because from these data, the conclusions for the study will be drawn. The manipulations of the data are the link between the original observations and the conclusions. Consistency between the data and the result is controlled by monitoring all transcription, manipulation, and correlations of the data in generation of the final manuscript.

Reporting of Results and Conclusions

Finally, a draft final report is provided for review, to the client and/or their agent.

It will receive critical review before acceptance. The final version will then be provided to others and again will receive critical review by other scientists or some skeptical governmental or public audience. In all cases, it will be essential to be able to justify the integrity of the data. Additionally, the methods, the initial data, the calculations and statistical analysis, and the conclusions must be defensible, meaning complete, accurate, internally consistent, and repeatable to withstand scientific criticism.

Types of Data

Earlier we mentioned different elements of the study record research plan or protocol, observations, calculations and statistical output, and conclusions. For ease of explanation, the terminology from the GLPs, GMPs, and GCPs (here on GLPs will be used to stand for all three in the general case) – protocol, raw data, statistical analysis, and final report – will be used to describe the components of the study record.

According to the GLPs, the protocol is a written document that is approved by the study director, the person responsible for the technical conduct of the study and sponsoring organization. The protocol is the research plan or the project plan in a management sense. It clearly indicates the objectives of the research project and describes all methods for the conduct of the work. It includes a complete description of the test system, the test article, the experimental design, the data to be collected, the type and frequency of tests executed, and the planned statistical analysis. Financial considerations should not be included in a protocol, which should be restricted to scientific details. An amendment may be included specifying important milestone dates, but this is not an essential feature, and such a schedule can be specified outside of the protocol.

The protocol needs to be strictly followed during research. "What," you say, "no experimental license, no free expression of scientific inquiry?" Of course there is, as long as the changes in procedures or methods are documented along the way as amendments to the protocol, leaving a written trail of what was done and why it was done. If the work you are doing is governed by strict contractual or regulatory guidelines, you may not be able to express much creativity, but remember the objective, in this case, is to provide consistent and reliable data for comparisons for regulatory purposes. Even the GLPs make provisions to amend the protocol and document any deviations from it. During all research, except perhaps during the most routine analysis, there may be changes in experimental methods and procedures, rethinking of design, decisions to analyze data in new or different ways, or unexpected occurrences that cause mistakes to be made. An important concept to apply here is that these variances from the plan must all be documented. Amendments to a protocol are "planned" changes to the protocol that are documented before they are implemented. Deviations address mistakes or events that are exceptions to the protocol and are documented after the fact.

Raw Data

"Raw data" is the term used to describe the most basic element of experimental observations. It is important to understand fully the concept of raw data. There are unique standards for recording raw data that do not apply to other types of data. These will be discussed later in the chapter. For now, let us look at what constitutes raw data. As regards the FDA and EPA GLPs, (FDA 2002a) raw data means any laboratory worksheets, records, memoranda, notes, or exact copies thereof that are the result of original observation and activities of the study and are necessary for the reconstruction and evaluation of the report of that study. All terms must be taken in the most literal sense and must be interpreted collectively to apply this definition to the data generated during a study or experiment. There are two key phrases: "are the result of original observations and activities of the study" and "are necessary for the reconstruction and evaluation of the report of that study." Raw data includes visual observations, direct measurements, output of instrumental measurements, and any activity (room temperature, room humidity, room airflow, light period, etc.) that describes or has an impact on the observations. Indeed, anything that is produced or observed during the study that is necessary to exactly reconstruct (know what happened) the study and evaluate (analyze or, for regulatory purposes, assess the quality of) the reported results of the study and its conclusions is raw data. This definition of raw data has been carefully designed to encourage the development of data that is defensible and reproducible.

Included in the scope of raw data may be data that result from calculations that allow the data to be analyzed, for example, the results of gas chromatography where the raw data are defined as the curve that was fitted by the instrument software from individual points. The individual points on the curve are essentially meaningless by themselves, but the curve provides the needed basic information. The area under the curve, which is used to calculate the concentration, is an interpretation of the curve based on decisions made about the position of the baseline and the height of the peak. This is not "raw data" since it is not the original observation and may be calculated later and, practically, may be recalculated. For the researcher to completely understand the results, the curve with the baseline, the area under the curve, and the calculations are required to be performed and recorded, but only the curve itself is "raw data." The distinction is that the curve is the original observation and must be recorded promptly. The current advance of the "section" of the GLP, governing how electronic (automated) data is collected, manipulated, audited, verified, stored, and provided to the FDA (section 11), adds another entire dimension to consideration of their issues.

Other Types of Data

Other types of data that are not typically viewed as raw data may be included with the study or experimental records. For example, correspondence, memoranda, and notes that may include information that is necessary to reconstruct and evaluate the reported results and conclusions. While these are not records of original experimental observations, they do represent documentation of the activities of the study and can help with its reconstruction. They often contain approvals for method changes by study management or sponsoring organizations, instructions to laboratory staff for performing procedures, or ideas recorded during the work. Here are some examples of raw data that are generated during a toxicology study:

Test article receipt documents	Equipment use and calibration
Animal receipt documents	Equipment maintenance
Records of quarantine	Transfer of sample custody
Dose formulation records	Sample randomization
Sample collection records	Animal or sample identification
Dosing records	Assignment to study
Animal observations	Necropsy records
Blood collections and analysis	Analytical results
Euthanasia records	Histology records
Pathologist's findings	

For government-regulated research, all electronic or written records that are documentation of the study conduct and results are treated as raw data. From the perspective of the scientific historian, the original notes, correspondence, and observations tell the story of the life and thought processes of the scientist being studied. From the mundane to the extreme, these records are important, a fact which will more than be appreciated when an audit might occur or challenge to the data might develop.

Computerized Data Collection

Special attention must be dedicated to computer-generated raw data. Automated laboratory instrumentation has come into widespread use, usually employing an integrated laboratory information management system (LIMS). In hand-recorded data, the record of the original observation is raw data. But what is considered raw data in computerized systems? In this case, raw data are the first recorded occurrence of the original observation that is readable by a human. This definition treats computer-generated data as hand-recorded data. It documents the "original observations and activities of the study and is necessary for reconstruction and evaluation of the report of that study" (EPA 1989a, 1989b; FDA 1979/1987). However, we must pay special attention to this type of data. The validity of hand-recorded data is based on the reliability of the observer and on well-developed and validated standards of measurement. For computer-generated data, the observer is a computerized data collection system, and the measurements are controlled by a computer program. These are complex systems that may contain complex flaws. Just as the principles behind measurements with a standard thermometer were validated centuries ago and are verified with each thermometer produced today, so must modern computerized instrumentation be validated and its operation verified. This causes a real dilemma for many scientists who are proficient in biomedical research but not in computer science. Because of the size and scope of this issue, we can only call your attention to the problem and refer you to the literature for additional guidance.

Finally moving to promulgation and clarification of requirements of GLP section 11 (21 CFR 11) compliance, multiple points must be considered. Though it is still not completely clear exactly what all will be required, seven elements are certainly involved: software validation, log-on security, existence of audit trails, authority controls (over entries and changes), storage of data, backup and archival, and training for users and administration. Again, this is a very complex area, and no more than a superficial perspective is presented here.

Statistical Data

Statistical data result from descriptive processes, summarization of raw data, and statistical analysis. Simply put, these data are not raw data but represent manipulation of the data. However, during this analysis process, a number of situations may affect the raw data and the final conclusions. For example, certain data may be rejected because they are shown to be experimentally flawed, an outlier believed to have resulted from an error, or not be plausible. We will leave it to other texts to discuss the criteria by which decisions like these are made. Here, we will say only that any manipulation of raw data is itself raw data. For example, a series of organ weights is analyzed. One of the weights is clearly out of the usual range for the species, and no necropsy observations indicated the organ was of unusual size. The preserved tissues are checked, and the organ appears to be the same size as others in the group. The statistician then may decide to remove that organ weight from the set of weights. The record of this action is raw data. The analysis is not, because it can be replicated by simple data handling techniques. It is a fine distinction that matters only to QA people in the context of recording requirements for raw data since both the analyses and record of the data change are required to reconstruct the report.

Statistical analysis is part of the study record. Documentation of the methods of statistical analysis, statistical parameters, and calculations is important. Critical evaluation of conclusions often involves discussion of the statistical methods employed. Complete documentation and reporting of these methods, calculations, and results allow for constructive, useful critical review. In most cases, such analysis is built into LIMS and follows a set pattern or decision tree approach (such as – and in many cases following – as presented in Gad and Weil 1988).

Results and Conclusions

The study record includes the results and conclusions made from review of the data produced during the scientific investigation. The data are summarized in abstracts, presented at meetings, published in journals, and, with all previously discussed types of data, are reported to government agencies. However, it is the scientist's interpretation of the data that communicates the significance of the experimentation. In all scientific forums, scientists present their interpretation of the data as results and conclusions. Results and conclusions are separate concepts. This is an important distinction not only because it is the required format for journal articles and reports but because it is important to separate them. Results are a literal, objective description of the observations made during the study, a statement of the facts. Conclusions, on the other hand, represent the analysis of the significance of these observations. They state the researcher's interpretation of the results. If results are presented clearly and objectively, they can be analyzed by any knowledgeable scientist, thereby testing the conclusions drawn. This is the process by which the body of scientific knowledge is refined and perfected.

For regulatory purposes, the results presented to the regulatory agencies (FDA or equivalent) must be complete. Included in such regulatory reports for submission must be tables of raw data, all factors that affect the data, and summaries of the data. In journals, the results section usually is a discussion with tabular or graphical presentations of what the researcher considers relevant data to support the conclusions. Conclusions presented in either case interpret the data, discuss the significance of the data, and describe the rationale for reaching the stated conclusions. In both bases, the results are reviewed and the conclusions evaluated by scientific peers. The function of the peer review process is to question and dispute or confirms the information gained from the experiment. Objective reporting of results and clear discussion of conclusions are required to successfully communicate the scientist's perspective to the scientific community.

Development of Study Data

Above we have discussed the types of data that make up the study record. The following discussion addresses quality characteristics for the study record, requirements for recording raw data, and methods for fulfilling the quality characteristics and raw data requirements by using various record keeping formats.

Quality Characteristics

There are four characteristics the study record must have: completeness, consistency, accuracy, and reconstructability. *Completeness* means the information is totally there, self-explanatory, and whole. *Consistency* in the study record means that there is "reasonable agreement between different records containing the same information" (DeWoskin 1995). *Accuracy* is agreement between what is observed and what is recorded. The final characteristic is *reconstructability*. Can the data record guide the researcher or someone else sufficiently so as to reproduce the events of the study? These characteristics are goals to meet in developing the study record and will be used in Chap. 4 to evaluate the quality of these records. They must be built into the study from the beginning, and considerable attention to these goals will be required as the study progresses to produce a complete, consistent, accurate, and reconstructable study record. Quality cannot be put in at the end of the study or experiment.

Recording Raw Data

Raw data may be recorded by hand in laboratory notebooks and worksheets or entered into a computerized data management system. Today, more and more data are computer generated and recorded as paper outputs or are electronically written to magnetic media and stored on microfiche or other electronic storage media. This section will discuss how raw data in both forms are recorded.

General Requirements for Raw Data Recording

Raw data must be recorded properly to preserve and protect them. The following is excerpted from the FDA GLPs:

> All data generated during the conduct of a study, except those that are generated by automated data collection systems, shall be recorded *directly, promptly,* and *legibly in ink.* All data entries shall be *dated on the date of entry* and *signed or initialed by the person entering the data.*

All introductory laboratory courses teach the basic techniques for the recording of raw data. Even though these standards are published as regulations for only certain types of research, we believe that there is never an instance when these minimum standards do not apply. There may be researchers who "get by" writing in pencil or scribbling data on paper towels, but they often ultimately suffer the consequences of their carelessness when data are lost or their records are unintelligible. Too, if these same researchers attempt to patent a product or method, or to submit their data to regulatory agencies, their submissions are simply not acceptable, because their data is flawed. In fact, if the regulatory data are incomplete or obscured in some way, the scientist involved may even be subject to civil or criminal penalties. It is always best to establish good habits early, especially for scientific record keeping.

For hand-recorded data, the phrase "directly, promptly, and legibly in ink" means to write it down in the notebook or on the worksheet as soon as you see it, so it is readable and in ink. The purpose is to accurately preserve the observation. Notes on paper towels, post-it notes, or scratch paper may be lost. Prompt recording promotes accuracy and chronologically correct records. Legibility assures that at a later time, you will understand what is written. This does not necessarily mean neat. If you are recording directly and promptly, neatness may have to be forgone. It does, however, mean readable and understandable.

The use of ink preserves the record from being erased or smeared illegibly. It is commonly understood that the ink should be indelible, meaning it cannot be erased and can withstand water or solvent spills. Some organizations may require a specific color of ink to be used, usually black or dark blue. This requirement originated because black ink was the most permanent and could be readily photocopied. Even without such requirements, the ink used in the lab should be tested to see how it withstands common spills and to see if imaged copies from a standard photocopier are of good quality. Some colors of ink and some thin line pens may not copy completely. There are a number of reasons why data may need to be copied, and that they are copied exactly becomes a very practical issue. Inks should not fade with time. Some analytical instruments produce printed data on heat-sensitive paper, which tends to fade in time. To preserve these data, laboratories will make photocopies. This is an issue that will be discussed more fully in Chap. 3.

The requirements to sign and date the data was recorded flow from practical and legal considerations; it is often useful to know who made and recorded the observation. In many research labs, graduate assistants or research technicians are responsible for recording the raw data. If questions arise later, the individual responsible may be sought out and asked to clarify an entry. For GLP studies, the signature represents a legal declaration, meaning the data recorded here are correct and complete. The data must be dated at the time of entry. This attests to the date of the recording of the observation and the progression in time of the study conduct. Some lab work is time dependent, and in this case, the time and date must be recorded. There is never any instance when data or signatures may be backdated or dated in advance.

Signatures and dates are crucial when documenting discovery and in supporting a patent claim and in intellectual property litigation. For studies conducted under the GLPs, the signature and date are legal requirements for the reconstruction of the study conduct. Falsely reported data may accordingly result in civil or criminal penalties to the person recording the data and his/her management for making false and misleading statements.

In some types of research, additional signatures and dates may be required. Data used to support a patent and data generated during the manufacture of drugs or medical devices must be signed and dated by an additional person – a witness or reviewer thus corroborating the stated information. An important point here is that the witness or reviewer can in the simplest form attest to nothing more than the signing and dating of the data entry and not to the integrity of the data collection methods or the data itself unless marked "read and understood," in which case the witness or reviewer is actually attesting to the integrity of the data as it has been generated.

Error Correction in Data Recording

What happens when there is a mistake in recording data or an addition that must be made to the data at a later time? Well the FDA GLPs address this:

> Any changes to entries shall be made so as not to obscure the original entry, shall indicate the reason for such change, and shall be dated and signed at the time of the change.

All changes to the written record of data must be explained and signed and dated. Doing so provides justification for the correction and again provides testimony as to who made the change and when it was done. To make corrections to the data, the original entry is not obscured. A single line is drawn through the entry. Then, the reason for the change is recorded with the date the change is made and the initials of the person making the change. For simplicity and ease of recording, a code may be established and documented to explain common reasons for making corrections to data. A simple example may be a circled letter designation like:

S = sentence error
E = entry error
C = calculation error

This is easy to remember and use. Any other types of errors or corrections must be described in sufficient detail to justify the change. A compendium of these symbols and abbreviations must be a matter of record, like in a suitable and relevant SOP.

Raw data may be generated by computer programs and stored on paper or magnetic material. Most laboratories approach this kind of data as they would hand-generated data. The GLPs state:

> In automated data collection systems, the individual responsible for direct data input shall be identified at the time of the data input. Any changes to automated data entries shall be made so as not to obscure the original entry, shall indicate the reason for the change, shall be dated and the responsible individual shall be identified.

For automated data collection systems, there are similar standards to hand-recorded data (FDA 1979/1987). All raw data should be recorded promptly and directly. Whereas the requirement for hand-collected data is that the records be written legibly and in ink, but the requirement for computer-collected data is permanence and security. However, there may be special considerations for how signatures and dates are recorded. The physical signature of data may not be possible when using electronic storage media. Electronic signature or the recording of the operator's name and the date is often a function provided in the software and is recorded and embedded with the data. When the data are printed in a paper copy, this information should be included. Some labs have adopted a policy requiring that the paper printout must be signed and dated by the operator. Some instruments produce a continuous printout or strip chart. In this case, the chart should be signed by the operator and dated on the date the data are retrieved. If the data are maintained on electronic media, the operator's name and date must be recorded on that medium.

Because computer security and risk of corruption or destruction of computer-stored data are a major concern, many laboratories maintain computer-generated data in paper printouts because the means for maintaining this data are traditional and easy to implement. As long as the printout represents a verified exact copy of the original raw data, it is acceptable and often even preferable to designate the printout as the raw data. This point should emphasize again the importance of proper validation of information technology systems and software, so that there is confidence in a printout being an exact copy of the electronic files.

When changes to the electronically stored raw data are made, the original observation must be maintained. This is accomplished in several ways. Newer software packages allow these changes to be made and properly documented at the same time. To do this, the original entry is not erased, and there is a way of recording the reason for the change along with the electronic signature of the person authorized to make the change and the date of the change. However, some data collection systems still do not have this capability. If this is the case, the original printout may be retained with the new printout that contains the change, the reason for the change, the signature of the person authorized to make the change, and the date of the change. Some computer programs allow for footnotes and addenda to be added to the record. These additions to the record, if made later, should also include a handwritten or computer-recorded signature and date.

Formats for Recording Data

As is discussed in Chap. 10 ("Electronic Reporting Requirements (SEND & eCTD)"), the requirement is for the toxicology data for drugs to be recorded in a specified electronic format (SEND). We will now begin to construct the study record. The format for the study record may be determined by the preferences of the researcher. Some researchers prefer to maintain all study records in laboratory notebooks. In private industry, research and development labs may be required to use lab notebooks because of potential patent documentation requirements. Many chemists have become accustomed to the use of lab notebooks. However, handwritten data may be maintained in laboratory notebooks and on worksheets and forms, or one may use computer-generated printouts and electronic storage media. The remainder of this section discusses guidelines for recording data using all formats.

Laboratory Notebooks

Laboratory notebooks are usually bound books with ruled or grid-lined pages that are used to record the events of an experiment or study. Organizations may order specially prepared notebooks that are uniquely numbered on the cover and spine. They have consecutively numbered pages, and some come with additional carbonless pages to make exact copies of the entries. Organizations may have strict procedures in place for issuing notebooks to individuals for use on specific research projects. After the glassware is cleaned, all that remains of a study is the notebook; its value is in the cost of repeating all the work because it could not be recreated. Therefore, SOPs should be written to control the assignment, use, and location of these records.

The pages may be designed to contain formats for recording information. In the header, there may be space for the title and date. In the footer, space may be allocated for signature and date of the recorder and signature and date of a reviewer or witness. When beginning to use a laboratory notebook, set aside the first few pages for the table of contents. Then a few pages may be held in reserve for notes, explanations, and definitions that are generally applicable to the contents.

The remainder of this section discusses the rules for recording data in the notebook. First, each page should contain a descriptive title of the experiment that includes the study designation and the experimental procedure to be performed. The date the procedure was performed is also recorded. Often a complete description of the experiment will require several pages. After the first page, subsequent pages should indicate, at least, an abbreviated title and cross-reference to the page from which it was continued.

The body of the experimental record should include the following sections:

- Purpose of the experiment
- Materials needed, including instruments, equipment, reagents, animals used, etc.
- Reagent and sample preparation
- Methods and procedures

Results

The *purpose* may be recorded in a few sentences. The *materials section* is a list of all the things you need for the experiment – the instruments to be used, equipment, and chemicals. When recording the analytical instruments, include the make, model, and serial numbers, the location of the instrument, and all settings and conditions for the use of the instrument. Remember, one needs to be able to provide sufficient detail that the experiment or study can be reproduced at any time in the future by someone minimally skilled in the art. The description of the chemical used should include a complete description including name, manufacturer, lot or serial number, concentration, expiry date if applicable, and stability profile. *Reagent and solution* preparation must be described in detail with a record of all weights and measurements. It is extremely important that sample identification and sample preparation be completely documented in detail. The *methods and procedures* section is a step-by-step description of the conduct of the experiment.

If SOPs are in place that describe any of the above information in sufficient detail, they may be referenced rather than writing or entering all of the tedium of the procedure again. Information recorded in the notebook is all weights and measurements and any information that is unique to this experiment or not specifically discussed in the SOP. SOPs often are written for more general applications. A SOP may state that the pH will be adjusted using a buffer or acid as required. The notebook should indicate what tool and substance were used to adjust the pH and the volume that was used. A SOP may describe the formulation of a compound in a certain amount, when the experiment requires a different amount. The mixing procedures may be cross-referenced, but it will be necessary to describe in detail the conversion of the SOP quantities and any changes in procedure resulting from the change in quantity. Study-specific SOPs can be very useful when properly written, used, and referenced.

The *experimental results* section must contain all observations and any information relating to those results. It should include any deviation from established methods, from SOPs, and from the protocol. Failed experiments must be reported even though the procedure was successfully repeated. Justification for repeating the procedure and a description of what may have gone wrong are recorded. All calculations should be shown in detail and include a description of the formula used.

Remember, all entries are recorded directly and promptly into the notebook at the appropriate time in the experiment and are recorded legibly and in indelible ink. Some information may be entered at the beginning of the day, some entered at the end of the day, but all weights, measurements, and recorded observations must be entered into the notebook directly and promptly as the information is generated.

For a complete record, it is often necessary to insert such information as shipping receipts, photographs, and printouts into the lab notebook. In doing so, do not obscure any writing on the page. The following are tips for inserting information into the notebook:

- Glue (e.g., "glue stick") the loose paper in place. (The use of tape is not recommended because tape over time loses its holding power.)
- Inserts may be signed, dated, stapled, and cross-referenced to the notebook and page so that they can be replaced if they become loose.

- Make verified (stamped: "Exact copy") copies of data that is too large for the page, shrinking it to fit the notebook page. Reference the location of the original.
- If, by some chance, data are accidentally recorded on a paper towel or other handy scrap of paper, these should be signed, dated, and glued into the notebook. It is not wise to transcribe data, thereby introducing the possibility of error or opening oneself to the criticism of potential of data tampering.

The bottom of each page must be signed by the person entering the data and dated at the time of entry. The date at the top of the page and the date of the activity in most cases will be the same as the date at the bottom of the page. A few exceptions are appropriate. The most legitimate exception to this rule occurs when a page is reserved for the results printout. The printout may not be available to insert until the following day. The printout should indicate the date when the data were first recorded which should in turn match the top date. The date at the bottom of the page indicates when it was glued into the notebook.

Occasionally, a scientist will forget to sign and date the page. When this happens, there is no quick fix. The only remedy is to add a notation: "This page was not signed and dated on ____, the time of entry," then, sign and date this statement using the date that this entry was made.

This discussion has been detailed because the signature and dates on the pages are very important. They are legally required for regulatory purposes. Data used to support patents and specified data produced under the FDA current Good Manufacturing Practices (GMPs) and Good Clinical Practices (GCPs) require the signature and date of a witness or reviewer. For example, the GMPs require that all materials weighed or measured in the preparation of the drug be witnessed, signed, and dated. Patent applications are supported by witnessed experimental records. Some institutions may require supervisory review of notebook entries with accompanying signature and date. This is to say that you should be aware of the uses of your data and any requirements for this additional signature. These additional signatures should be embedded in the following statement: "Read and understood by ----- on -----."

An important concept to remember is that bound, consecutively page-numbered notebooks are used to demonstrate the progression of the research and to document the dates of data entry and the chronological nature of the work performed. To prevent the corruption of this record, unused and partially used pages may be marked out so no additions may be made. A suggested method is to draw a "Z" through the page or portion of the page not used. At the end of the project, there may be unused notebook pages. These may be "Z'd," or the last page may indicate that this is the end of the experimental record and no additional pages will be used.

Forms and Worksheets

While many analytical laboratories continue to use lab notebooks, other labs may use forms and worksheets to record their data. The purpose is to provide an efficient format for recording data that are routine in nature. The basic concept is that forms and worksheets should be designed to be easy to use and to provide a complete record of all relevant data. They may be used in combination with lab notebooks as described above or kept in files or loose-leaf binders. Explanatory footnotes may be preprinted or added to explain abbreviations and/ or the meaning of symbols. Additional space for comments and notes should be incorporated into the format.

Computer spreadsheets and word processing make forms and worksheets easy to design and produce.

The advantages of using forms and worksheets include the following:

- They may be customized and formatted to prompt for all necessary information.
- They are easy to follow, complete, and well-organized.
- Header information, title, study designation, sample numbers, etc. may be filled out in advance, thus saving time.
- Cross-references to applicable SOPs may be included on the worksheet.
- They help to standardize data collection.

Disadvantages of using forms and worksheets include the following:

- They must be carefully designed and should be pretested for completeness and ease of use.
- They may encourage a tendency not to write more information than is specifically requested when designed space is allotted for notes and comments only.
- Forms and worksheets that are designed for general use may contain blanks that are not necessary for the current study. Yet all blanks must be com-

pleted. If not needed, "n/a" (not applicable) should be written in the blank or a dash put in the space or when the form is printed "blacked out."

- Forms and worksheets create a routine that can become mindless; individuals need to take care to properly complete the form.
- Example 1: Necropsy forms often contain a complete list of tissues to be checked by the technician. When only some tissues are inspected or retrieved, it may be too easy to check inappropriate boxes.
- Example 2: Animal behavioral observation forms contain blanks to record all observations. The observer must record something in the blank space. A check or "OK" may be used to describe normal behavior if such is defined on the form or in an SOP. A problem occurs when these designations are used automatically without proper attention being paid to observing and recording the behavior of each animal, particularly when most animals are behaving normally.

In discussing the above disadvantages, we are not trying to discourage the use of worksheets. However, one must be careful to institute procedures and practices that assure that forms and worksheets are properly used.

As in any data record, the signature and the date of entry are recorded at the time of the entry and represent and attest to the accuracy of the information. Any changes to the data or additional notes made after completion of the form or worksheet are made as previously described. Any unused lines on the form or worksheet should be crossed or "Z'd" out. If the signature of a witness or reviewer is required, there should be a line allocated for this purpose.

Forms and worksheets can be a useful and practical way to record and preserve raw data – if you pay attention to the rules of data recording. Most automated data systems have intake/input screens consisting of a series of forms.

Automated Data Collection Systems (LIMS – Laboratory Information Management System)

This is the hottest, most fluid and most difficult topic in this book. Application of data collection rules to computer systems has been the topic of numerous seminars, books, journal articles, government policy committees, and regulatory interpretation. As an example of the difficulties surrounding the proper implementation of an electronic data policy, the FDA has spent several years trying to reach a consensus on a policy for electronic signatures (Freudenthal

1997; FDA 1997a, b). However, the new CSEND standards became mandatory for data submission in May of 2018 and other types of studies ae being added to the list of requirements (see Chap. 11 for a detailed discussion).

Two major issues surround automated data collection systems: validation of the system and verification of the system's proper operation.

Validation asks whether the system is properly designed and tested so that it performs as it should to measure and record data accurately, completely, and consistently. In other words, are all the bugs worked out so that the system does not lose, change, or misrepresent the data you wish to obtain? We recollect, from many years ago, a software program for recording animal weights. If a particular animal had died on study and was not weighed at a weigh session, a "0" was entered for the weight. It was discovered that the software would automatically reject the 0 and record in its place the next animal's weight. This was totally unacceptable. The system was inadequately designed to properly handle commonly occurring data collection exceptions.

The second issue is the verification of the system's operation. Have you tested and proven that the data produced and recorded by the system are accurate, complete, and consistent, meeting all the date quality standards discussed under handwritten data?

Validation and verification are processes that involve hardware and software development and acceptance testing, laboratory installation procedures and testing, computer security, and special record keeping procedures, to name a few. There are numerous publications on this topic. If you are working in a research area subject to the authority of the FDA or its equivalents, we suggest starting with the following reference: the FDA Computerized Data Systems for Nonclinical Safety Assessment: Current Concepts and Quality Assurance, known as the Red Apple Book and the FDA Technical Reference on Software Development Activities.

The following sections will discuss the defining raw data for automated data collection systems, what should be recorded in the raw data, electronic signatures, and report formats and spreadsheets. It should be noted that most (but not all) GLP compliant testing utilize LIMS data capture systems.

Computer-Generated Raw Data

It was Dr. Gad's privilege to work with a team of experts during the later stages of finalization of the GALPs (Good Automated Laboratory Practices). One of the most difficult tasks was deciding how to define raw data for laboratory information management system (LIMS). Hours and days were spent on this issue alone. Here is the definition that was ultimately adapted:

LIMS Raw Data are original observations recorded by the LIMS that are needed to verify, calculate, or derive data that are or may be reported. LIMS raw data storage media are the media to which LIMS Raw Data are first recorded.

From these discussions, we have developed a broader-based alternative definition of computer-generated raw data. For automated data collection systems, "raw data" means the first record on the system of original observations that are human readable and that are needed to verify, calculate, or derive data that are or may be reported. The GALP definition above was designed to fit the scope of the GALPs.

The real issue is how to apply the definition. Hand-recorded raw data is easy to define. What you see is what you write. Automated systems are much more complex. Analytical instruments may perform several functions. For example, the transmittance of a light beam is measured and then converted into an electronic signal; this signal is transmitted to a computer, the software on the computer converts the signal to a machine-readable representation, this representation is translated into a value, this value is recorded into a reporting format that performs calculations and a summary of the input data, and the reported number or numbers are sent to an electronic file or to a printer.

The question is when do we have raw data? It is when an understandable value is first recorded. If the human-readable value is saved to a file prior to formatting, this is raw data. If the first recording of the data is in the report format, this is raw data. Some labs have declared the signal from the instrument to the computer to be raw data, but it is then very difficult to use the signal as a means for verification of the report of the data. This example represents only one situation of the possible variations in instrumentation. Each automated data collection system must be assessed to determine when the output is "raw data." What exactly is raw data for electronic instruments and computers needs to be openly and unambiguously stated and defined in order to avoid any misuse or misinterpretation.

Why is the definition of raw data for computer applications so important? One obvious reason is to meet regulatory requirements. Behind these requirements are the same data quality characteristics that apply to hand-recorded data: accuracy, completeness, consistency, and the ability to reconstruct the study. As mentioned earlier, transcription of data can cause errors. Each time data are translated or reformatted by a software application, there is the potential for the data to be corrupted or, even worse, lost. When the data are recorded and human readable *before* these downstream operations, these "raw data" can then be used to verify any subsequent iterations.

Here is the type of information that should be included in the automated raw data record:

- The instrument used to collect the data
- The person operating the instrument
- The date (and time) of the operation
- All conditions or settings for the instrument
- The person entering the data (if different from the operator)
- The date and time entered or reported
- The study title or code
- Cross-reference to a notebook or worksheet
- The measurements with associated sample identification
- All system-calculated results

If the system does not allow the input of any of the above information, it may be recorded by hand on the printout or on cross-referenced notebook pages or worksheets.

Automated raw data may be stored in soft copy (e.g., magnetic media) or in hard copy (e.g., paper printout, microfiche, and microfilm). However soft copy storage of raw data presents a unique set of problems that are often avoided by printing it in hard copy. Many labs choose to printout raw data, because it assures the data are available and unchanged. More about storage on magnetic media is discussed in Chap. 3.

Many software applications for instruments record the data in a worksheet format. The same rules as those for hand-generated worksheets should apply for automated formats. However, some raw data may not yet be formatted when they are first recorded. In this case, a key to the formatting of the raw data must accompany the data.

Why do we not designate the final formatted report as raw data in all cases? Remember, in the definition of raw data, the phrase, "first recorded occurrence of the original observation." Because steps occur between the collection of the data and the final reporting of the data in a final report, the final report cannot be raw data. This is important because the data should have undergone as little manipulation and transfer as possible over different software applications. This prevents corruption and loss and allows the raw data to be used to verify additional operations performed on it. Also, why not designate the signal read by the instrument or transmitted by the instrument as the raw data? This is because this event cannot be understood by humans and therefore is not useful to verify the results and conclusions. Testing should be performed on this signal, however, to validate the operation of the instrument and its communication functions (e.g., positive controls or adequate standards).

Electronic Signatures

Electronic signatures (FDA 1997a, b) are the recorded identity of the individual entering data and are input through log-in procedures that are presumed to be secure. One of the issues regarding electronic signatures is the validity of a computer-entered signature, because it is not traceable by handwriting analysis to the person signing and presumably anyone could type in a name. One of the charges years ago against Craven Labs was that the laboratory changed the clock on the computer to make it appear that samples were analyzed on an earlier date. Currently the FDA is accepting electronically recorded names or initials as signatures although the policy has not been made official as of this writing.

Until a policy statement is made, two criteria may be used to justify the use of electronic signatures. All individuals who operate the instruments or associated software must be aware of the meaning and importance of the entry of their name or unique personal code and the computerized date stamp. That is what constitutes a legal signature. Second, the electronic signature is best justified when access to the system is strictly controlled. Controlled access usually involves some sort of password or user identification system that must be activated before an authorized person may perform an operation. Some automated systems have levels of access that may control different operations by allowing only certain individuals to perform certain tasks. Access levels may include read only, data entry, data change authorization, and system level entry or change. When these controls are in place, the system may automatically record the person's name into the file based on the password entered. Some systems use voice recognition, fingerprint, or other biometric recognition. This discussion only begins to touch on the complexities of computer security-related issues.

Spreadsheets

Spreadsheet use to the modern lab is what invention of the printing press was to publication. Although spreadsheets make recording, processing, and reporting data easy and quick, some special considerations are important to the use of these powerful programs. Whether data are keyed into spreadsheets or electronically transferred to them from existing data files, the entry of the data must be checked to assure the data record is complete and correct. Commonly, mistakes occur in calculations and formulae in designating data fields and in performing inappropriate operations on the data. Because of the versatility of spreadsheets, one needs to take special care in validating the spreadsheet. When one performs calculations in the spreadsheet, check the spreadsheet formulae and be sure that the arithmetic formula is defined on the spreadsheet. The way the program rounds numbers and reports significant digits is important to the calculation of results and the reporting of the data. When you try to recalculate or evaluate the processes performed by the spreadsheet program, be sure to define all functions used.

Most recently, FDA has announced plans to promulgate a standard (CSEND – Current Standard for Exchange of Nonclinical Data) for the electronic submission of such data in support of regulatory submissions. This is part of the efforts by the CDISC (Clinical Data Interchange Standards Consortium) team.

Reporting the Data

This final section suggests ways to generate data tables and figures for the final report or manuscript. Here are some guidelines:

- The title of the table or figure should be descriptive of the data.
- Column and row headings should be understandable, avoiding undefined abbreviations.
- Units of measure should be included in the column headings or axes of charts.
- For individual data, all missing values must be footnoted and explained.
- All calculations used to derive the data should be defined stepwise and, when the calculation is complex or nonstandard, given in a footnote.

- Statistical summaries or analyses should be clearly defined including the type of process performed. Statistically significant values may be identified with a unique symbol that is footnoted.
- All abbreviations or acronyms should be clearly defined.
- Continuing pages should contain at least a descriptive portion of the title and indicate "continued."
- The data should be easy to read and be uncluttered. The font should not be too small.
- Charts should contain a legend of any symbols or colors used, and the labels of the axes should be descriptive and easily understood. Keep in mind that black and white copies of these charts and graphs may be made at some time and a method to identify the colored components as black and white components should be identified and stated.
- The text of the report should include references to the tables or figures when the data is presented.
- The text of the report should exactly match the data in the tables or figures. Any generalization, summarization, or significant rounding should be designated as such in the text.

Distinguishing Essential from Negotiable Study Elements

An important step in managing and executing studies and experiments is to determine which parts of the study or experiment must be included and how they should be included. It is desirable to maximize the amount of information to be obtained, while also considering time, numbers of animals, cost, potential statistical significance, hard drive space when appropriate, and the use of other resources. It may not be realistic to try to accomplish all the objectives which can be stated during the early stages of study design. Remember the "KISS" principle (keep it simple, stupid). Simple experiments provide simple results. Complex experiments produce chaos. This distinction of essential and negotiable study elements is a critical step which will enable the study sponsor to select a suitable laboratory as well as to negotiate the specific components of the study. Also keep in mind the fact that regulated science is different than science performed for science-sake. Each experiment/study should incorporate components that can answer the questions that a potential reviewer at the agency might ask. Adding study components that are interesting or neat can potentially create problems down the line in generating data that cannot be adequately explained to the agency.

Designating the Study Monitor

Another important aspect that needs to be considered early in the process of external placement of a study concerns personnel. Of the individuals involved with a given study, the study director is probably the most important. In the past, it was not uncommon that the employee or consultant who functions as a study monitor on behalf of the sponsor would be called the "study director." This is now a difficult concept to grasp, since the responsibilities of the study director imply being intimately involved with and overseeing the day-to-day activities of the study. These actions can only be discharged by an employee of the laboratory contracted to perform the study. Regardless of what the on-site study director is called, the sponsor needs to provide sufficient authority to allow important decisions to be made without prolonged discussions on the telephone or, worse yet, emergency site visits by the sponsor and for clean lines of authority for any potential changes. For example, if an animal is judged by the veterinary staff to be in pain, the study director needs to be able to consult with the attending veterinarian to make a timely decision with regard to the fate of the animal and not be delayed by time zone differences or lack of availability of the sponsor via phone or email. This is a very important animal welfare issue.

For complex or long-term studies, the laboratory should provide an alternate or deputy study director to ensure both continuing internal oversight and a contact for the sponsor if the primary study director is unavailable.

Having defined the work to be done, ranked the elements of the study as essential or negotiable, and selected a study monitor from within the sponsor's organization, a laboratory must be found which can do the necessary work.

Shifting Paradigms

From the turn of the century up until 2007 was the third golden age of contract toxicology, the first two having been in the mid-1970s until the early 1980s and the second having been from the early until the mid-1990s. To a degree, for all contract research organizations, each of these has seen expansion of facilities, marked prosperity, and changes in practice services offered and technology utilized. The first and last of these also saw both new ("green grass") facilities built and opened. Each has also been followed by an economic contraction, with reductions in costs charged to clients along with corresponding reductions in profit, merging of CROs, reductions in staff, and closing of some facilities and terminations of some services.

As this is written, we are still in the period of contraction of the economy and of spending in R&D, especially by the many smaller pharmaceutical companies which are the bread and butter of the work stream for CROs.

These changes from the perspective of those seeking the services of CROs have been viewed as generally positive changes. (1) Pricing by CROs is quite competitive, and (2) study start times are quite short.

There are also negative aspects of the current situation primarily that staffing and organizations are frequently changing (Snyder 2009a, 2009b, 2010). Contributing to this state of change is the entry of multiple new CROs in China, India, and the broader world. This is further discussed in Chap. 6.

References

DeWoskin, R. S. (1995). *Quality assurance SOPs for GLP compliance*. Buffalo Grove: Interpharm Press.

DIA. (2018). *2018 contract service organization directory*. Fort Washington: Drug Information Association (DIA).

EPA. (1989a). *FIFRA good laboratory practice standards*. Environmental Protection Agency (EPA), Final Rule, Fed.Reg. 54:34052–34074.

EPA (1989b). *FIFRA good laboratory practice standards*. Environmental Protection Agency (EPA), Final Rule, Fed. Reg. 52:48933–48946.

FDA. (1979/1987). *Good laboratory practice regulations*, Final Rule, Fed. Reg. 52:33768–33782.

FDA. (1984). *Compliance Program Guidance Manual*, Chapter 48, Human drugs and biologics: Bio research monitoring. Washington, DC, Food and Drug Administration.

FDA. (1997a). *Electronic signatures; electronic records*; Final Rule, 21 CFR Part 11.

FDA. (1997b). *Electronic submissions, establishment of public docket; Notice*, 21 CFR Part 11.

FDA. (2002a). *Code of federal regulations*, Title 21, Part 58 (Food, Drug and Cosmetic Act).

FDA. (2002b). *To obtain inspection reports from FDA, one can call their FOI office at (301) 443-6310 or online at*. The mail address for such is: Department of Health and Human Services, 200 Independence Ave., SW, Washington, DC 20201.

FDA. (2015). *Food and Drug Administration's 2002 Code of Federal Regulations* are available on-line at http://www.gmppublications.com.

Freudenthal, R. I. (1997). *Directory of toxicology laboratories offering contract service.* West Palm Beach: Aribel Books.

Gad, S. C. (2010). *International guidelines for the nonclinical safety evaluation of drugs and devices.* New York: Springer.

Gad, S. C. (2018). *Regulatory toxicology* (3rd ed.). Philadelphia: Taylor & Frances.

Gad, S. C., & Weil, C. S. (1988). *Statistics and experimental design for toxicologists* (2nd ed.). Caldwell: Telford Press.

Jackson, E. M. (1985). *International directory of contract laboratories.* New York: Marcel Dekker, Inc.

Texas Research Institute. (1986). *Directory of toxicology testing institutions.* Texas Research Institute: Houston.

Additional Reading

DIA. (1988). *Computerized data systems for non-clinical safety assessments: Current concepts and quality assurance.* Drug Information Association (DIA), Maple Glen, September 1988.

FDA. (1976). Food and Drug Administration's Good Laboratory Practice Regulations original proposal, *Fed. Reg. 41:*51206–51230. This details the reasons for the proposed GLPs and includes a catalog of deficiencies found in laboratories which performed studies in support of FDA regulated products.

FDA. (1987). *Good laboratory practice regulations*, Final Rule, *Fed. Reg.* 52:33768–33782, September 4, 1987.

FDA. (1993a). Good clinical practices: *CFR*, Title 21, Part 50, 56, 312, April 1, 1993.

FDA. (1993b). *Guide for detecting fraud in bioresearch monitoring inspections*, Office of Regulatory Affairs, U.S. FDA, April 1993.

FDA. (1994). Electronic Signatures; Electronic Records; Proposed Rule, *Fed. Reg.* 59:13200, August 31, 1994.

FDA. (n.d.-a). Current good manufacturing practices for finished pharmaceuticals, *CFR*, Title 21, Part 211.

FDA. (n.d.-b). Current good manufacturing practices for medical devices, General, *CFR*, Title 21, Part 820.

Gad, S. C., & Taulbee, S. M. (1996). *Handbook of data recording, maintenance, and management for the biomedical sciences.* Boca Raton: CRC Press.

Grall, J. (Ed.). (1981). *Scientific considerations in monitoring and evaluating toxicological research.* Washington, DC: Hemisphere Publishing Corporation.

Hoover, B. K., Baldwin, J. K., Uelner, A. F., Whitmire, C. E., Davies, C. L., & Bristol DW. (Eds.). (1986). *Managing conduct and data quality of toxicology studies.* Princeton: Princeton Scientific Publishing Co., Inc.

Jackson, E. M. (1984). How to choose a contract laboratory: Utilizing a laboratory clearance procedure. *Journal of Toxicology: Cutaneous and Ocular Toxicology, 3,* 83–92.

James, J. W. (1982). *Good laboratory practice*, ChemTech, 1962–1965, March 1982.

NIH. (1985). *Guide for the care and use of laboratory animals*, DHEW Publ. No. (NIH) 78–23, revised 1985.

NIH. (1986). *Guide to the care and use of laboratory animals* (pp. 1985–1986). Bethesda: National Institutes of Health.

NIH. *Institutional animal care and use committee guidebook*, NIH Pub. No. 92-3415. U.S. Department of Health and Human Services, E33–37.

Paget, G. E., & Thompson, R. (Eds.). (1979a). *Standard operating procedures in toxicology.* University Park Press: Baltimore.

Paget, G. E., & Thompson, R. (Eds.). (1979b). *Standard operating procedures in pathology.* University Park Press: Baltimore.

Paget, G. E. (1977). *Quality control in toxicology.* Baltimore: University Park Press.

Paget, G. E. (1979). *Good laboratory practice.* Baltimore: University Park Press.

Snyder, S. (2009a). Buzzwords, *Contract Pharma,* April, 2009, 32–34.

Snyder, S. (2009b). Working with study directors. *Contract Pharma,* July/August: 28–30.

Snyder, S. (2010). Welcome to the Toxies. *Contract Pharma,* April: 32–34.

Taulbee, S. M., & DeWoskin, R. S. (1993). *Taulbee's pocket companion: U.S. FDA and EPA GLPs in parallel.* Buffalo Grove: Interpharm Press.

The History of CROs: Including CRO Snapshots

David G. Serota with section by Shayne C. Gad and Charles B. Spainhour

Note: This chapter was prepared by the author based on both his personal knowledge of the preclinical Contract Research Organization industry referred to as CRO throughout this chapter and from information provided by a number of other professionals who are currently employed at or had previously been employed at the various organizations discussed in this chapter (contributors are listed at the end of the chapter). The information presented focuses mainly on CROs in North America where it is estimated that around 100 different CROs have existed over time, but many of these have either terminated operations or have been acquired by other organizations, primarily larger CROs. In addition, with the passing of so many key players from those organizations over time, it was almost impossible to gather information for many CROs. Furthermore, some larger CROs declined the opportunity of sharing the requested historical information about their organizations due to confidential issues which the author found to be disappointing. Nevertheless, the author believes that in the absence of any previously published history of the CRO industry, the information presented in this chapter is useful and portrays a meaningful history of this industry. While the author acknowledges that there may be gaps and errors in some of the information presented, this should not be unexpected in the absence of any previously written history and the availability of professionals who lived the history.

D. G. Serota
7th Inning Stretch Consulting LLC, Kalamazoo, MI, USA

© Springer Nature Switzerland AG 2020
S. C. Gad et al., *Contract Research and Development Organizations-Their History, Selection, and Utilization*, https://doi.org/10.1007/978-3-030-43073-3_2

Appendix I presents a genealogy chart of toxicology CROs – historical, name changes, mergers, and other organizational changes. It will most likely be out of date by the time this volume is published.

Introduction

The Contract Research Industry is an integral part of the toxicology community and has been for almost 100 years. In many ways, the growth of this industry has mirrored the growth of toxicology in the twentieth century as toxicology was not developed as a pure science but rather one that grew out of other sciences such as pharmacology, physiology, anatomy, and biochemistry. Indeed, many have described toxicology as "pharmacology, but at higher doses," and this has not been an unfair characterization. CROs have served multiple functions over the years beyond that of just conducting contracted toxicology studies. They have served as a primary source in the development of new and novel technical procedures involving all commonly used research animal models, they have been at the forefront in testing better animal housing and caging advancements, they have been leaders in the introduction of more efficient and scientifically improved technical procedures, and they have served as a significant training ground for the development and training of a vast number of toxicologists who later went on to hold senior leadership positions in the industrial, governmental, and regulatory sectors of the toxicology industry.

The first recognized CRO that was not considered an extension of a chemical or pharmaceutical organization was most likely Food and Drug Research Laboratory (FDRL) which was formed in 1926. This was followed by the Illinois Institute of Technology Research Institute (IITRI) in 1936, Southern Research Institute (SRI) in 1941, Hazleton Laboratories and SRI International in 1946, and Lovelace Biomedical in 1947. During those early years, there were no standard toxicology testing study designs, no published regulatory requirements for toxicology testing, and no associations or societies that represented toxicology and where the toxicologists of the day could convene to share ideas and concerns. Indeed toxicology was not even recognized as a true scientific discipline. There were only a few independent CROs in operation as a significant amount of toxicology testing at that time was performed at either company laboratories such as Dow, DuPont, and Eastman Kodak or at university laboratories such as Kettering of the University of Cincinnati, the

University of Miami (Florida), New York University, Rutgers University (in association with Esso Research), and the Carnegie Mellon Institute Chemical Hygiene Laboratory (in association with Union Carbide). Toxicology at that time was mostly descriptive in nature with little knowledge or interest in mechanisms. Study designs, laboratory techniques, and the interpretation of study results differed among the various laboratories that were conducting the toxicology testing. Studies were generally conducted according to the inclinations of the investigator, and pathological evaluations were almost never performed.

During the 1960s, several key events occurred which stimulated greater dialogue and discussion involving the role and future of toxicology. The first key event was the worldwide reported incidence of babies being born with a condition by the name of phocomelia, which manifested itself as shortened, absent, or flipper-like limbs. This was first reported in 1961 and was traced back to women who had been prescribed and taken the drug thalidomide for morning sickness during their first trimester of pregnancy, while the incidence of phocomelia was less in the United States than in Europe due to the resistance of FDA scientist Dr. Frances Kelsey, who refused to grant approval for thalidomide use in the United States. This event though helped lead to profound changes in FDA approval procedures by the passage of the Kefauver-Harris Drug Amendment Act in 1962. This Act tightened restrictions surrounding the surveillance and approval process for drugs to be marketed and sold in the United States. This act required that drug manufacturers prove that a drug was both safe and effective before it could be marketed. The other key event that occurred during the same year was the publication of Rachel Carson's book, *Silent Spring*, which alerted the public to the detrimental effects on the environment of the widespread and indiscriminate use of pesticides. This in turn led to discussions in Congress about the need for implementing a national environmental policy, culminating with the creation of the Environmental Protection Agency in December of 1970.

The 1960s represented a major turning point in the history of toxicology, as a significant emphasis was now being placed on drug and environmental safety, resulting in the critical need for toxicologists trained in both applied and regulatory toxicology. It also resulted in the need for a significant increased capacity for conducting toxicology studies to support drug and environmental safety, leading to the creation of new CROs to meet that demand. These new CROs included such companies as Gulf South Research Institute, Litton Bionetics,

Bio/dynamics, International Research and Development Corporation (IRDC), and Bio-Research Laboratories (in Canada), in the early 1960s, and Calvert Laboratories and Centre International de Toxicologie (CIT) in France in the late 1960s.

During the 1970s, several significant governmental organizations were created to monitor and foster a greater control over issues associated with worker safety with the passage of the Occupational Safety and Health Act in December of 1970, which led to the creation of NIOSH (National Institute for Occupational Safety and Health). In addition with the passage of this act, Issues associated with the rising use of pesticide products led to the creation of the Environmental Protection Agency (EPA) in December of 1970. In 1972, the administration of the Federal Insecticide, Fungicide, and Rodenticide Act (FIFRA) that was first established in 1947 was moved from the authority of the Department of Agriculture to the newly created EPA, where a new emphasis was placed on the preservation of human health and protection of the environment by strengthening the registration process by shifting the burden of proof to the chemical manufacturer, enforcing compliance against banned products, and creating a regulatory framework that was missing from the original law. The primary objectives of the original act were to register pesticides distributed in interstate commerce with the Department of Agriculture and to protect farmers by requiring accurate labeling of pesticide contents, which enabled farmers to make informed choices regarding the product's effectiveness. However, concerns regarding the toxic effects of pesticide and residues on applicators, non-target species, and the environment resulted in significant changes in the 1972 revision. In 1976, the Toxic Substance Control Act (TSCA) became law which required industry reporting, record keeping, and testing of chemicals substances in commerce. In 1978, the National Toxicology Program (NTP) was established as part of the National Institute of Environmental Health (NIEHS) whose mission resulted from congressional concerns about the health effects of chemical agents in the environment, especially as it related to carcinogenic concerns. A significant number of long-term chronic toxicity/carcinogenicity studies were contracted to select CROs that met the room and housing requirements of NTP (with, e.g., facilities designed as clean-dirty facilities), these included Southern Research Institute, Midwest Research Institute (founded in 1944), and Battelle Memorial Institute (founded in 1929). The impact of these new initiatives, which required an increased number of toxicology studies to be conducted, resulted in a significant increase in the number of new CROs to meet that demand. These new CROs included MB Research Labs, Stillmeadow, TPS, WIL Research, Springborn, Borriston Laboratories, and Argus Research Laboratories. However, this decade also saw the closing of several CROs, such as Cannon Laboratories, as a result of the introduction of Good Laboratory Practices (GLPs) into the industry by the FDA and as a result of poor and/or dishonest practices in some existing CROs and in some in-house company laboratories, leading some organizations to opt out of the industry due to the significant effort and cost to become GLP compliant.

The CRO landscape remained fairly constant during the 1980s and 1990s although several new CROs were created during this time to meet the increasing need of outsourced toxicology testing as the larger pharmaceutical companies began to downsize their in-house testing capabilities along with the rapid rise of the biotech industry. These included Sinclair Research, R.O.W. Sciences, Sierra Biomedical, and ITR (Canada). Portending the future of acquisitions in the industry, Hazleton Laboratories became the largest CRO in the world during that time through a series of acquisitions, buying the Tobacco Research Council Laboratories in Harrogate, England in 1974, Affenzucht Munster in Munster, Germany in 1980, the Institut Merieux site in Lyon, France in 1981, RALTECH (owned by Ralston Purina) in Madison, Wisconsin in 1982, and Litton Bionetics in Rockville and Gaithersburg, Maryland, in 1985.

A new and aggressive player joined the CRO industry when Charles River Laboratories (CRL) entered the preclinical CRO field with the acquisition of Sierra Biomedical in 1999. Formed in 1947 as a rodent breeding company, CRL changed the landscape of the industry with a bold and aggressive acquisition strategy over the next 20 years, including the purchase of Argus Research and Pathology Associates in 2001; Springborn Laboratories in 2002; ClinTrials BioResearch (CTBR) in 2004; Argenta, BioFocus, and ChanTest Laboratories in 2014; WIL Research in 2016; MPI Research in 2018; and CiToxLab in 2019 – making CRL the world's largest preclinical CRO. In 2019, LabCorp (parent company of Covance) and Envigo executed a merger between Huntington Life Sciences and Harland Laboratories in 2015 and entered into an agreement whereby Covance purchased Envigo's preclinical capabilities while Envigo purchased Covance's research animal model capabilities.

As the CRO industry enters into the third decade of this century, there is no reason to expect that the level of acquisitions will slow as larger organizations look to increase their portfolios and profitability in the face of a continuing bullish outsourcing demand of toxicology and related services and since the cost and timing of building new CROs remain both expensive and difficult.

The Early Years

Food Drug Research Laboratories

The first recognized private CRO was Food Drug Research Laboratories (FDRL), created in 1926 by Philip Hawk and Bernard Oser as Food Research Laboratories in Philadelphia, Pennsylvania. Oser, a biochemist by training, received his doctorate from Fordham University and worked at FDRL for 47 years. He served in numerous senior scientist and management roles, culminating in his serving as president from 1957 to 1970 and then as chairman until 1973. He was a founding member of the Institute of Food Technologies and in the 1950s he was a significant voice in alerting the food industry of the need for toxicological studies and safety evaluations on food additives. He also served as the chairman of the First Gordon Conference on Toxicology and Safety Evaluation in 1956, which brought together many of the scientists who later formed the Society of Toxicology and served on the editorial board of *Toxicology and Applied Pharmacology*. In the mid-1930s, the company changed its name to Food Drug Research Laboratories with Kenneth Morgaridge joining the organization as vice president in the late 1930s. In 1956, the company relocated to Maspeth, New York, and set up operations in an old dance hall. Noted toxicologists there at that time included Harold Schwartz and Steve Carson. In the early 1970s, the company again relocated, this time to East Orange, New Jersey, where the corporate headquarters were located and clinical studies were conducted, and Waverly, New York, where approximately 60 people were employed and rodent, dog, and nonhuman primate studies were conducted and where the FDRL Wistar rat strain was developed. Noted toxicologists at the Waverly site included Mike Gallo, Kent Stevens, Peter Becci, Tom Re, John Babish, and Richard Parent. In the early 1990s, the company was renamed Liberty Laboratories, which refocused its activities almost completely on feline breeding and sales.

Lakeside Laboratories

Lakeside Laboratories was established is 1925 and was part of the ethical drug division of Colgate Palmolive Company. It was headquartered in Milwaukee, Wisconsin very close to Lake Michigan and that is how it got its name. In a sense it was not a true CRO, since it belonged to a pharmaceutical company. However, it did conduct some contract work for other companies. The vivarium consisted of about ten animal rooms in which specialty work such as placental transfer, metabolism (using various radiolabeled compounds), and PK studies was conducted. The group was headed by Jim Tom Hill who was supported by Patricia Frank, Claude Judd, and Norm Jefferson. In 1975, it was purchased by Merrill Dow National, and shortly afterward the facility was closed.

Illinois Institute of Technology Research Institute

The Illinois Institute of Technology Research Institute (IITRI) was established in 1936. It was originally founded as the Armour Research Foundation by the Armour Institute of Technology (a doctorate-granting university whose name was later changed to the Illinois Institute of Technology), and in 1963 the organization changed its name to IITRI. Based in Chicago, Illinois, the facility consisted of 50 animal rooms which included both standard vivarium space and specialized facilities for containment at BSL-2 and BSL-3 levels. In addition, over the past 40 years, IITRI has been a premier provider of inhalation toxicology services. David McCormick has had a long-standing career there as a toxicologist and company leader. It was the first CRO to develop and validate murine models for the identification of immunotoxic agents as part of a tripartite program performed in collaboration with NIEHS and the Medical College of Virginia, and it was the largest provider of preclinical pharmacology and toxicology drug development services for the National Cancer Institute over the past 20 years. It has extensive experience in bioelectromagnetics and conducted programs for NIEHS and NTP to evaluate the possible carcinogenicity of magnetic fields and radiofrequency fields emitted by cell phones and other wireless devises. Noted toxicologists at IITRI included David McCormick and Nabil Hatoum.

Chemical Hygiene Fellowship (Bushy Run Research Center)

The Chemical Hygiene Fellowship was established in November of 1937 under a contract between the Mellon Institute and the Carbide and Carbon Chemical Company (Union Carbide). Its beginning was modest, with a staff of two and two rooms totaling 500 square feet at the Mellon Institute in Pittsburgh, Pennsylvania, that is now part of the Pittsburgh Medical School. Over the next 22 years, the laboratory grew to a staff of 25 and approximately 11,000 square feet of space. In 1959, the laboratory moved to a 30,000 square foot building in Murrysville, Pennsylvania, about 15 miles east of Pittsburgh, which had originally been used as a radiation laboratory as part of the Manhattan Project, and by 1976 had grown to a staff of 110 with 65,000 square feet of space. This building was located on 230 acres on what was called the Bushy Run Campus. Up until 1980, the laboratory was managed by Mellon Institute, but in 1980 Union Carbide assumed the duties of managing the laboratory, and the name was changed to the Bushy Run Research Center (BRRC). Most studies were conducted to support Union Carbide chemicals. Henry Smyth served as the first director of the laboratory and held that position for 30 years, passing away in 1957 on the actual day of the laboratory's 50th anniversary. He was followed by Charles Carpenter and then Carol Weil. The laboratory was especially known for its expertise in inhalation and dermal carcinogenesis studies which would be consistent with their mission of testing chemical compounds development by Union Carbide. BRRC was the first laboratory to adopt rigid specifications for standardized toxicity testing, especially for range-finding studies, and other laboratories soon followed their lead. BRRC was also the first laboratory to test chemicals for skin penetration as previously this route of administration had generally been ignored. They were also one of the first laboratories that placed a significant emphasis on collecting clinical and anatomical pathology data on the kidney and liver as an important measurement of toxicity. Noted toxicologists at BRRC included Henry Smyth, Carol Weil, Shayne Gad, Ray Yang, Daryl Dodd, and Steve Frantz. In 1998, the laboratory was closed.

Southern Research Institute

Southern Research Institute (SRI) was established in 1941 as a nonprofit organization to foster research and technology development as an economic engine for Birmingham, Alabama, and the Southern United States. Thomas W. Martin, an attorney and president of the Alabama Power Company, was the primary founder. Martin, with the cooperation of other business leaders in Birmingham, established SRI to help make the city a major research center in the South and to develop the South's agricultural, mineral, and forest resources. In the early years, biological research was not a focus area for the laboratory. The first director of SRI was Wilbur Lazier, an organic chemist who previously worked at DuPont and who had an important role in the development of nylon and other polymers. Research into oncology became a major part of SRI in 1974 when Howard Skipper became president. Skipper was a veteran of the US Army's Chemical Warfare Service and had an established reputation as a researcher in the field of oncology. Toxicology at SRI began in earnest in 1976 with the establishment of a contract with what would ultimately become the National Toxicology Program (NTP). Paul Denine became the head of the new preclinical pharmacology and toxicology division in 1978, and he was followed by J. David Prejean who held that position for over 10 years. SRI had sites in Birmingham and in Fredrick, Maryland. The Fredrick site opened in 1990 and primarily conducted infectious disease studies in 19 animal rooms and 43,000 square feet of space. The Birmingham site supported numerous other capabilities unrelated to biological testing, such as engineering and environmental research. For toxicology testing, the Birmingham site consisted of 54 animal rooms and approximately 63,000 square feet of space, including several BSL-3 rooms. While noted mostly for conducting programs for governmental agencies such as NTP, NCI, and NIDA, SRI is also a full-service provider for drug development services, with a strong experience in testing biologics, especially vaccines, oncolytic viral vectors, and gene therapy vectors. Noted toxicologists at SRI include Paul Bushdid, Alan Stokes, Tina Rogers, David Serota, John Page, Charles Lindamood, and Charles Hebert, with Eric Morinello and Vince Torti receiving their initial CRO training at SRI.

Hazleton Laboratories

Hazleton Laboratories was established in 1946 by Lloyd Hazleton who previously had been on the faculty of both Georgetown Medical School and George Washington University Medical School. He received his doctorate in pharmacology from the University of Washington and established Hazleton Laboratories outside of Vienna, Virginia, on the grounds of an old schoolhouse. Hazleton was well respected within the toxicology community and was known for his philosophy of mentoring and training young toxicologists, receiving the Society of Toxicology's Education Award in 1982 in recognition of his company's training of numerous young toxicologists that went on to successful careers in other organizations. At its zenith, the Vienna campus was on 90 acres of prime real estate and consisted of around 80 animal rooms that housed rodents, rabbits, dogs, and nonhuman primates. Lloyd Hazleton sold the company in 1970 to TRW Corporation who renamed it TRW Science Center. In 1972, TRW Corporation sold the company to Environmental Sciences Corporation, headed by Donald Nielsen and Kirby Cramer, who returned the Hazleton name. In 1976, Hazleton opened a new, state-of-the-art, rodent facility in Reston, Virginia, that had over 60 animal rooms. Through a series of acquisitions and through organic growth, Hazleton, in 1982, had become the world's largest independent biological testing laboratory in the world. These acquisitions included the Tobacco Research Council Laboratories in Harrogate, England, in 1974; Affenzucht Munster in Munster, Germany, in 1980; the Institut Merieux site in Lyon, France, in 1981; and RALTECH in Madison, Wisconsin, in 1982. In 1985, Hazleton purchased Litton Bionetics in Rockville and Kensington, Maryland. In 1987, the company was sold to Corning, Inc. and renamed Corning Hazleton, and in 1996 Corning, Inc. spun off its toxicology testing segment as an independent company which was subsequently named Covance, Inc. In 2010, Covance, Inc. announced that it was closing the Vienna site and several years later the buildings were demolished and the site sold for real estate development. Noted toxicologists at the Hazleton Vienna site include Lloyd Hazleton, Cliff Jessup, Gene Paynter, Bill Knapp, Robert Weir, Bob Scala, James Gargus, Bill Olsen, Bill Coate, Fred Reno, Tom Mulligan, Dan Dalgard, Ray Cox, Sandra Morseth, Sidney Green, David Brusick, Steve Haworth, and Brian Myhr. Among those who received their initial training in toxicology at Hazleton were Geoffrey Hogan, Robert Kapp, Vince Piccirillo, David Serota, Gary Wolfe, Debra Pence, Joy Cavagnaro, Merrill Osheroff, Alan Hoberman, Vicki Markiewicz, Jan Trutter, and Tracey Zoetis.

SRI International

SRI International was established in 1946 by a group at Stanford University as an independent, nonprofit, non-endowed corporation chartered by the State of California and was originally named Stanford Research Institute. It formally separated from Stanford University in 1970 and became knowns as SRI

International in 1977. Gordon Newell created the toxicology group at SRI International in the early 1950s. Newell received his doctorate in biochemistry from the University of Wisconsin and was at SRI International for over 25 years. The main facility was located in Menlo Park, California, but there were several additional satellite facilities including Plymouth, Michigan, and Harrisonburg, Virginia. The Menlo Park facility included 40 buildings encompassing over 1.3 million square feet of space on a 63-acre site. The Bioscience Division included approximately 250,000 square feet of animal areas, laboratory space, and support areas. SRI International was one of the pioneers of genetic toxicology testing, inventing the pKM101 plasmid in Ames strains and in vivo unscheduled DNA syntheses tests and validating the Ames test, the repeat-dose micronucleus test, the mouse lymphoma test, and the in vitro and in vivo unscheduled DNA tests. Noted toxicologists at SRI International included Gordon Newell, Robert Baldwin, Rick Becker, Jon Reid, Jon Mirsalis, James MacGregor, Karen Steinmetz, Hanna Ng, Gordon Pryor, and Carol Green.

Lovelace Biomedical

Lovelace Biomedical was established in 1947 by William "Randy" Lovelace II, a Harvard trained surgeon, as a needed specialty medicine clinical and nonprofit medical foundation in Albuquerque, New Mexico. Originally known as the Lovelace Foundation for Medical Education and Research, over the years the organization's research operations expanded in size and scope that was parallel with the advances of the medical and healthcare industries. Initially funded predominantly by government contracts to execute cutting-edge projects related to public health, Lovelace Biomedical is known as a place of medical firsts. With a strong tie to the aviation community during its earliest days, in the period between 1950 and 1970, Lovelace Biomedical became known as the nation's premier center for aviation and space medicine research and, in 1959, under contract with NASA, tested 32 candidate pilots which culminated in the selection of the first 7 Mercury astronauts. In 1964, Randy Lovelace was appointed Director of Space Medicine for NASA. During the period from 1962 through 1993, Lovelace Biomedical entered into a cooperative agreement with the Atomic Energy Commission in the areas of toxicology, with an emphasis in inhalation toxicology. During the 1980s the company changed its name to the

Inhalation Toxicology Research Institute. They were the first organization to demonstrate that cigarette smoking caused cancer in laboratory animals. They developed many innovative measurement devices in the area of aerosol sciences, including the Lovelace multi-jet impactor, the Lovelace nebulizer for delivery of fine particles, and Lovelace particle separator, and a parallel plate diffusion battery measuring particle size in aerosols. In 1996, the company became privatized under the leadership of Robert Rubin as the not for profit Lovelace Respiratory Research Institute and over the next 20 years sponsored research that combined basic science in the areas of respiratory disease, contract sciences in toxicology, infectious diseases, and medical countermeasures. In 2016, under the leadership of Jacob McDonald, the organization again changed its name to Lovelace Biomedical with a strong focus and emphasis on commercial toxicology testing. The company is still based in Albuquerque and sits on 100 acres of land with 300,000 square feet of laboratory space and 80 animal rooms. Noted toxicologists that have worked there include Roger McClellan, Joe Mauderly, Charles Hobbs, Steve Belinsky, Janet Benson, Rogene Henderson, Ron Wolf, Matt Campen, Chet Leach, and Jacob McDonald.

Charles River

Chares River was founded in 1947 as Charles River Breeding Laboratories when Henry Foster purchased one thousand rat cages from a Virginia farm and set up a one-man laboratory in Boston, Massachusetts, that overlooked the Charles River. Over the next 50 years, Charles River Breeding Laboratories became one of the world's largest breeders of quality laboratory animals for basic and applied research. In 1955, the company's headquarters was relocated to Wilmington, Massachusetts, and began the commercial production of pathogen-free rodents by using the industry's first barrier-type production building. In 1956, the first Caesarean Originated Barrier Sustained (COBS®) rodents were introduced and became the new industry standard for animal production. In 1966, the company became international with the opening of a new animal production facility in France, and in 1981 it instituted the first commercial comprehensive genetic monitoring program. Virus antibody-free (VAF/Plus®) animals were introduced in 1984, and during the same year the company was purchased by Bausch & Lomb with the Foster Family still running the company. In 1988, Charles River entered the field of transgenic services with the arrival of the first transgenic mice for breeding. In 1992, Charles River began to expand its services by entering the specialty services area with the purchase of Specific Pathogen Antigen Free Avian Services (specializing in the production of eggs and poultry and serologic diagnostic services) and the 1996 purchase of Endosafe, Inc., a manufacturer of Limulus Amebocyte Lysate products and services. In 1997, James Foster bought the company back from Bausch & Lomb, and in 1998, the company expanded its portfolio by entering the biopharmaceutical services industry. Over the next 20 years, an aggressive acquisition strategy made Charles River the largest company of its type in the world. These acquisitions included Sierra Biomedical in 1999; Primedica in 2001; Inveresk Research in 2004; Piedmont Research Center in 2009; Accugenix in 2012; Argenta, BioFocus, and ChanTest in 2014; Celsis International and Oncotest GmgH in 2015; WIL Research and Agilux Laboratories in 2016; MPI Research in 2018; and CiToxLab in 2019. These sites were in addition to a 412,000 square foot laboratory facility in Shrewsbury, Massachusetts, that Charles River opened in 2007, closed in 2010, and reopened in 2016 (with 80,000 square feet of vivarium space).

The Middle Years

Industrial Biotest

Industrial Biotest (IBT) was founded in 1953 by Joseph Calandra who was a professor of pathology and biochemistry at Northwestern University. The facilities were located at a site in Northbrook, Illinois, and had up to 350 employees employed there. In 1966, it was sold to Nalco Holding Company. During the early 1970s, it was the largest preclinical CRO in the world and conducted more than one third of all contracted toxicology testing in the United States. In the mid-1970s, IBT was accused of conducting fraudulent and tainted toxicology testing and was investigated by both FDA and EPA staff, leading to many reported studies being rejected by regulatory agencies and the expensive re-testing of many compounds. Three senior executives of IBT were tried and convicted by a jury of conducting and submitting fraudulent studies and in the cover-up of those activities, and in 1978 IBT closed. Much of the negative events identified at IBT led to the promulgation of the Good Laboratory Practices (GLP) in 1976.

Woodard Research

Woodard Research was founded in 1956 by Geoffrey Woodard and his wife Marie Woodard. Geoffrey Woodard was a former FDA pharmacologist and who also taught at George Washington University. The facility was located in Herndon, Virginia, with approximately 100,000 square feet of space spread among various research buildings. Woodard Research conducted studies in rodents, rabbits, dogs, cats, nonhuman primates, quail, ducks, and fish, along with farm animals such as cattle and pigs. Along with the Geoffrey Woodard, other noted toxicologists that worked there include Robert Belilies and William Scott. In 1972, the laboratory closed.

Gulf South Research Institute

Gulf South Research Institute (GSRI) was established in the early 1960s in New Iberia, Louisiana, at an old naval base by the Louisiana Partnership for Technology. GSRI was located on a 118-acre site which included 440,000 square feet of vivarium space. Most of the work conducted there was related to a significant nonhuman primate colony population that was involved in viral studies, but there were also approximately ten rooms that were used to conduct carcinogenicity studies for the NTP. In addition, there was also the capability for conducting both acute and inhalation studies. Jim Clinton was the corporate director of GSRI and Richard Parent also worked there for several years. GSRI closed in 1984 and the site was taken over by the University of Louisiana at Lafayette, renamed the New Iberia Research Center with its role was redefined as a nonhuman primate center to provide nonhuman primates to support contract research. In 1990, it expanded its mission to provide preclinical safety testing services.

Bio/Dynamics

Bio/dynamics was founded in 1961 by two faulty members from Rutgers University Bureau of Biologic Research, Thomas Russell, a biochemist, and John McCoy, a pathologist (one of the founders of the Society of Toxicologic Pathologists). The first facility was housed in rented space in a veterinary clinic in Edison, New Jersey. In 1963, the 55-acre Mettler farm in East Millstone, New Jersey, was purchased as the new site for Bio/dynamics, and Thomas Russell left Rutgers to devote his full attention to building the company. By 1964, the staff had grown to 12 employees. The farmhouse became the company headquarters office, the milk house a small animal laboratory/ necropsy area, and the dairy barn a dog kennel. Getting to work in the morning occasionally involved traffic jams of cattle being herded down Mettler Lane with grazing on the lawn outside of the headquarters building. In 1973, the company was acquired by IMS International, a market research organization serving the international pharmaceutical industry. At that time, the staff had grown to approximately 100 employees with 9 buildings on site. In 1978, IMS International purchased Life Science Research (LSR), a UK-based contract toxicology laboratory and the two laboratories became the Life Sciences Division of IMS International. In 1976, a state-of-the-art inhalation facility was constructed and by 1980, there were approximately 300 employees with 15 buildings on site. In 1983, Thomas Russell left the company to pursue other ventures and Geoffrey Hogan became the President of Bio/dynamics. In 1987, Applied Bioscience International (APBI) was formed when IMS International divested itself of its life science division. Over the next several years, continued mergers and acquisitions produced a family of companies that included CANTAB, ENVIRON International Corporation, Environmental Testing and Certification Corporation (ECT), Landis International, and Pharmaco Dynamics Research, a clinical organization. In 1993, Pharmaco LSR was formed by the union of three APBI-owned companies, Bio/dynamics, LSR, and Pharmaco. At that time Bio/dynamics had 340 employees and 18 buildings on site. In 1995, Huntington International Holdings purchased APBI's two toxicology companies (Bio/dynamics and LSR), and these companies were united with the Huntington International Holdings facility in Cambridge, England, to become Huntington Life Sciences (HLS). The group was originally led by Christopher Cliffe who was followed by Brian Cass in 1999, both being former executives of the Hazleton Laboratories site in Harrogate, England. Michael Caulfield, who began his career as an archivist at Bio/dynamics in 1985, became general manager of the HLS site in East Millstone. In 2014, HLS acquired Harlan Laboratories, a major supplier of rodents for biological testing and owner of several CROs in Europe, including the former SafePharm Laboratories in England and RCC Laboratories in Switzerland. Two divisions were established, Rodent Models and Services (RMS) and Contract Research Services (CRS), with Bio/dynamics becoming

Princeton CRS. In 2015, the company was re-branded as Envigo, and the East Millstone site had 350 employees and 95 animal rooms in facilities consisting of almost 200,000 square feet. In 2019, Envigo and LabCorp (the parent company of Covance, Inc.) entered into an agreement by which LabCorp purchased Envigo's contract research service business, while Envigo purchased LabCorp's animal research models and service business. Noted toxicologists that have worked there included Andrew Sivak, William Strauss, Ted King, Jerry Smith, William Rinehart, Sylvie Gosselin, Geoffrey Hogan, Carol Auletta, Gary Hoffman, Cathy Kelly, Robert Parker, Rosemary Mandella, John Atkinson, Debra Barrett, Diann Blanset, Dan Cerven, David Compton, Ira Daly, Paul Newton, George Rusch, Jim Killen, Lee Grotz, Oscar Moreno, John Mitchell, Robert Sabol, Raymond Schroeder, William Tierney, and Deborah Novicki.

Litton Bionetics, Inc.

Bionetics Research Laboratories was founded in 1961, with a small toxicology facility in Falls Church, Virginia, and a larger facility in Kensington, Maryland. During these early years, most of the toxicology work conducted there was under government contracts, especially for the National Cancer Institute, involving cancer bioassays in rodents for dyes that were being used as food additives. Ross Hart served as Director of Toxicology during those times. In 1968, the company was purchased by Litton Industries and changed its name to Litton Bionetics, Inc. In the early 1970s, a new, state-of-the-art facility was built in Rockville, Maryland (approximately 100,000 square feet of space), and all toxicology units and analytical chemistry were consolidated in this facility, along with a section of the facility designed to conduct inhalation studies. It was also at the Rockville facility that Robert Gallo housed his animals that were used in his research program that identified the retrovirus that was the cause of AIDS. Genetic and molecular toxicology functions remained at the Kensington site. Following the retirement of Ross Hart in the early 1970s, Robert Weir became Director of Toxicology and in 1972; Litton Bionetics was awarded the first government contract to manage and operate the Frederick Cancer Research Laboratory in Frederick, Maryland. In 1973, the first commercial genetic toxicology testing facility in the United States was opened in the Kensington facility under the leadership of David Brusick, and a second site opened in Veenendal, The Netherlands, in 1980 under the direction of Fred Hoorn. In 1985, Hazleton Laboratories purchased the toxicology testing business of Litton Bionetics (Rockville and Kensington sites), and at that time there were approximately 200 employees at both sites. Noted mammalian toxicologists at Litton Bionetics included Robert Weir, John Keller, Les Goldsmith, Robet Belilies, Ron Filler, and Michael Moore. Noted genetic toxicologists include David Brusick, Brian Myhr, James Ivett, Robert Young, Hema Murli, Maria Cifone, Michael Cimono, Devara Jaganath, Tim Lawlor, and Steve Haworth.

International Research and Development Corporation

International Research and Development Corporation (IRDC) was founded in 1962 by Francis Wazeter, who had a doctorate in pharmacology and had formerly worked at the FDA. The facility was located in Mattawan, Michigan, and began its existence with approximately 140,000 square feet of space and 140 animal rooms. At its zenith, it consisted of over 300,000 square feet of space containing approximately 240 animal rooms and with over 400 employees. It serviced a full range of clients representing the pharmaceutical, chemical, cosmetic, and food industries both domestically and internationally, with 75% of its business associated with human and animal health products, 10% of its business associated with both petrochemicals/agrichemicals and food and consumer products, and 5% of its business associated with medical devices. For several years, it also owned a clinical research company called IRAD that was in Florida. In the early 1990s, at the time that Francis Wazeter selected his son, Francis Wazeter, Jr., to run IRDC, the company fell on financial troubles. In 1990, a skin care products company in California, Carme, Inc., was acquired and financed mostly with bank debt. This acquisition proved to be a disastrous endeavor, and the company fell into bankruptcy and went into receivership in September 1995. The bankruptcy was the result of unethical business practices including a serious accounting fraud at the skin care products unit. In November 1995, the residual assets of IRDC were purchased by an investing group led by William Parfet to create a private company called MPI Research. Noted toxicologists at IRDC included Edwin Goldenthal, Cliff Jessup, James Schardein, Ray York, Dean Rodwell, Gerald Shafer, Malcolm Blair, Eric Spicer, James Laveglia, and Richard Slauter.

Bio-Research Laboratories (Canada)

Bio-Research Laboratories was founded in 1965 by Clifford Chappel, a former medical director at Wyeth Pharmaceuticals. It was originally located in a mini laboratory housed at MacDonald College in Montreal, Canada, and later moved to Pointe Claire in Montreal. It offered clinical patch testing, preclinical drug development, and aquatic toxicology services. It was here that the "great bacon study" was conducted where large amounts of bacon were fried daily and fed to animal test subjects to ascertain the effects of nitrosamines. In 1976, the company was purchased by Canada Development Corporation (CDC) as part of a strategy to build a Canadian owned healthcare company with other members of the group including Connaught Laboratories, Nordic Pharma, and Raylo – this new company was named Connlab. With the advent of Good Laboratory Practices (GLPs) making the Pointe Claire facility unacceptable for conducting studies, CDC in 1977 purchased the former Smith, Kline & French site in Senneville, Montreal, which consisted of 30 acres and a laboratory building. A new vivarium was added in 1978, there were 83 employees, and F. Fried was appointed president. In 1978, Fried retired and Michael Ankcorn was appointed president and CEO. In 1984, CDC decided to spin off Connlab as a public company which was renamed CDC Life Sciences. In 1985, a new, purpose-built 60,000 square foot building to support additional toxicology work was opened. In 1989, CDC Life Sciences was subject to a successful hostile takeover by Institut Merieux of France who put the toxicology divisions up for sale. The uncertainty and insecurity of this action resulted in both the loss of a significant amount of business and the departure of many senior leaders and technical staff. However, during this same time, the expertise of conducting infusion toxicology was developed and the site became a center for excellence of this technology. In 1991, Institut Merieux sold the company to CAI Capital who in turn sold the company to ClinTrials in 1997, renaming the company CTBR. In 2001, the CTBR/ClinTrials group was sold to Inveresk Research in Scotland and renamed CTBR/Inveresk, and an additional new vivarium facility was opened. In 2004, CTBR/Inveresk was sold to Charles River, at that time CTBR had over 1600 employees and approximately 350 animal rooms.

There were at least two other CROs named BioResearch – one in Philadelphia (started and managed by Karl Gabriel) and the other in Cambridge, MA, operated by Frederick Homburger and specializing in hamster studies.

Ricera

Ricera began as Diamond Shamrock in 1967 with the merger of Shamrock Oil and Diamond Alkali Chemical, a maker of heavy chemicals. The original president was William Bricker. Some year later, they went into a joint venture with Showa Denko and became SDS Biotech. They were then purchased by Fermeta, an Italian company, and changed the name to Ricera in 1986; Ricera was the Italian word for research. In 2007, Ricera became Concord Biosciences. The facility was n Concord Township near Painesville, Ohio, and consisted of 110,000 square feet and 20 animal rooms. Noted toxicologists who worked there include James Killeen, James Laveglia, Larry Powers, William Ford, and Darren Warren.

Calvert Laboratories

Calvert Laboratories was founded in 1969 as Pharmakon Laboratories in Scranton, Pennsylvania, by Richard Matthews who was a pharmacologist who had previously worked at Upjohn and Union Carbide. Matthews had an entrepreneurial spirit who saw the vision of the upcoming boom in biotechnology. Pharmakon Laboratories initially offered classic in vivo pharmacology studies. In 1980, the company moved to Waverly, Pennsylvania, and over the next ten years the company introduced additional testing services that included acute toxicology, cytogenetics and genetic toxicology, immunology, pharmacokinetics, and full-service general toxicology. In 1990, the company was purchased by the biotechnology company DNX (Princeton, NJ), which a a few years later purchased the Hazleton site in Lyon, France, with the resulting company calling itself Pharmakon Research International. In 1996, Pharmakon merged with Bioclin, a clinical CRO to form a new publicly held company called Chrysalis, which was subdivided into nonclinical and clinical portions in the United States and Europe, which now covered a complete range of preclinical and clinical (phases I–IV) studies. In 1998, a large pharmaceutical company discontinued the development of a potential major cardiovascular drug, and as the clinical arm of Chrysalis 1 had been scaling up and incurring substantial expenses to conduct this project, the clinical part of Chrysalis found itself in bankruptcy. The nonclinical portion of Chrysalis remained solvent, but these events led to the purchase of Chrysalis by Phoenix International Life Sciences (PILS), which was based in Montreal, Canada. However, PILS soon found itself in bankruptcy after the very same large pharmaceutical company that sank the clinical arm of Chrysalis cancelled the performance of a large bioanalytical program in support of a phase III study. This in turn led to MDS of Toronto, Canada, to acquire PILS in 1999. The many assets of PILS were dissected and sold, spun off as independent units, or absorbed within MDS. A small company in Cary, North Carolina, composed of former pharmaceutical executives and consultants to the pharmaceutical industry in general called Calvert Holdings acquired Chrysalis in 2000 and changed its name to Calvert Preclinical Services. The executive chairman of the board and majority owner of Calvert Preclinical Services was Russell McLauchlan, formerly of Lederle. In 2002, Calvert Preclinical Services changed its name to Calvert Laboratories. The services offered by Pharmakon-Chrysalis-Phoenix-MDS-Calvert remained the same: acute through chronic toxicology studies, carcinogenicity studies, DART studies, discovery and safety pharmacology studies, pharmacokinetics and ADME studies, and immunology studies at the Waverly facility that included approximately 40,000 square feet and 40 animal rooms. It became the first CRO to offer GLP contract services in safety pharmacology and immunology. Noted toxicologists at Pharmakon-Chrysalis-Calvert include Robert Naismith, Charles B. Spainhour, Joan Chapdelaine, Vincent Ciofalo, Roger Toothaker, Leon Stankowski, Juan SanSebastian, Michal Virat, Francois Verdier, and Bernard Regnier.

Experimental Pathology Laboratories

Experimental Pathology Laboratories (EPL) was founded in 1971 by John (Jack) Ferrell and William Busey, two pathologists who had previously worked at Hazleton Laboratories in Vienna, Virginia. Early pioneers in the profession of toxicologic pathology, they recognized the need for independent contract pathology services in the coming years and created a small business consisting of two pathologists, three technicians, and one secretary in Herndon, Virginia. Over the years, EPL has grown to be one of the largest leading independent pathology companies in the world, with sites in several states and in Europe. EPL has two main laboratories, one site in Sterling, Virginia, where the corporate headquarters are located, and one site in Research Triangle Park, North Carolina. The Sterling site occupies over 28,000 square feet of space which includes 8600 square feet of space dedicated for histological processing. This site includes complete facilities for the histologic processing and microscopic evaluation of mammalian and aquatic animal tissues, and it was designed specifically with attention placed on the orderly and effective flow of work and employee safety. The site in Research Triangle Park comprises approximately 43,000 square feet of space, and it is where EPL manages the NTP Archives and NTP Frozen Tissue Bank to store pathology materials, frozen specimens, and data from government-sponsored toxicity and carcinogenicity studies. EPL also manages the NIEHS Data and Specimen Repository at this site. EPL was instrumental in designing and developing a pathology peer review system for verifying the pathology data generated by the National Cancer Institute's Carcinogenesis Program, later called the National Toxicology Program. This system of pathology peer review is widely used by pharmaceutical companies and toxicology laboratories to resolve difficult pathology issues when the data are to be submitted to regulatory agencies. After John Ferrell and William Busey retired in 1998, Jerry Hardisty became President of EPL, and following Hardisty's retirement in 2015, Kathleen Funk became EPL President. Noted pathologists at EPL include John Ferrell, William Busey, Jerry Hardisty, Robert Maronpot, Paul Snyder, Kathleen Funk, Gerald Long, Peter Mann, Thomas Steinbach, and Paul Snyder.

MB Research Laboratories

MB Research Laboratories was founded in 1972 by Oscar Moreno and Terry Bannon in Spinnerstown, Pennsylvania. The original site consisted of 14,000 square feet of space and 12 animal rooms, with the mission of the company to provide rapid, accurate, and reproducible acute toxicity assays. While still fulfilling that role, MB Research Laboratories has been at the forefront in the development of alternative assays since 1989. The validation of alternatives has been supported by numerous governmental and industry grants. Today, MB Research Laboratories offers GLP in vitro and ex vivo alternatives for cytotoxicity, dermal irritation, ocular irritation, dermal sensitization, and dermal corrosivity studies while continuing to provide expertise in in vivo acute animal assays. Noted toxicologists at MB Research Laboratories include Oscar Moreno, Daniel Cerven, George DeGeorge, Albert Gilotti, Edward Yurknow, Dee Kim Tessler, John Mitchell, and Bennett Varsho.

Pacific BioLabs

Pacific BioLabs was founded in 1972 as Northview Biosciences in Northbrook, Illinois, by Martin Spalding, a chemist at the Murine Company (a maker of eye drops) that was acquired by Abbott Laboratories in 1970. In 1982, Northview Biolabs acquired E.S. Unilabs in Berkeley, California, a small contract laboratory that offered microbiology and small science services with a staff of 18, and reincorporated in California as Northview Pacific Laboratories, Inc. At the request of large client that was a contract sterilizer, Northview Biolabs opened in new facility in 1991 in Spartanburg, South Carolina. All of these business units were part of Northview Biosciences, Inc. (NVB), which served as a corporate holding company. In 2006, SGS acquired NVB and the facilities in Illinois (offering analytical chemistry and microbiology services for pharmaceutical companies) and South Carolina (offering medical device microbiology services), but not the California site. At that time, the Illinois site had 21,000 square feet of space and 90 employees, while the South Carolina site had 10,000 square feet of space and 13 employees. In 2006 Northview Pacific Laboratories, Inc. (now located in Hercules, California) was renamed Pacific BioLabs, Inc. The facility consists of 34,000 square feet of space with 29 animal rooms and 90 employees and offers analytical chemistry, bioanalysis, microbiology, and toxicology services. Noted toxicologists at Pacific BioLabs include Timothy Doherty, Dennis Chapman, Michael Yakes, and Gurpreet Ratra.

Utah Biomedical Toxicology Laboratories

Utah Biomedical Toxicology Laboratories (UTBL) was founded around 1973. Originally funded by NIH money to serve as a center for pursing artificial heart replacement research, it was purchased by the Sorenson family of Salt Lake City and led by James Sorenson. The facility was in Salt Lake City, Utah in the University of Utah Research Park. The laboratory contained approximately 20,000 square feet of space with 20 animal rooms, including 3 surgical suites with observation decks. Studies were conducted in rodents, rabbits, dogs, pigs, sheep, cattle, and horses. The laboratory specialized in surgical studies and medical device biocompatibility studies, and it was one of a few laboratories at that time conducting biocompatibility studies for medical devices. Noted toxicologists at UTBL include Randy White, Jerry Nelson, Russell Eyre, Steve Beck, Wayne Ball, and William Ford. In 1986, the company was divided into two groups, toxicology and medical, and sold to HeartPort who closed the toxicology group. In 1992, HeartPort was purchased by a large pharmaceutical company, and the facility was taken over by the University of Utah in 1994.

Stillmeadow, Inc.

Stillmeadow, Inc. was founded in 1975 in Sugar Land Texas by Robert Sabol, who had a degree in animal sciences from Delaware Valley College and had previously served as a laboratory manager at Bio/dynamics. The original location consisted of 600 square feet of space and reached 5000 square feet of space by 1990 when it moved to its current location and expended to 50,000 square feet in 1995. In 1997, it acquired ENSR's bio-monitoring laboratory and added a 10,000 square aquatic toxicology laboratory. In 2008, it added an additional 15,000 square foot building. Stillmeadow conducts mammalian toxicology studies but is especially known in the industry as one of the few CROs that conducts aquatic, entomology, and environmental toxicology studies. Noted toxicologists at Stillmeadow, Inc. included Vince Murphy, Kenneth Washburn, Jan Kuhn, Mark Holbert, Warner Phelps, Andres Doig, and Cole Younger.

Toxicology Pathology Services, Inc.

Toxicology Pathology Services, Inc. (TPS) was founded in 1976 by James Botta, an Auburn University-trained veterinarian. The laboratory, located in Mount Vernon, Indiana, consisted of 90,000 square feet of space with 44 animal rooms. In 1989, TPS was acquired by BASi, and in 2018, BASi was acquired by Seventh Wave. Noted toxicologists at TPS included James Botta, Gina Gratz, and Phillip Downing.

WIL Research

WIL Research was founded in 1976 as Welcome Independent Laboratories in Cincinnati, Ohio, by G. Bruce Briggs, a veterinary toxicologist and Ralph Hodgdon, a business administrator. Prior to establishing WIL Research, Briggs had held senior leadership roles at Pfizer; Smith, Kline & French, and Hill Top

Research. The original site in Cincinnati comprised 24,000 square feet of space with approximately 30 animal rooms. In 1978, WIL Research was acquired by Great Lakes Chemical Corporation and in 1980 WIL Research acquired the Hess and Clark Research Farm in Ashland, Ohio from Rhone Poulenc. During 1982–1983, the operations in Cincinnati were all transitioned to the Ashland site which was located on 40 acres comprising 7 research buildings and approximately 70,000 square feet of space. Currently this site occupies 300,000 square feet of laboratory space. WIL Research was the first CRO to develop, validate, install, and market an electronic data capture system for in-life and post-life toxicology measurements, including developmental and reproductive studies, statistics, and report generation. It was also the first CRO to install and operate BioClean animal rooms for conducting chronic toxicity studies in rodents. Noted toxicologists at WIL research included Bruce Briggs, James Laveglia, Dean Rodwell, Mark Nemec, Chris Chengelis, and Dale Mayhew.

Springborn Institute for Bioresearch

Springborn Institute for Bioresearch was founded in 1976 by Robert Springborn, a chemist who had previously been at Monsanto and W. R. Grace. The 26-acre site in Spencerville, Ohio, had previously been a veterinary research business created in 1965 called Bio-Tox Labs, which had been purchased by Diamond Shamrock in 1969 to perform large animal research. At the time of the Springborn purchase, the site encompassed 27,000 square feet of space with 18 animal rooms. In 2001, the organization changed its name to Springborn Life Sciences, and in 2002, Springborn Life Sciences was purchased by Charles River. Currently the site contains 117,000 square feet of laboratory space and approximately 250 employees. Noted toxicologists at Springborn included Richard Hiles, Dean Rodwell, Peter Becci, Malcolm Bair, Joseph Siglin, and Rusty Rush.

Hazleton Munster

Hazleton Munster was originally founded as Affenucht Munster (AZM) in Munster, Germany, in 1976 by Rainhart Korte, a reproductive toxicologist you had previously been at Schering AG, to serve as a primate breeding facility for use in the vaccine industry. In 1980, Rainhart Korte sold AZM to Hazleton

Laboratories, and the breeding facility was turned into a toxicology laboratory in 1981 to focus on reproductive toxicology in rodents, rabbits, and nonhuman primates. In 1982, acute and general toxicology services were added, but acute services were discontinued in 1984. In 1997, the site became a nonhuman primate only facility. Rainhart Korte served as Managing Director through 2002, and he was followed by Friedhelm Vogel who served in that position through 2019. Following the Hazleton history, the facility became part of Corning in 1987, was renamed Covance in 1996, and became part of LabCorp in 2015. It was considered the first CRO to offer nonhuman primate reproduction studies (conducted approximately 80 such studies), and over the years it has initialed many new and innovative housing and technical procedures to enhance the quality of toxicology studies performed in nonhuman primates. Currently the facility has over 200 employees and 117 animal rooms with an ability to house over 2000 macaques and 200 marmosets. Noted toxicologists at Hazleton Munster included Rainhart Korte, Friedhelm Vogler, Gerhard Weinbauer, Wolfgang Mueller, and Sven Korte.

Borriston Laboratories

Borriston Laboratories was founded by the Dynamic Corporation in 1977 in Temple Hills, Maryland. The laboratory was initially started to house and continue a 7-year cigarette smoking study in dogs for the NCI after the initial contractor decided to not continue the study. In 1978, Borriston Laboratories decided to expand its services and began offering a full set of standard acute, subchronic, and chronic/carcinogenicity studies in rodents and dogs and developmental and reproduction studies in rodents and rabbits. At its peak, it had over 100 employees and 40 animal rooms, used mostly for rodents and rabbits. Noted toxicologists at Borriston Laboratories included Tom Mulligan, Vine Piccirillo, and Richard Costlow. In 1985, Borriston Laboratories were sold to Andrew Tegeris and merged with Pharmacopathics Laboratories to become Tegeris Laboratories in Laurel, Maryland, but Tegeris Laboratories closed in 1988.

Argus Research Laboratories

Argus Research Laboratories was founded in 1979 by Mildred Christian, E. Marshall Johnson, and Gerald Lightkep in a modified barn on Buckshire Farm in Perkasie, Pennsylvania. The idea to form a CRO that focused on reproductive and developmental toxicology came from Mildred Christian who had just completed her doctorate at Jefferson University (E. Marshall Johnson had been her major professor) and who felt that no existing US CRO could conduct scientifically adequate and GLP compliant studies of this type. The original laboratory had six animal rooms and four employees. In 1982, Argus Research Laboratories began leasing and modifying warehouse space in Horsham, Pennsylvania, and in 1990 it left the Perkasie site to grow and develop the Horsham site. In 1987, it purchased the Center for Photobiology from Temple University and began offering phototoxicity capabilities. In 1991, the TSI Corporation purchased Argus Research Laboratories allowing Johnson and Lightkep to retire. TSI Corporation had previously purchased EG&G Mason Laboratories in Worcester, Massachusetts and a small CRO in Redfield, Arkansas, but had overextended itself and sold these assets to the Genzyme Transgenic Company (GTC) a few years later. GTC was 42% owned by Genzyme, and it had been formed to produce drugs in goat milk on a GMP farm in Charlton, Massachusetts. The concept was that the CRO business would generate the income necessary to support the production of drugs, but when that strategy failed, GTC formed a company called Primedica so that the CRO business could be sold. Charles River purchased Primedica in 2001, closed the Redfield site in 2008, moved the Worcester site to Shrewsbury, Massachusetts, and renamed the Horsham site Charles River Horsham. Currently the Horsham site has 65 animal rooms in a 124,000 square foot laboratory with a staff of 230. Noted toxicologists at Argus Research Laboratories included Mildred Christian, Don Forbes, Chris Sambuco, and Alan Hoberman.

The Later Years

Toxicology Research Laboratory at the University of Illinois at Chicago

The Toxicology Research Laboratory at the University of Illinois Chicago (UIC) in Chicago, Illinois, was established in 1987 by Barry Levine who had previously worked in both the CRO and pharmaceutical industries. The facility consisted of approximately 110,000 square feet of space encompassing slightly more than 100 animal rooms. Most of the testing was conducted in support of government contracts, but studies for the pharmaceutical industry were also performed. Noted toxicologists at UIC included Barry Levine, Debra Kirchner, Alan Brown, Ashraf Youssef, and Peter Korytko.

International Toxicology Research

International Toxicology Research (ITR) was created in Montreal, Canada, in 1989 as a subsidiary research facility of the Japanese Bozo Research Center by Kumi Yamanouchi. The facility encompasses 185,000 square feet of laboratory space with 72 animal rooms and 15 inhalation exposure rooms. It is a full service CRO conducting toxicology studies in all common animal species with an expertise in large molecule programs and immunology endpoints. Noted toxicologists at ITR included Colin Bier and Joseph Younan.

Smithers Avanza

Smithers Avanza was established in 1992 in Gaithersburg, Maryland, by Roy O. Williams, as R.O.W. Sciences, Inc. to support NTP reproductive and developmental studies. Williams began his career as an inhalation technician at Hazleton Laboratories and later founded R.O.W. Sciences as a company to support NIH in managing animal facilities. He then decided to build his own facility in Gaithersburg and hired Bruce Briggs as the first toxicologist there. The original facility had 35,000 square feet of space with 35 animal rooms. In 1998, TherImmune purchased the site, doubled the size of the facility, and expanded the staff from 35 to 250 and began offering full toxicology services to the pharmaceutical and biotechnology industries. Over the next 20 years, the company was sold several times with a number of name changes: GeneLogic Laboratories (2003–2006), Bridge Laboratories (2006–2009), Avanza Laboratories (2009–2011), and Smithers Avanza (2011–2019). In 2019, Smithers Avanza was acquired by BASi. Noted toxicologists who worked at this facility included Bruce Briggs, Gary Wolfe, Ric Stanulis, Steve Godin, Eias Zahalka, Scott Manetz, Michael Dorato, and Florence Caputo.

Sinclair Research

Sinclair Research was originally established in 1964 as the Sinclair Comparative Medical Research Farm as part of the University of Missouri, with its primary function to provide laboratory animal research support for the university's environmental health surveillance center and environmental trace substance research center. Over the years, its role expanded to become a resource for a wide variety of animal and health-related research and become very involved in the development and use of animal models. In 1992, Sinclair Comparative Medical Research was privatized and Sinclair Research was established in 1994. The current site, located about 15 miles east of Columbia, Missouri, sits on 200 acres and contains both a swine breeding facility and a contract toxicology testing facility. The company is owned and led by Guy Bouchard, who received his veterinary degree from the University of Montreal. The contract testing facility consists of 250,000 square feet of vivarium and ancillary space with 70 animal rooms. Sinclair Research is a leader in the area of miniature swine and has conducted and published numerous research articles pertaining to swine, but it also conducts toxicology studies in all commonly used animal species. Noted toxicologists at Sinclair Research include Scott Boley, Jeffrey Klein, and Jason Liu.

Sierra Biomedical

Sierra Biomedical was founded in Sparks, Nevada, in 1992 by William Hobson who had previously worked at Primate Research Institute in Alamogordo, New Mexico. The company business model was to offer high-quality toxicology testing in nonhuman primates to support the growing biotechnology industry on the West coast. The original facility was in leased space and housed 200 nonhuman primates. In 2007, a new 465,000 square foot purpose-built facility was erected in Reno, Nevada, and the laboratory functions were moved from the Sparks facility. In 1994, there were 35 employees, but currently there are over 1000 employees. The new facility can house over 3000 nonhuman primates and is the largest nonhuman primate CRO in North America. In 1999, Sierra Biomedical was purchased by Charles River. Noted toxicologist at Sierra Biomedical included Doug Kornbrust, Jon Kapeghian, Gary Chellman, and Tom Zanardi.

Northern Biomedical Research

Northern Biomedical Research (NBR) was founded in 1993 by Robert Boyd, a veterinarian. The 60,000 square foot facility is located in Norton Shores, Michigan, and contains 19 animal rooms and two surgical suites. The laboratory specializes in surgical studies in most species of laboratory animals and pioneered several surgical techniques and postoperative animal care practices for targeted drug delivery to numerous organ systems, especially the central nervous system, utilizing a state-of-the-art custom built 3T MRI for imaging and stereotaxic administration to the central nervous system.

MPI Research

MPI Research was founded by William Parfet and Jerry Michell in 1995, having bought the remaining assets of International Research and Development Corporation (IRDC). Parfet, the great grandson of W. E. Upjohn, the founder of the Upjohn Company in Kalamazoo, Michigan, was a businessman, while Mitchell was a medical research doctor and former head of research and development at the Upjohn Company. Michell sold his interests in MPI Research in 1998, and Parfet put together an executive team that served together for over 10 years and led the company to great success. That team consisted of William Harrison as President, James Laveglia as Director of Research, Andy Dumpis as Director of Finance, and David Serota as Director of Toxicology. Starting with about 300,000 square feet of space comprising 125 animal rooms and a staff of around 175 at the time of purchase, by 2008 MPI Research had grown to over 1,000,000 square feet of space comprising over 550 animal rooms and a staff of over 1800. Several small acquisitions were made during this period but the company's growth was based on expansion of the existing facility in Mattawan, Michigan, through a concentrated and successful effort to market to biotechnology organizations. In 2008, Parfet sold a minority interest in the company to TA Associates of Boston, Massachusetts, and in 2015 the company was sold to Avista Capital Holdings, a private equity firm. In 2018, the company was sold to Charles River. Noted toxicologists at MPI Research included Edwin Goldenthal, James Laveglia, David Serota, Paul Newton, Richard Slauter, Ray Schroder, Ali Faqi, Theodore Baird, David Gauvin, Christopher Papagiannis, Scott Boley, and Mark Johnson.

Covance, Inc.

Covance, Inc. evolved from Hazleton Laboratories after Corning spun off Corning Pharmaceutical Services in 1996 as an independent, full-service publicly traded company. Covance, Inc. consisted of preclinical testing sites in Vienna, Virginia; Madison, Wisconsin; Harrogate, England; and Munster, Germany. The Vienna site was closed in 2010. The Madison site has just under 1,000,000 square feet of space and provides both in vivo and in vitro metabolism, general toxicology, safety pharmacology, large animal DART, and small molecule bioanalysis services. The Harrogate site has slightly over 500,000 square feet of space and supports general toxicology, safety pharmacology, immunotoxicology, genetic toxicology, and small animal DART studies. The Munster site has approximately 150,000 square feet of space and supports primate studies for general toxicology and DART studies. In 2008, Covance, Inc. purchased the 450-acre Greenfield, Indiana, site from Eli Lilly and Company. The Greenfield site has just over 1,000,000 square feet of space and supports general toxicology, small animal DART studies, in vivo and PK screening, and molecular and anatomical imaging. In 2011, the Greenfield site added a stand-alone building for conducting small animal DART studies. In 2009, Covance opened a 288,000 square foot facility on 77 acres of land in Chandler, Arizona, but due to economic conditions, this facility was closed in 2012. In 2015, the Laboratory Corporation of America (LabCorp) acquired Covance. In 2019, LabCorp entered into an agreement with Envigo by which LabCorp purchased Envigo's contract research service business while Envigo purchased LabCorp's animal research models and service business. Noted toxicologists at Covance Madison include Karen MacKenzie, Anthony Kiorpes, Matt Palazzolo, Suzanne Wolford, and Susan Henwood.

Burleson Research Technologies, Inc.

Burleson Research Technologies, Inc. (BRT) was founded in 1996 in Morrisville, North Carolina, by Gary and Florence Burleson, both who had strong backgrounds in immunology and immunotoxicology. The facility consists of 10,000 square feet of space and has 35 employees. BRT specializes in immunology and immunotoxicology services and offers services in infectious disease models, and host resistance hypersensitivity, and immune response assays. In 2014, BRT has held to NTP immunotoxicology contract. Noted toxicologists at BRT include Gary Burleson and Florence Burleson.

SNBL USA

SNBL USA was founded in 1996 as a subsidiary of SNBL Japan by Ryoichi Nagata, the son of the founder of SNBL Japan which was established in 1957. The site, located in Everett, Washington, encompasses 210,000 square feet of space and 130 animal rooms. SNBL USA was known for its nonhuman primate experience in conducting general toxicology and reproductive studies and through its passive restraint cages that were designed by Ryoichi Nagata to reduce the stress of study procedures. In 2018, SNBL USA was acquired by Altasciences, a clinical research company based in Montreal, Canada. Noted toxicologists at SNBL USA included Tina Rogers, Christopher Slater, Darren Warren, and Mark Osier.

Experimur

Experimur was founded in Chicago, Illinois, in 2000 by Nabil Hatoum and Bernadette Ryan who had both previously worked at ITTRI. The current facility was opened in 2010 with 54,000 square feet of space and 40 animal rooms. It offers full general toxicology and reproductive/developmental toxicology services. Noted toxicologists at Experimur include Nabil Hatoum, Bernadette Ryan, Christopher Slater, Bjorn Thorsrud, John Devine, Anne Doyle, Edward Mallett, and Supida Monaikul.

Wuxi

Wuxi was founded in 2001 by four co-founders including Ge Li who was a chemist and worked for seven years at Pharmacopeia before becoming CEO of Wuxi. The company started from a single chemistry site but through growth and acquisition now has over 30 sites worldwide with over 22,000 employees. The toxicology facility is located in Suzhou, China, and occupies 314,000 square feet of space encompassing 120 animal rooms. A major expansion of this facility was completed in late 2019, enlarging the facility to 580,000 square feet of space with 220 animal rooms. In 2008, Wuxi merged with Apptec to create a more global presence. Noted toxicologists at Wuxi include Sue McPherson, Anthony Kiorpis, and Yi Jin.

Xenometrics

Xenometrics was founded in 2006 by Alfred Botchway and Tom Haymaker in Stillwell, Kansas. They had previously been with the Quintiles preclinical unit in Kansas City, Kansas, which had been purchased by Aptuit in 2005, but which was closed a year later. They handpicked numerous staff who had previously been with Quintiles/Aptuit to join them in this new company. They rented space from Bayer Crop Science, which opened in 1979, and began offering PK and safety pharmacology services. In 2009, Xenometrics acquired the 78,000 square foot Bayer facility, and in 2017, Xenometrics was acquired by Citoxlab, renaming itself Citoxlab USA in 2018.

CiToxLAB

CiToxLAB was established in 2011 as a conglomeration of international CROs, comprising 1300 employees at 9 sites. These CROs included CIT-France (Centre International de Toxicologie), founded in 1969 and located in Evreux, France, with 200,000 square feet of space; LAB (now Citox NA), founded in 1998 and located in Laval, Canada, with 176,000 square feet of space; Scantox (now Citox Denmark), founded in 1977 and located in Koge, Denmark, with 93,000 square feet of space; a Hungarian site (now Citox Hungary) located in Veszprem, Hungary, with 164,000 square feet of space; Atlanbio, founded in 2004 and located in Normandy, France, with 19,999 square feet of space; AccelLab founded in 2004 and located in Boisbriand, Canada; Xenometrics (now Citox USA) founded in 2006 and located in Stillwell, Kansas, with 78,000 square feet of space; Solvo Biotechnology founded in 1999 and located in Budapest, Hungary; and Experimental Pharmacology & Oncology (EPO) founded in 1999 and located in Berlin, Germany, with 12,000 square feet of space. Each of these sites generally offered a different area(s) of expertise as follows: CIT-France, full service toxicology capabilities including genomics; Citox NA, full service toxicology capabilities, specializing in DART, safety pharmacology, inhalation, and irradiation safety; Citox Denmark, toxicology specializing in pig studies, especially the Gottingen minipig for juvenile, reproductive, and wound healing studies; Citox Hungary, general and inhalation toxicology; Atlanbio, analytical/bioanalytical support through all phases of the drug development process; AccelLab, specializing in medical device testing; Citox USA, full service toxicology capabilities; and EPO, specializing in preclinical assessment of new anti-cancer drugs. Based on the planned business strategy of CiToxLAB, the wide geographic nature of this group of laboratories along with their diverse areas of expertise would make them a major player in the CRO world. In 2016, the company was purchased by Ardian, and in 2019 the company was purchased by Charles River Laboratories.

Acknowledgment of Contributors

The author wishes to thank and acknowledge those professionals in the field of toxicology who provided historical information that was included in this chapter. Without their participation, this chapter could never have been written.

Ralph Anderson, Carol Auletta, Guy Bouchard, David Brusick, Gary Burleson, Daniel Cerven, Any Cianciaruso, Heather Dale, George DeGeorge, John Devine, Phillip Dowling, William Ford, Roy Forster, Patricia Frank, Shayne C. Gad, Michael Gallo, Carol Green, Dean Haan, Jerry Hardisty, Ryan Harper, Nabil Hatoum, Tom Haymaker, Charles Hebert, Alan Hoberman, Mark Holbert, Dave Howard, Doug Kornbrust, Sven Korte, James Laveglia, Barry Levine, David McCormick, Jacob McDonald, Sue McPherson, Richard Parent, Chris Perkins, Vince Piccirillo, Fred Reno, Tina Rogers, Rusty Rush, Janice Schinder-Horvat, Charles B. Spainhour, Matt Spalding, Bonnie Stuut, Friedhelm Vogel, Randy White, Gary Wolfe, Joseph Younan.

Trends and the Dark Side of the Story

Shayne C. Gad and Charles B. Spainhour

As reflected in this chapter, commercial toxicology service organizations (CROs) have significantly evolved since their first appearance more than 80 years ago. These 'ages' are reflected in the lists of existing CRO's and their histories as reflected in the front section of this chapter, in the earlier edition of this book, in Appendices A and B, and in Freudenthal 1997, Texas Research Institute 1986, and Gralla 1981.

In the modern decade, it is generally accepted that there have been four major cycles in the in the history of the CRO industry. These are commonly referred to as the "golden ages," because there was great demand for services from CROs, expansion of existing CRO facilities, and the appearance of new CRO organizations.

Each of these booms was followed by periods of economic setbacks and financial downturns.

The first occurred in the 1970s, when environmental concerns lead to the increased regulation of products. Particularly fueled by expectations of vast demand due to the Toxic Substance Control Act, this led to expansion of CROs and the initiation of formal academic programs in the field of toxicology. This came to an end in the early 1980s as regulatory testing requirements did not expand as much as expected.

The second period started in the late 1980s, as a significant increase in the amount of required testing of food additives and pharmaceuticals fueled expansion (Jackson 1984). This period faded away at the turn of the century when there was an economic downturn.

The third golden age came about out of the appearance of many small pharmaceutical "start-ups" appearing and needing regulatory toxicology testing of their candidate drugs. This era also was ended by the economic downturn in 2007/2008.

We are currently in the fourth "golden age" fueled by both major domestic pharmaceutical and medical device companies outsourcing most of their testing and increasing companies seeking to bring their products into the US and European markets and a surge of new companies seeking to develop new drugs and devices. The end of this period is not yet in sight, but certainly the COVID-19 pandemic has adversely effected the industry.

At the same time, we should capture here at least some of the history of failures in maintaining ethics and quality in testing operations.

Good Laboratory Practices (GLP) as law have been with us since 1977, with the primary purpose being need that they were intended to meet safety assessments both preceding that date by many years and continuing to the present and beyond.

Good recording of data, plans, and procedures in the laboratory has always been essential to the conduct of both scientific research and the entire self-modifying/evolutionary process by which science as a whole operates. The documentation of the fact that proper procedures were followed is an unfortunate reflection of the need to insure against everything from sloppiness to dishonesty. Furthermore in many areas of biomedical research and testing, such guidelines are now also a requirement of law. To understand the need both for all of these procedures and for the laws requiring then, we must review the history of problems in the area.

A complete history of the problems associated with biomedical data recording and management is a book in itself. In fact, a number of books have been published on this very matter (Broad and Wade 1982; Hoover et al. 1986; Huber 1991). Though the problem of data falsification or the suspicion of such dates back to Ptolemy and is not limited in the biomedical sciences, our overview of history will be limited to the period from 1960 on and to the biomedical sciences.

In the period 1960–1961, a graduate student at Yale who went on to become a postdoc at Rockefeller performed a series of brilliant experiments on cytochrome c and glutathione with well-respected senior investigators (Broad and Wade 1982). These results were widely published, but the work was soon found to not be repeatable. The publications and work were retracted, and the junior individual involved resigned and left research altogether. This episode received no press attention. The first widely publicized case to come to the public's attention, starting the erosion of the public's faith in science, was that of the "patchwork mouse" in 1974 (Hixson 1976). William T. Summerlin was a junior researcher working at Sloan-Kettering in a large lab with Robert Good, who was the laboratory supervisor. Good's lab had published almost 700 well-regarded papers in immunology with Good as a co-author on all of them over the preceding 5 years. Summerlin reported a number of successful transplantations in animals, which could not be replicated by others. Finally, he used a black felt tip pen to enhance the appearance of successful transplantation of skin patches on some mice. A technician, who was working the laboratory (but not Dr. Good), detected the alteration in what became a well-publicized case.

In 1978 an entire team of researchers working for Dr. Marc Straus at Boston University were working as part of a clinical trial sponsored by the Eastern Cooperative Oncology Group. The team reported that they had "falsified" nearly 15% of all the data entered from the trial, under direction from Dr. Straus. The falsification consisted of everything ranging from concealing errors made by the team in following the specific study protocol to allowing physicians to diverge from the study treatment without having to exclude the patients form the trial (Carlfield 1988). This situation was repeated with much wider publicity by a Canadian research team that was part of the breast cancer trials in 1994, leading to the well-respected overall head of the trial having to resign (Anderson 1994).

Industry also has had its share of problems, both real and suspected. During the1970s the largest industry biological testing lab in the country was Industrial Biotest. In 1975 an FDA investigator stumbled by accident on problems in the data from testing on Naprosyn. As investigators dug deeper into the data on studies on the safety of more than 600 drugs, chemicals, and food additives evaluated by IBT, they found enough fraud to lead to the indictment and conviction of four senior officers of the company (Anon 1981a, 1981b, 1983a, 1983c). The of greater impact was that the documentation of study procedures and data recording could not be verified. Given the already known problems with the data and the conduct of some studies (e.g., animals that were recorded as having died on study not being necropsied until after autolysis had set in, etc.), the results of all the studies were suspect. Studies either had to be repeated or validated if possible. This case and others in the same time frame led to the adoption of the Good Laboratory Practice (GLP) regulations, which now govern all preclinical (i.e., nonhuman) studies performed to establish the safety of a drug, medical device, or chemical regulated by the United States and most foreign governments.

The GLP regulations, which are discussed in a later section of this book, call for regular inspections of all laboratories (i.e., industry, contract, and university) involved in the generation of such data. This program of regular unannounced inspection has continued to identify problems involving some actual fraud,

Table 2.1 Industry and Contract Lab Violations of the GLPs (1980–1984)

Organization	Year	Violation	Penalty
Litton	1980	Deviations from protocols and SOPs	Warning letter
		Mix-up or misidentification of test materials	
		Inadequate SOPs (Anon 1980)	
Gulf South Research	1983	Poor data keeping on NTP carcinogenicity studies (Marcus 1983)	Lab went out of business
Biodynamics	1980	Timeliness of postmortem exams	None
		Reporting of tumors	
		Poor husbandry (Anon 1983)	
		Late reporting	
	1983	Pathologist not present at necropsy	
		Poor husbandry	
SAIC	1986	Backdating of Superfund data (Anon 1983d; Zurer 1991)	$750,000 fine
Carter Wallace/AMA Laboratories	1992	No study protocols	$132,000 fine
		Failure to sign data entries	
		No study personnel files	
BioTek Industries/ Microbac Laboratories	1992	No QA unit	$100,000 fine
		Lack of written protocols and SOPs	
		Missing items and inconsistencies in raw data and report	
Craven Laboratories	1992	"Tweaking" of pesticide residue data	Prison terms
Twelve pesticide firms	1993	Inadequate documentation and records (Anon 1994)	$183,000 in fines

Table 2.2 Purported recent cases of academic and government scientific misconduct

Institution	Year	Allegations	Outcome
Tufts	1986	Fraudulent data in *Cell* paper	Secret service involved Five years of investigations NIH finding of fraud
Vanderbilt	1982	Fraud, poor record keeping	Discrediting of research on alcoholism (and of researchers)
Caltech	1989	Fraudulent and missing data (Roberts 1991)	Paper retracted Responsible postdocs dismissed
University of Pittsburgh	1979	Misanalysis of lead data	Office of Scientific Integrity investigation
University of California, San Diego	1986	Publishing false data	Faculty member resigned
University of Alabama, Birmingham	1989	Plagiarism False claims to the government	$2MM civil suit verdict
St. Luc Hospital/ Montreal	1994	Not following protocol Falsifying ineligible patient enrollment	Overall breast cancer study head removed

invention of data, deletion of data, alteration of data, and other activities that are in violation of procedural/documentation requirements of the regulations. A few examples spanning the first 15 years since the regulation became effective are provided in Table 2.1.

Also see Anon 1991; Cohen 1991; Hall 1991; Hamilton 1991; Placa 1991; Tifft 1991; Kumar 1991; Stone 1994. The problems which have led to a decrease in the creditability of science have not been limited to industry. As shown in Table 2.2, academic and government labs and researchers have also had problems on a continuing basis. These problems have not been just cases of suspected or real fraud, but also of plagiarism and various other forms of scientific misconduct. Scientific misconduct has a variety of forms (Kyburg 1968; Stone 1991; Taubes 1995):

Plagiarism Presenting work done by another as your own

Misallocation of Credit Claiming (or accepting) credit for work done by another. This includes a lack of adequate acknowledgment of the work of one's intellectual predecessors

Bias Uneven, unbalanced, or one-sided collection, analysis, or reporting of data

Trimming Improving the appearance of quality of work or of clarity of outcome by removing or failing to report some data or observations

Sloppy/Poor Records and Methods The most honest of intentions, but the documentation of what has been done and seen is either so incomplete, unclear, or disorganized that the value of the work is at best suspect and discounted

Wholesale Fraud Complete invention of some or all of the work done and resulting data

Junk Science That which supports adversarial opinions and is not supported by the work of others or accepted by the scientific community (Huber 1991)

References

Anderson, C. (1994). How not to publicize a misconduct finding. *Science, 262*, 1679.

Anon. (1980). FDA tells Litton to bring three facilities into GLP compliance, *Food Chem. News*, May 12, pp. 19–20.

Anon. (1981a). Nalco Chemical unit ex-officials charged with faking lab data. *Wall Street J.*, June 23.

Anon. (1981b). Lab execs indicted for faking toxicity data. *Chemical & Engineering News, 59*(26), 5.

Anon. (1983). Bio/Dynamics defends permethrin studies; House subcommittee may investigate. *Pestic. Toxic Chem. News*, September 21, 31–32.

Anon. (1983a). The darker side of a laboratory. *Chem. Week*, May 18.

Anon. (1983c). Tighter controls on toxics testing. *Chem. Week*, August 24, 32–39.

Anon. (1983d). There are no plaudits for EPA laboratory audits, *Ind C hem. News*, Juen, 30–33.

Anon. (1991). NIH finds misconduct at Georgetown. *Science, 363*, 35.

Anon. (1994). Twelve companies violated FIFRA Good Lab Standards. EPA says, *Pestic. Toxic Chem. News*, October 5, 13–14.

Broad, W., & Wade, N. (1982). *Betrayers of the truth*. New York: Simon & Schuster.

Carlfield, E. (1988). The international school of professional ethics: or, How to succeed in science without really trying. *Current Contents, 8*, 3–5.

Cohen, J. (1991). What next in the Gallo Case? *Science, 254*, 944–949.

Freudenthal, R. I. (1997). *Directory of toxicology laboratories offering contract service*. West Palm Beach: Aribel Books.

Gralla, E. J. (Ed.). (1981). *Scientific considerations in monitoring and evaluating toxicological research*. Washington, DC: Hemisphere Publishing Corporation.

Hall, S. S. (1991). Baltimore resigns at Rockefeller. *Science, 254*, 1447.

Hamilton, D. P. (1991). Verdict in sight in the "Baltimore Case". *Science, 251*, 1168–1172.

Hixson, J. (1976). *The patchwork mouse*. New York: Doubleday.

Hoover, B. K., Baldwin, J. K., Uelner, A. F., Whitmire, C. E., Davies, C. L., & Bristol, D. W. (Eds.). (1986). *Managing conduct and data quality of toxicology studies*. Princeton: Princeton Scientific Publishing Co., Inc..

Huber, P. W. (1991). *Galileo's revenge* (p. 274). New York: Harper Collins.

Jackson, E. M. (1984). How to choose a contract laboratory: Utilizing a laboratory clearance procedure. *Journal of Toxicology: Cutaneous and Ocular Toxicology, 3*, 83–92.

Kumar, V. (1991). Hood Lab investigation. *Science, 254*, 1090–1091.

Kyburg, H. E. (1968). *Philosophy of science*. New York: Macmillan.

Marcus, F. F. (1983). U.S. says sloppy drug tests at laboratory in south prompt wide review. *Wall Street J.*, October 24, D12.

Placa, J. (1991). Draft of Gallo report sees the light of day. *Science, 253*, 1347–1348.

Roberts, L. (1991). Misconduct: Caltech's trial by fire. *Science, 253*, 1344–1347.

Stone, R. (1991). Court test for plagiarism detector? *Science, 254*, 1448.

Stone, R., & Marshall, E. (1994). Imanishi-Kari case: ORI find fraud. *Science, 266*, 2468–1469.

Taubes, G. (1995). Plagiarism suit wins; experts hope it won't set a trend. *Science, 268*, 115.

Texas Research Institute. (1986). *Directory of toxicology testing institutions*. Houston: Texas Research Institute.

Tifft, S. (1991). Scandal in the laboratories. *Time*, March 18, 74–75.

Tokay, B. A. (1984). Keeping tabs on the toxicology labs. *Chem. Bus.*, February, 12–20.

Zurer, P. S. (1991). Contract labs charged with fraud in analysis of Superfund samples. *Chemical & Engineering News, 69*(8), 14–16.

Pharmaceutical Development

3

The process by which a new therapeutic entity is discovered and developed to the point that it is available to patients in the marketplace is complex, expensive, and long. We will not pretend to present or analyze this process in any detail here, but rather to give a basic understanding of the process and of the components which may be outsourced to a contract organization. There are no current or comprehensive volumes describing this process, though there are some volumes on the area (Guarino 1987; Mathieu 2000; Smith 1992; Sneader 1986; Spilker 1994).

As explained at the beginning of this volume, the pharmaceutical development process is a long (perhaps from 10–16 years from drug inception to market approval) and costly ($250–1,300 million, depending on how one allocates costs) process, even when successful. It is shaped by medical needs, regulatory requirements, economics, finances, ethics, legal considerations, our understanding of sciences and diseases, and limitations of technology. All of these interact to shape a process which serves to iteratively reduce risks (to both economic and human safety), with the probability of failure being reduced in a stepwise fashion (Matoren 1984; Zbinden 1992). Figure 3.1 briefly summarizes this process, while Fig. 3.2 presents a more detailed summary of the process and activities up to the filing of an INDA (Investigative New Drug Application) and Fig. 3.3 an alternative presentation. We will use the six categories of activities in Fig. 3.2 (safety, pharmaceutical development, pharmacology, analytical, clinical and regulatory) as a framework to discuss activities

© Springer Nature Switzerland AG 2020
S. C. Gad et al., *Contract Research and Development Organizations-Their History, Selection, and Utilization*, https://doi.org/10.1007/978-3-030-43073-3_3

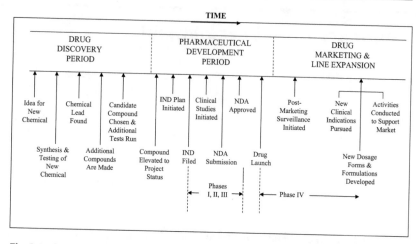

Fig. 3.1 Generalized flow of pharmaceutical development

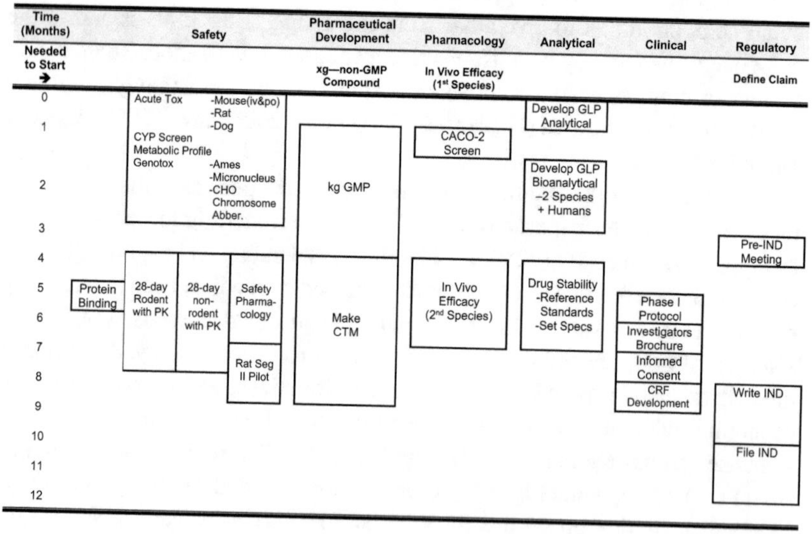

Fig. 3.2 Components of development to the filing and opening of an IND

throughout the development process. The major pharmaceutical companies have their research and development expenses well documented (Tables 3.1 and 3.2). These figures are impressive, as are the sales of their products

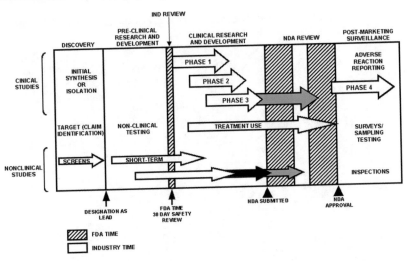

Fig. 3.3 The pharmaceutical development process, viewed as four stages (discovery, pre-clinical development, clinical development, and NDA review) as well as the important post-market surveillance phase

(Table 3.3). It should be kept in mind, however, that there are more than 2500 smaller pharmaceutical development companies (both "small molecule" and biotech) in the United States which have an even higher proportion of their budgets invested annually in research and development.

For our purposes (i.e., from the development to market perspective), the purpose of all nonclinical (animal and in vitro) development is to reduce the risks and probability of adverse events while optimizing the potential for therapeutic efficiency in humans. But between initial nonclinical testing (and concurrent with additional animal testing) and a drug's reaching the marketplace, the potential for having adverse effects in the general patient population it is intended for is further guarded against by a scheme of increasingly more powerful human ("clinical") trials (Piantadosi 1997; Nylen 2000). How a drug is moved through this process is the subject of this chapter.

Safety

The safety component of the development of a new drug has both a nonclinical (i.e., not in human beings) and a clinical component. Until an IND is opened, all safety evaluation is classified as nonclinical (also properly called, to this

Table 3.1   R&D, PhRMA member companies. Growth in domestic R&D and R&D abroad, ethical pharmaceuticals, PhRMA member companies, 1970–2009

Year	Domestic R&D	Annual percentage change	R&D abroad[a]	Annual percentage change	Total R&D	Annual percentage change
2009[b]	$34,306.0	−2.2%	$10,976.1	−7.1%	$45,782.1	−3.496
2008	35,571.1	−2.8	11,812.0	4.6	47,383.1	−1.1
2007	36,608.4	7.8	11,294.8	25.4	47,903.1	11.5
2006	33,967,9	9.7	9005.6	1.3	42,973.5	7.8
2005	30,969.0	4.8	8888.9	19.1	39,857.9	7.7
2004	29,555.5	9.2	7462.6	1.0	37,018.1	7.4
2003	27,064.9	5.5	7388.4	37.9	34,453.3	11.1
2002	25,655.1	9.2	5357.2	−13.9	31,012.2	4.2
2001	23,502.0	10.0	6220.6	33.3	20,772.7	14.4
2000	21,363.7	15.7	4667.1	10.6	26,030.8	14.7
1999	18,471.1	7.4	4219.6	9.9	22,690.7	8.2
1998	17,127.9	11.0	3839.0	9.9	20,966.9	10.8
1997	15,466.0	13.9	3492.1	6.5	18,958.1	12.4
1996	13,627.1	14.8	3278.5	−1.6	16,905.6	11.2
1995	11,874.0	7.0	3333.5	not reported	15,207.4	not reported
1994	11,101.6	6.0	2347.8	3.8	13,449.4	5.6
1993	10,477.1	12.5	2262.9	5.0	12,740.0	11.1
1992	9312.1	17.4	2155.8	21.3	11,467.9	18.2
1991	7928.6	16.5	1776.8	9.9	9705.4	15.3
1990	6802.9	13.0	1617.4	23.6	8420.3	14.9
1989	6021.4	15.0	1308.6	0.4	7330.0	12.1
1988	5233.9	16.2	1303.6	30.6	6537.5	18.8
1987	4504.1	16.2	998.1	15.4	5502.2	16.1
1986	3875.0	14.7	865.1	23.8	4740.1	16.2
1985	3378.7	13.3	698.9	17.2	4077.6	13.9
1984	2982.4	11.6	596.4	9.2	3578.8	11.2
1983	2671.3	17.7	546.3	8.2	3217.6	16.0
1982	2268.7	21.3	505.0	7.7	2773.7	18.6
1981	1870.4	20.7	469.1	9.7	2339.5	18.4
1980	1549.2	16.7	427.5	42.8	1976.7	21.5
1979	1327.4	13.8	299.4	25.9	1626.8	15.9
1978	1166.1	9.7	237.9	11.6	1404.0	10.0
1977	1063.0	8.1	213.1	18.2	1276.1	9.7
1976	983.4	8.8	180.3	14.1	1163.7	9.6
1975	903.5	13.9	158.0	7.0	1061.5	12.8
1974	793.1	12.0	147.7	26.3	940.8	14.0

(continued)

Table 3.1 (continued)

Year	Domestic R&D	Annual percentage change	R&D abroad[a]	Annual percentage change	Total R&D	Annual percentage change
1973	708.1	8.1	116.9	64.0	825.0	13.6
1972	654.8	4.5	71.3	24.9	726.1	6.2
1971	626.7	10.7	57.1	9.2	683.8	10.6
1970	566.2	—	52.3	—	618.5	—
Average		11.6%		15.5%		12.2%

Source: Pharmaceutical Research and Manufacturers of America, PhRMA Annual Membership Survey, 2009
Notes: 1. R&D expenditures for ethical pharmaceuticals only
2. Domestic R&D includes expenditures within the United States by PhRMA member companies
3. R&D abroad includes expenditures outside the United States by US-owned PhRMA member companies and R&D conducted abroad by US divisions of foreign-owned PhRMA member companies
4. Increases in R&D expenditures are likely due to a more rigorous data collection methodology
[a]Estimated
[b]R&D abroad affected by merger and acquisition activity

point, preclinical). After an IND is opened, both clinical and nonclinical components of safety evaluation are required. The timing of the nonclinical components, particularly after an IND is opened, is susceptible to a fair degree of judgment. The details of the components of this process are beyond the scope of this volume (see Gad 2016, for such details).

All the safety evaluation components have in common that they are heavily regulated and subject to either GLPs (Good Laboratory Practices) or GCPs (Good Clinical Practices). The nonclinical components include genotoxicity (a minimum of three studies, usually an *Ames* assay (in vitro) and CHO chromosome aberration or unscheduled DNA synthesis in vitro and a mouse micronucleus in vivo), safety pharmacology (with evaluations of cardiovascular, central nervous system, and respiratory pharmacologic activities being required prior to the filing of the IND (pre-IND) and others before large clinical trials in patients are initiated), immunotoxicology (just now coming into being specifically required), systemic toxicity (single- and multiple-dose studies in two or more species with a pharmacokinetic (PK) component or arm to the multi-dose pre-IND, then longer multiple-dose studies in concert with clinical develop-

Table 3.2 Domestic R&D by function, Ethical pharmaceuticals, PhRMA member companies, 1998–2000 (dollar figures in millions)

Function	1998		1999		2000	
	Dollars	Share (%)	Dollars	Share (%)	Dollars	Share (%)
Synthesis and extraction	$2066.7	12.07	$1763.1	10.0	$987.7	9.3
Biological screening and pharmacological testing	$2600.5	15.1	$2508.1	14.2	$2582.9	12.1
Toxicology and safety testing	$895.5	5.2	$802.1	4.5	$872.1	4.1
Pharmaceutical dosage formulation and stability testing	$1550.0	9.0	$1290.6	7.3	$1081.3	5.1
Clinical evaluation: phases I, II, and III	$4873.9	28.3	$5139.5	29.1	$5464.6	25.6
Clinical evaluation: phase IV	$998.9	5.8	$2060.5	11.7	$1882.3	8.8
Process development for manufacturing and quality control	$1705.0	9.9	$1463.4	8.3	$1499.9	7.0
Regulatory: IND and NDA	$757.7	4.4	$730.3	4.1	$644.2	3.0
Bioavailability	$413.4	2.4	$321.6	1.8	$327.8	1.5
Other R&D	$1265.9	7.9	$1594.3	9.0	$2693.7	12.6
Uncategorized ethical pharmaceutical R&D[a]	$0.4	0.0	$797.6	4.3	$2327.2	10.9
Total	$17,127.9	100	$18,471.1	100	$21,363.7	100

Source: Pharmaceutical Research and Manufacturers of America, PhRMA Annual Membership Survey, 2002

Notes: 1. Company-financed R&D expenditures for ethical pharmaceuticals only

2. Domestic R&D includes expenditures within the Unites States by PhRMA member companies

[a]Represents companies that provided total R&D expenditure figures, but not individual details

ment), developmental and reproductive toxicities, carcinogenicity evaluations (if the drug is intended to be for chronic use), and any special studies that may be of interest to the reviewing agency or specific to the class of drugs or the intended use of the potential drug. Also generally required are determinations of degree of protein binding, the pharmacokinetics and disposition of the drug in animals and man, metabolic activation and inhibition, and the nature and level of significant metabolites in man (Ozdemir et al. 2001).

Table 3.3 Top pharmaceutical companies

Company	Annual revenue (2009 global pharma sales)	R&D expenditures (2009)
Pfizer	$44.2 billion	$7.9 billion
GlaxoSmithKline	$43.0 billion	$5.2 billion
Sanofi-Aventis	$38.7 billion	$6.5 billion
Novartis	$36.0 billion	$7.2 billion
AstraZeneca	$31.6 billion	$5.1 billion
Johnson&Johnson	$24.6 billion	$5.1 billion
Merck	$23.6 billion	$4.8 billion
Roche	$21.0 billion	$7.2 billion
Eli Lilly	$19.3 billion	$3.8 billion
Wyeth	$19.0 billion	$3.4 billion
Bristol-Myers Squibb	$17.7 billion	$3.6 billion
Abbott	$16.7 billion	$2.7 billion
Bayer	$15.1 billion	$2.5 billion
Amgen[a]	$14.7 billion	$3.0 billion
Schering-Plough	$14.2 billion	$3.5 billion
Boehringer Ingelheim	$13.6 billion	$2.9 billion
Takeda	$12.2 billion	$2.7 billion
Teva	$11.1 billion	$786 million
Genentech[a]	$10.5 billion	$2.8 billion
Astellas	$9.7 billion	$1.3 billion
Daiichi Sankyo	$8.8 billion	$1.6 billion
Novo Nordisk	$8.6 billion	$1.5 billion
Merck KGaA	$7.6 billion	$1.5 billion
Eisai	$7.2 billion	$2.2 billion
Otsuka	$6.5 billion	$1.0 billion
Baxter international	$5.3 billion	$868 million
Servier	$5.2 billion	N/A
Gilead Sciences	$5.1 billion	$722 million
Mylan	$4.3 billion	$317 million
UCB	$4.3 billion	$1.1 billion

[a]Indicates biopharmaceutical companies

Pharmaceutical Development

The chemical development process also stretches through most of the length of the pharmaceutical development process. The needs to be met include:

- Manufacture of increasing amounts of quantities of active pharmaceutical ingredient of suitable purity and stability. Early lots are in gram (or tens of grams) quantities for small molecules. Such are produced under GLPs but not GMPs. Frequently the first upscale produces lots of hundreds of grams. Finally, lots of kilo or greater sizes are produced. Keep in mind that the purities of these different lots are important. There are no specific guidelines written with regard to the levels of purity of test article material for nonclinical studies. Do not under any circumstances produce material that is of extremely high purity for nonclinical studies. You can back yourself into a corner. If the material that is used in preclinical studies is of higher purity than that used in clinical studies, then the preclinical studies will have to repeated, because of the unfavorable impurity difference. This does not mean that the purities of preclinical and clinical lots have to be the same or identical. Typically the purity of any preclinical material should be about 95% or within 5% of the intended purity of the clinical trial material (CTM). It is acceptable and desirable to use material in nonclinical studies that is of lesser purity than the CTM. As synthetic scale-up proceeds, the impurity profile of the test article will more than likely adversely change as a direct result of the scale-up and the kinetic qualities of side reactions. While such problems can be addressed, such activity consumes money, time, and resources and can readily be avoided with proper planning. Somewhere in here (typically late in the process), the most stable (and possibly soluble) form (frequently a salt) is produced under GMPs. Later efforts still may seek to identify and optimize the most economical production process.

- Human dosage form(s) must be developed and produced. When used in clinical trials, these are labeled CTM (clinical test material). If for an oral drug, a simple formulation (such as a stable, simple capsule) may be used for phase I studies, more elegant formulations are produced for later studies. If the route is parenteral simple sterile, stable and isotonic solutions are explored.
- Formulations must be developed, first for preclinical studies and then for clinical studies. Lots of considerations come into such formulations including bioavailability, stability, use of allowed excipients, and patient acceptability.

Swarbrick and Boylan (2002) provide an excellent overview of the range of skills and technology involve here.

Pharmacology

Pharmacology studies (other than safety pharmacology) initially serve to identify candidate compounds for development, that is, identify and optimize "leads." Such studies (particularly in appropriate "gold standard" models of the specific disease to be treated – or predictive of efficacy) are essential both in making decisions to go forward with development of a compound and in helping estimate or model the dose to be used in the clinic. Dose selection or "target identification" for clinical trials is best performed based on achieving an effective concentration of therapeutic entity at the target site (receptors or organs in vivo), but should also at least have achieved plasma levels at efficient doses driving the target concentration for clinical studies.

Additionally, it is important to evaluate the specificity of action at the target sites. This means that activity and/or binding at other receptor sites must be characterized quantitatively (e.g., K_i, K_d, K_a, etc.), as such may limit the actual target concentration and potential utility of a drug.

Since 2006, the FDA has started to require formal laboratory evaluation (with formal reports) to support the claims and/or assumptions of pertinent pharmacodynamics – that is, desired therapeutic activity in a suitable animal model.

Analytical

It is clearly essential to be able to both identify and quantitate the actual drug entity itself in a range of biological and nonbiological milieu. These include the lots of drug produced (where purity and the identity of any accompanying impurities also is important), stability study samples, dosage preparations for preclinical studies, and fluid and tissue samples from in vivo studies.

The last of these tasks usually means being able to accurately and sensitively quantitate the levels of the drug entity in serum, blood or plasma and urine, and possibly target tissues. Such methods need to be developed and validated not only for humans but also for the principal species used in nonclinical studies (usually rats and either dogs or nonhuman primates (NHP), plus in rabbits to verify exposure in developmental toxicology studies).

It also becomes important at some point to be able to identify and quantitate the levels of significant metabolites, particularly if they are pharmacologically active. The limit of detection (LOD) needs to be in the picogram (pg/ml) range to satisfy regulatory agencies. This limit of detection is not documented in any guideline, but has slowly evolved over the recent years as analytical technology has increased to permit such a level of detection. What exactly does a pictogram level of detection mean? Well certainly 1 pg/ml is a highly desirable level, and 1000 pg/ml is not ideal. In method development, try to get as close as one can to the 1 pg/ml level, but if the final result is 495 pg/ml, that will be acceptable to the agency. A level such as 500 ng/ml will not be acceptable, providing that there is not sufficient documentation to *prove* and support that number as a methodological endpoint.

Clinical

Generally the single most expensive (and time consuming) portion of any pharmaceutical development timeline is the clinical evaluation portion (Gad 2009; Spilker 1994). Initially these studies (Phase I) are intended primarily to evaluate the safety (tolerance) and pharmacokinetics of a drug, and unless the drug is intended to treat life-threatening conditions, such studies are performed in healthy volunteers and not patients. Patients can be used in life-threatening conditions. While it should generally be possible to perform such work with just three (single-dose escalating, multi-dose tolerance, and a single-dose escalating) or four studies (validation of achieved dose by an optimized formulation/dosage form), many more may need to be performed.

Subsequent to the completion of the phase I studies, a series of phase II studies are generally performed in patients, first and very importantly to give confidence in efficacy. Finally, it should be noted that regulatory approval generally requires the completion of two successful "pivotal" studies. These are generally phase III studies, but may be phase II studies. The requirements are adequate numbers of patients to achieve unequivocal statistical proof of efficacy of an accepted a priori endpoint and adequate numbers and exposure of a representative patient population to identify the potential occurrence of any significant safety concerns when the drug is on the market. All this is done while protecting trial subject safety and confidentiality to the fullest extent possible (Willman 2000; Wechsler 2001).

The phase III testing phase is almost always both the longest and most expensive segment of the drug development process. From the earliest point, sponsors/investigators seek to gain first any reliable hint that the drug works (see Biomarkers Definitions Working Group 2001) while also worrying about previously undetected safety concerns such as hepatic damage (Kaplowilz 2001).

Regulatory

In parallel with all of the technical activities in the pharmaceutical development process, there is an accompanying string of activities which must be conducted to fulfill the regulatory requirements for successfully completing the market approval (NDA) process (Gad 2010; Gad 2018). Such usually start with bringing about a successful pre-IND meeting with FDA. Subsequent to this interaction, the following generally must occur:

- An INDA (investigational new drug application) must be assembled, paginated, and submitted. Any resulting questions raised by the FDA must be answered effectively and in a very timely manner.
- The "opening" of the IND (investigational new drug (application)) must be verified (the FDA does not usually provide any such verification).
- Necessary IND amendments (documenting changes in formulation; significant findings as to safety; changes in clinical study protocols, facilities or personnel or new protocols) must be to the FDA submitted in a timely manner.
- An end of phase II meeting with FDA should be effectively executed.
- Assembly and submission of an NDA, with effective and timely response to any subsequent FDA queries.
- An effective quality monitoring and auditing program of vendors performing GLP, GMP, and/or GCP regulated tasks.

Except for those cases where there is substantial potential to save or extend lives (such as anticancer and anti-AIDS drugs) or where the intended target diseases are chronic and severe (e.g., Parkinson's or MS) or the routes of administration are invasive (e.g., intrathecal), the initial evaluations in humans are performed in "normal," healthy volunteer with the primary objective being limited to defining the limits of tolerance (safety) of the potential drug and its pharmacokinetic characteristics. These trials may also seek to detect limited (usually surrogate or indirect) indicators of efficacy, but are severely limited in doing so (Biomarker Definitions Working Group 2001). Later trials look at the drug's actions on carefully defined and selected groups of patients.

With the number of drugs withdrawn from the marketplace since 1990 (or, perhaps, the degree of media coverage of such withdrawals), public concern with and media coverage of the workings of the drug safety evaluation aspects of the development process have risen sharply (Granter 1999; Wechsler 2001). It is currently estimated that in the United States, adverse drug reactions (ADRs) rank between the fourth to sixth leading cause of death (Eikelbom et al. 2001). While improvements in the nonclinical procedures of drug safety assessments are possible and even likely, clearly the clinical aspects are likely to be where the most relevant improvements in trials and a better understanding of individual or subpopulation differences in human responses to drugs are to be found.

While there is much press about the concern that the "increased pace of drug approval" has caused the release onto the market of less safe drugs (Willman 2000), the causes are more mundane and of much longer standing. The most common "unexpected" (from nonclinical trial results) safety findings in initial trials involve the skin (dermatitis of one form or another) and the liver (Kaplowilz 2001).

An important reason for the high incidence of serious and fatal ADRs is that the existing drug development paradigms do not generate adequate information on the mechanistic sources of marked variability in pharmacokinetics and pharmacodynamics of new therapeutic candidates, precluding treatments from being tailored for individual patients with their physiologic, biochemical, and genetic idiosyncrasies (Ozdemir et al. 2001).

Pharmacogenetics is the study of the hereditary basis of person-to-person variation in drug response. The initial focus of pharmacogenetic investigations has traditionally been unusual and extreme drug responses resulting from a single gene effect. The Human Genome Project and recent advancements in molecular genetics now present an unprecedented opportunity to study all genes in the human genome, including genes for drug metabolism, drug targets, and post-receptor second messenger mechanisms, in relation to variability in drug safety and efficacy. In addition to sequence variations in the genome, high-throughput and genome-wide transcript profiling for differentially regulated mRNA species before and during drug treatment will serve as important tools to uncover novel mechanisms of drug action. Pharmacogenetic-guided drug discovery and development represent a departure for the conventional approach, which markets drugs for broad patient populations, rather than smaller specifically targeted groups of patients in whom drugs may work more effectively and optimally. To date, these new tools have not brought a product to market. But their use is in demand, as are the older receptor – binding screening services intended to determine the specificity of action of a potential drug.

Putting It All Together

While not a separate or distinct segment of pharmaceutical development, the need for integrative project management services to ensure that all of the pieces fit together in a coherent fashion (whether of clinical trials or the entire development process) is clearly essential and in an area where extensive contract services are necessary and available. In the large pharmaceutical companies (Table 3.3), these skills historically have been to a large part internal. For the vast majority of the smaller 3500 pharmaceutical/biotech companies (in the United States and Canada), this is not the case, and the services must be contracted at least in part or more commonly in the whole from either a large ("meta") CRO, a smaller CRO, a provider specializing in niche services, or a "fatigue" organization which serves only a few clients at a time. There are, it must be noted, an equal number of drug companies not in the United States or Canada.

References

Biomarkers Definitions Working Group. (2001). Biomarkers and surrogate endpoints: Preferred definitions and conceptual frameworks. *Clinical Pharmacology and Therapeutics, 69*, 89–95.

Eikelbom, J. W., Mehta, S. R., Pogue, J., & Yusuf, S. (2001). Safety outcomes in meta-analyses of phase II versus phase III randomized trials. *JAMA, 285*, 444–450.

Gad, S. C. (2009). *Clinical trials handbook*. Hoboken, NJ: Wiley Interscience.

Gad, S. C. (2016). *Drug safety evaluation* (3rd ed.). New York: Wiley.

Gad, S. C. (2010). *International regulatory safety evaluation of pharmaceuticals and medical devices*. Berlin: Springer.

Gad, S. C. (2018). *Regulatory Toxicology* (3rd ed.). Boca Raton, FL: Taylor and Francis.

Granter, J. (1999). Responding to industry critics: If the industry doesn't address concerns raised by the consumer press, who will? *Applied Clinical Trials, 10*, 18–22.

Guarino, R. A. (1987). *New drug approval process*. New York: Marcel Dekker.

Kaplowilz, N. (2001). Drug induced liver disorders: Implications for drug development and regulation. *Drug Information Journal, 35*, 347–400.

Mathieu, M. (2000). *New drug development: A regulatory overview*. Waltham: Parexel.

Matoren, G. M. (1984). *The clinical research process in the pharmaceutical industry.* New York: Marcel Dekker.

Nylen, R. A. (2000). *The ultimate step-by-step guide to conducting pharmaceutical clinical trials in the USA.* Tampa: RAN Institute.

Ozdemir, V., Shear, N. H., & Kalow, W. (2001). What will be the role of pharmacokinetics in evaluating drug safety and minimizing adverse effects? *Drug Safety, 24,* 75–85.

Piantadosi, S. (1997). *Clinical trials: A methadoligic perspective.* New York: Wiley.

Smith, C. G. (1992). *The process of new drug discovery and development.* Boca Raton: CRC Press.

Sneader, W. (1986). *Drug development: From laboratory to clinic.* New York: Wiley.

Spilker, B. (1994). *Multinational pharmaceutical companies.* New York: Raven Press.

Swarbrick, J., & Boylan, J. C. (2002). *Encyclopedia of pharmaceutical technology* (2nd ed.). New York: Marcel Dekker.

Wechsler, J. (2001). Clinical trial safety and oversight top policy agenda. *Applied Clinical Trials, 1,* 18–21.

Willman, D. (2000, December 28). Quickened pace of drug approvals by FDA taking toll. *San Jose Mercury News,* p. 1A.

Zbinden, G. (1992). *The source of the River Po.* Frankfurt am Main: Haag + Herchen.

Medical Device Development

4

The medical device industry in the United States and worldwide is immense in its economic impact (sales in 2017 were $338 billion worldwide, $156 billion in the United States alone, $64 billion in the European Community, and $45 billion in Japan; in 1998 the US medical equipment trade surplus was $18.2 billion. Between 87,000 and 140,000 different devices are produced in the United States annually by approximately 8200 different manufacturers employing some 311,000 people. Furthermore, it is believed that more than 1000 of these manufacturers are development-stage only companies without products yet on the market. Medical devices are or extreme importance to the health of the citizens of the world (Nugent 1994; The Wilkerson Group 1999) (see Table 4.1). While it is true that the large companies dominate the market in terms of sales and revenue, just as with pharmaceuticals, it is the small companies that dominate innovation. The assessment of the safety to patients using the multitude of items produced by this industry is dependent on schemes and methods that are largely peculiar to these kinds of products; are not as rigorous as those employed for foods, drugs, and pesticides; and are in a persistent state of flux. Regulation of such devices is, in fact, relatively new. It is only with the Medical Device Amendments (to the Food, Drug, and Cosmetic Act of 1976) that devices have come to be explicitly regulated at all and with the Safe Medical Devices Act of 1990, the Medical Device Amendments Act of 1992, and subsequent laws that the regulation of devices for biocompatibility became rigorous (see Table 4.2). According to section 201(h) of the Food, Drug, and Cosmetic Act, a medical device is an instrument, apparatus,

© Springer Nature Switzerland AG 2020
S. C. Gad et al., *Contract Research and Development Organizations-Their History, Selection, and Utilization*, https://doi.org/10.1007/978-3-030-43073-3_4

Table 4.1 The largest US
medical device markets
(2001)

US$ in billions	
Diagnostics (in vitro)	$20.5
Surgery (min. invasive)	$16.4
Orthopedic	$14.7
Wound care	$13.0
Cardiovascular	$12.5

Table 4.2 FDA classification of preamendment medical devices

Part no.	Title	Date of publication
21 C.F.R. Part 862	Clinical chemistry and clinical toxicology	May 1, 1987
21 C.F.R. Part 864	Hematology and pathology devices	May 11, 1987
21 C.F.R. Part 866	Immunology and microbiology	November 9, 1982
21 C.F.R. Part 868	Anesthesiology devices	July 16, 1982
21 C.F.R. Part 870	Cardiovascular devices	February 5, 1980
21 C.F.R. Part 872	Dental devices	August 12, 1987
21 C.F.R. Part 874	Ear, nose and throat devices	November 6, 1986
21 C.F.R. Part 876	Gastroenterology-urology devices	November 23, 1983
21 C.F.R. Part 878	General and plastic surgery devices	June 24, 1988
21 C.F.R. Part 880	General hospital and personal use	October 21, 1980
21 C.F.R. Part 882	Neurological devices	November 4, 1979
21 C.F.R. Part 884	Obstetrical and gynecological devices	February 26, 1980
21 C.F.R Part 886	Opthalmic devices	September 2, 1987
21 C.F.R. Part 888	Orthopedic devices	September 4, 1987
21 C.F.R. Part 890	Physical medicine devices	November 23, 1983
21 C.F.R. Part 892	Radiological devices	January 20, 1988

implement, machine, contrivance, implant, in vitro reagent, or other similar or
related article, including a component, part, or accessory, that is:

Recognized in the official National Formulary, or the United States Pharmacopoeia
(USP 2020), or any supplement to them.
Intended for use in the diagnosis of disease, in man or other animals.
Intended to affect the structure or any function of the body of man or other animals,
and that does not achieve any of its primary intended purposes through chemical
action within or on the body of man or other animals, and that is not dependent upon
being metabolized for the achievement of any of its principal intended purposes.
(CDRH 1992)

- FDA determines that the devices is substantially equivalent to another device that was not in commercial distribution before such date but that has since been classified into class I or II (through the 510(k) process).
- FDA reclassifies the device into class I or II.

The procedures for reclassifying a "postamendment" class III device are codified in 21 C.F.R. Section 860.134(b) (1)–(7).

The device classification process continues to this day. As FDA becomes aware of new devices that require formal classification or pre-1976 devices that were somehow overlooked in the original classification procedures, the agency initiates new classification proceedings, again requesting the recommendation of one or more of the appropriate advisory panels.

Under this definition, devices might be considered as belonging to one of nine categories (North American industrial classification): surgical and medical instruments, ophthalmic, dental, laboratory apparatus, irradiation, specialty devices, medical/surgical supplies, in vitro diagnostics, and electromedical. There were (in 2000) 16,170 companies involved in these sectors – 6750 of them manufacturers worldwide. This is a global industry with a $260 billion annual market. The US market alone is $120 billion, or 42% of this (MDDI 2000) (see Table 4.3).

Table 4.3 Ten projected biggest growth device products (in 2000)

Rank	Product	Percentage revenue growth rate (years)	Specialty
1	Fibrin sealants	174.6 (95-02)	Wound care
2	Solid artificial organs	141.2 (95-02)	Transplant/implant
3	Left ventricular assist devices	96.0 (95-02)	Cardiovascular
4	Skin substitute products	63.1 (97-04)	Wound care
5	Refractive surgical devices	54.4 (98-05)	Opthalmic
6	Gynecologic fallopscopes	49.5 (95-00)	Endoscopic/MIS
7	PTMR products	47.8 (00-04)	Cardiovascular
8	Bone growth substitutes and growth factors	47.0 (97-04)	Orthopedics
9	Growth factor dressings	46.0 (97-04)	Wound care
10	Vascular stent grafts	46.0 (97-04)	Cardiovascular

The top 20 medical devices in terms of revenues in 1999 were the following:

1. Incontinence supplies
2. Home blood glucose-monitoring products
3. Wound closure products
4. Implantable defibrillators
5. Soft contact lenses
6. Orthopedic fixation devices
7. Pacemakers
8. Examination gloves
9. Interventional cardiovascular coronary stents
10. Arthroscopic accessory instruments
11. Prosthetic knee joint implants
12. Lens care products
13. Prosthetic hip joint implants
14. Multiparameter patient-monitoring equipment
15. Mechanical wound closure
16. Wound suture products
17. Absorbable polymers
18. Hearing aids
19. Wheelchair and scooter/mobility aids
20. Peritoneal dialysis sets (The Wilkerson Group 1999)

The steps and processes involved in developing and bringing to market a new medical device are significantly different than those in pharmaceutical development. This process, while less complex, less expensive, and shorter than that for a drug, is also less well-defined and less profitable if successful. But the fundamental objectives in development and approval are the same as for a drug – to have a product that can be profitably marketed with proven therapeutic efficacy and safety.

There are two significant routes to regulatory approval (and therefore development) for a device (Kahan 2000), 510(k) and PMA (premarket approval). The 510(k) route is less rigorous but requires that the device be either class I or II (the lower two categories of risks) and that there already be a similar ("predicate") device on the market. Such devices may or may not require clinical studies (efficacy and safety may be adequately established in nonclinical studies). Suitable materials must be utilized (and analytical data must be available to establish that the levels of purity and nature of impurities in said materials are acceptable), and the resulting actual product must be sterilized, packaged, and labeled in accordance with regulatory requirements. Also a 510(k) application must be assembled, submitted, and approved by CDRH (Center for Devices and Radiological Health). Such applications account for roughly 98% of new devices, with only 10% of such applications requiring some sort of clinical testing.

There are alternative routes such as the 510(j) route of approval, but it is very rare and will not be discussed here.

The other route for approval requires a PMA (premarket approval). Devices coming to market by this regulatory route include all of those in class III and also those in class II that either do not have a predicate or are of some specified category. Clinical studies must always be performed for these to both demonstrate efficacy and evaluate safety in clinical use.

Biocompatibility

The year 1990 saw the passage of the Safe Medical Devices Act, which made premarketing requirements and postmarketing surveillance more rigorous. The actual current guidelines for testing originated with the USP guidance on the biocompatibility of plastics. A formal regulatory approach springs from the tripartite agreement, which is a joint intergovernmental agreement between the United Kingdom, Canada, and the United States (with France having joined later). After lengthy consideration, the FDA announced acceptance of International Standards Organization (ISO) 10993 guidelines for testing (ASTM 1990; FAO 1991; MAPI 1992; O'Grady 1990; Spizizen 1992) under the rubric of harmonization. This is the second major trend operative in device regulation: the internationalization of the marketplace with accompanying efforts to harmonize regulations. Under the efforts of the ICH (International Conference on Harmonization), great strides have been made in this area.

Independent of FDA initiatives, the USP (United States Pharmacopoeia) has promulgated test methods and standards for various aspects of establishing the safety of drugs (e.g., the recent standards for inclusion of the levels of volatiles in formulated drug products), which were, in effect, regulations affecting the safety of both drugs and devices. Most of the actual current guidelines for the conduct of nonclinical safety evaluations of medical devices have evolved from such quasi-agency actions (e.g., the USP's 1965 promulgation of biological tests for plastics and ongoing American National Standards Institute (ANSI) standard promulgation).

A medical device that is adequately designed for its intended use should be safe for that use. The device should not release any harmful substances into the patient that can subsequently lead to any adverse biologic effects. Some manufacturers believe that biocompatibility is sufficiently indicated if their devices are made of medical grade material or materials approved by FDA as direct or indirect additives. The term medical grade does not have an accepted legal or regulatory definition and therefore can be misleading without appropriate biocompatibility testing.

There are no universally accepted definitions for biomaterial and biocompatibility, yet the manufacturer who ultimately markets a device will be required by the Parenteral Drug Association (PDA) to demonstrate biocompatibility of the product as part of the assurance of its safety and effectiveness. The manufacturer is responsible for understanding biocompatibility tests and selecting methods that best demonstrate the following:

- The lack of adverse biological response from the biomaterial
- The absence of adverse effects on patients

The diversity of the materials used, types of medical devices, intended uses, exposures, and potential harms present an enormous challenge to the design and conduct of well-designed biocompatibility testing programs. The experience gained in one application area is not necessarily transferable to another application. The same applies to different or sometimes slightly different (variable) materials. Biodegradation and interaction of materials complicates and confounds the assessment.

Biocompatibility describes the state of a biomaterial within a physiological environment without the material adversely affecting the tissue or the tissue adversely affecting the material. Biocompatibility is both a chemical and physical interaction between the material and the tissue and the biological response to these reactions.

Biocompatibility assays are used to predict and prevent adverse reactions and establish the absence of any harmful effects of the material. Such assays help to determine the potential risk that the material may pose to the patient. The proper use of biocompatibility tests can reject potentially harmful materials while permitting safe materials to be used for manufacturing the device.

Any biocompatibility statement is useful only when it is considered in the proper context. A statement such as "propylene is biocompatible" lacks precision and can lead to misunderstanding. Any statement of biocompatibility should include information on the type of device, the intended conditions of use, the degree of patient contact, and the potential of the device to cause harm. Manufacturers should avoid using the term "biocompatible" without clearly identifying the environment in which it is used and any limitations on such use.

The need for biocompatibility testing and the extent of such testing that should be performed depends on numerous factors. These factors include the type of device, intended use, liability, degree of patient contact, nature of the components, and potential of the device to cause harm. There are no universal tests to satisfy all situations, and there is no single test that can predict biological performance of the material or device and reliably predict the safety of the device. The types and intended uses of medical devices determine the types and number of tests required to establish biocompatibility. Biological tests should be performed under conditions that stimulate the actual use of the product or material as closely as possible and should demonstrate the biocompatibility of a material or device for the specifically intended use. These tests will be more extensive for a new material than for those materials that have an established history of long and safe uses.

All materials used in the manufacture of a medical device should be considered for an evaluation of their suitability for intended use. Consideration should always be given to the possibility of the release of toxic substances from the base material(s), as well as any contaminants that might remain after the manufacturing process or sterilization. The extent of these investigations will vary, depending on previously known information (prior art) and initial screening tests.

Fundamentals of Biocompatibility Tests

Biocompatibility is generally demonstrated by tests utilizing toxicological principles that provide information on the potential toxicity of materials in the clinical application (Gad and Gad-McDonald 2016). Many classical toxicological tests, however, were developed for a pure chemical agent and are not applicable to biocompatibility testing of materials. In addition, medical devices are an unusual test subject in toxicity testing. A biomaterial is a complex entity of multiple components, and the material toxicity is mediated by both its physical and chemical properties. The toxicity from a given biomaterial often comes from its leachable components, and the chemical composition of a material is often not known or not known with precision. Toxicological information on the material and its chemical composition is seldom available, and the possible interactions among the components in any given biological test system are seldom known.

Accordingly, biocompatibility should not be defined by a single test. It is highly unlikely that a single parameter will be able to ensure biocompatibility; therefore it is necessary to test as many biocompatibility parameters as appropriate. It is also important to test as many samples as possible; therefore suitable positive and negative controls should produce a standard response index for repeated tests.

Additionally, the use of exaggerated conditions, such as using higher-dose ranges and longer contact durations or multiple insults that are more severe by many factors than the actual condition(s) of use, is/are important. Adopting an acceptable clinical exposure level that is multiple factors below the lowest toxic level has been a general practice.

Most of the biocompatibility tests are short-term tests designed to establish acute toxicity. Data from these short-term tests should not be extrapolated to cover the areas with longer periods of exposure in which no test results are available.

Biocompatibility testing should be designed to assess the potential adverse effects under actual use conditions or specific conditions close to the actual use conditions. The physical and biological data obtained from biocompatibility tests should be correlated to the device and its use. Accuracy, reproducibility, and interpretability of tests depend on the method and the equipment used and the investigator's skill and experience.

There are several toxicological principles that the investigator must consider before planning biocompatibility testing programs. Biocompatibility depends on the tissue or tissues that contact the device. For example, the requirements for a blood-contacting device would be different from those applicable to a urethral catheter. Also, the degree of biocompatibility assurance depends on the involvement and the duration of contact with the human body.

Some materials, such as those used in orthopedic implants, are meant to last for a long period of time in the patient. In this case, a biocompatibility testing program needs to show that the implant does not adversely affect the body during the long period of use. The possibility of biodegradation of material or device should not be ignored. Biodegradation by the body can change an implant's safety and effectiveness. The leachables from plastic used during a hemodialysis procedure may be very low, but the patient who is dialyzed three times a week may be exposed to a total of several grams during his or her lifetime; therefore the cumulative effects (chronic exposure) should be assessed.

Two materials having the same chemical composition but different physical characteristics may not induce the same biological response. Also, past biological experiences with seemingly identical materials have their limits, too. Toxicity may come from leachable components of the material due to differences in formulation and manufacturing procedures.

Empirical correlation between biocompatibility testing results and actual toxic findings in humans and the extrapolation of the quantitative results from short-term in vitro testing to quantitative toxicity at the time of use are controversial. Such accumulation of data needs a thorough, cautious, careful, and scientifically sound interpretation and explanation within the boundaries of the information at hand. The control of variation in the assessment of biological susceptibility and resistance to obtain a biological response range for a toxic effect needs careful attention as does an assessment of the host factors that determine the variability of susceptibility in a toxicological response adjustment to susceptibility. The variability in human populations also needs careful attention.

The challenge of the assessment of biocompatibility is to create and use knowledge to reduce the degree of unknowns in the development process and in turn use this information to help make the best possible decisions pertaining to actual conditions of use. The hazard presented by a substance, with its inherent toxic potential, can only be manifested when fully exposed in a patient. Risk, which is actual or potential harm, is therefore a function of toxic hazard and exposure. The safety of any leachables contained in the device or on the surface can be evaluated by determining the total amount of potentially harmful substance, estimating the amount reaching the patient's tissues, assessing the risk of exposure, and then performing a risk versus benefit analysis. Then the potential harm from the use of biomaterial is completely identified from the biocompatibility analyses and data of an alternate material.

Clinical Testing

Current data indicate that large medical device developers are conducting fewer studies at fewer locations, but the sheer number of products in the pipeline is providing significant opportunities for investigative sites and CROs with experience conducting device trials. Indeed, spending on clinical medical device studies remains one of the fastest-growing segments (see Table 4.4).

Whereas spending for clinical studies of drug therapies grew 14% annually over the past several years, spending for devices grew by more than 20% annually in that same period. It is estimated that sponsors will spend more than half a billion dollars on clinical research for medical device trials in 2002. Sponsor usage of CROs to manage device trials is also growing substantially. The driver of growth in medical device trials is not regulatory pressure, as is often the case. It is the medical community. "Doctors are clearly the ones driving most of the research," said Charlie Whelan, an industry analyst in the medical device group of San Jose, California, based Frost & Sullivan. "They're conservative by nature and won't use something until they feel there's sufficient clinical evidence to support its use. Some doctors want more data than the FDA requires. They want longer-term data or want answers to more specific questions."

The persistent pattern of filings in this market is expected to continue and possibly grow with enhanced physician demand for clinical trial evidence and a rich pipeline of potential new devices (Table 4.5).

Table 4.4 Clinical grant spending for medical device trials in the United States

1994	$100
1998	$250
2002	$530

Table 4.5 Original IDEs and approved number of IDEs

1991	220
1993	248
1995	210
1997	272
1999	305
2001	284
2002	307
2003	246
2004	217
2005	238
2006	234
2007	214
2008	215

The number of original investigational device exemption (IDE) applications and the numbers of pre-market approvals (PMAs) and PMA supplements have been increasing steadily. These devices are novel and present potentially higher risk. They also require more pre- and post-marketing clinical research studies. "There is no shortage of opportunity in this market segment," said Whelan. "Many hundreds of new device companies have been created in each of the past five years, fueled by an aging population and new technologies."

Market Characteristics

The global medical device market, excluding imaging and clinical diagnostics, is valued at over $150 billion annually. Product lines are numerous and diverse, ranging from latex gloves and wheelchairs to hearing aids and artificial hearts. About 80% of the medical device market is composed of small companies with fewer than 50 employees. Nearly one fourth of the 13,000 plus medical device and diagnostics manufacturers are startup companies with no source of revenue. This fragmentation mirrors the multitude of small markets for a widely diverse range of devices used in medical interventions.

The strategy for most manufacturers is to get a 510(k) and then do a clinical study. It's not an "investigation device" anymore, and the FDA never sees the data. The studies are still subject to Part 56 and Part 50 regulations regarding IRB approval and informed consent, but the FDA has no tools or means to effectively monitor and ensure compliance.

Europe is again seeing a healthy portion of the activity, largely because devices are far less regulated across the Atlantic than in the United States. The only ethical regulatory strategy that makes sense is to first do a clinical study in Europe and get approval and then come to the United States. Most often clinical trials are conducted in Europe where they tend to be larger projects with an average of 531 subjects per study versus 172 on average in the United States. Companies specifically conduct five clinical studies to bring a device to market in Europe, more than twice the US average. Unlike the increasingly global nature of clinical trials for ethical pharmaceuticals, medical device trials are becoming less international.

Device companies are placing their studies in many of the same places where drug studies are conducted. Typically, clinical studies go to leading academic institutions where the prevalence of disease in the patient population is most representative.

Table 4.6 Increasing use of CROs for medical device trials

Percentage of device companies who report using CRO for...		
	1998 (%)	2001 (%)
Protocol design	0	11
CRF design	0	12
Monitoring services	13	29
Regulatory services	8	11
Statistical services	8	33

According to Frost & Sullivan, medical device companies contract out less than 5% of their clinical research projects to CROs (see Table 4.6). "They use CROs a lot less than drug companies," said Whelan. "Our forecast suggests that, in coming years, the medical device industry is likely to outsource more of its R&D, but not very much – i.e., up to maybe 7% by 2005." Most of the research that needs to be done can typically be done in-house. Doing research through a CRO also exposes the company to a lot of risk, including patent infringement. There are an estimated half dozen CROs in the United States and another half dozen in Europe that cater mostly, if not exclusively, to medical device companies. Many of them are boutique CROs that specialize in particular types of devices. All of them are fairly small, with between 5 and 30 employees. The big, multipurpose CROs, like Quintiles and Parexel, also assist sponsors with device trials. About 96% of medical device manufacturers utilize CROs most frequently for statistical and monitoring services.

Changing Focus, Changing Oversight

The US device industry is continuously developing new and innovative techniques in areas such as molecular diagnostics (including test for infectious diseases, inherited and metabolic diseases, and cancer), minimally invasive surgery, biocompatible materials used for cardiovascular purposes, and orthopedic implants.

Combination products, gene therapies, imaging technologies, and devices that can be linked to bioterrorism are among the hottest areas of medical device research currently.

A recent report by Frost & Sullivan named digital radiography and molecular diagnostics as two sectors worth watching for new developments in the

Table 4.7 Improving development performance

Percentage of IDEs approved by FDA in first review cycle	
1997	69%
1999	68%
2001	80%

months ahead. As healthcare providers shift to digital radiography techniques, image integration will gain in importance. Financial simulation will gain in importance. The simultaneous shift toward home healthcare and nursing home care is also bound to spur demand – and thus the launch of even more new products – ranging from ambulatory aids to orthopedic supports. "Products focusing on self-care, the geriatric population and women are likely to experience impressive growth," a recent report has stated.

Regulations are as stringent for devices as for drugs, claim FDA officials (see Table 4.7). Submission-to-decision review times, however, are now worse for original PMAs than for new drug applications – 411 versus 365 days – and the highest since the passage of FDAMA. Review times on 501(k)s, meanwhile, are falling. Third-party review of eligible class I and II 510(k) devices, paid for by the manufacturer, is very small – but growing – contributor to review spending. The Center for Devices and Radiological Health's (CDRH's) Office of Device Evaluation (ODE) received only 107,510(k)s reviewed by third-party organizations in FY 2001, which amounted to about 16% of all eligible 510(k). However, that's a 128% increase over the 47 such submissions received the prior year. Expansion of the pilot program in March 2001 more than tripled the number of eligible devices to 670.

As the FDA itself reports, the frequency and consequence of hazards resulting from medical use error far exceed those arising from device failures. So the FDA is paying far more attention to device design and labeling. The Office of Health and Industry Programs (OHIP) assists CDRH's ODE by providing "human factors reviews" for PMA and 510(k) devices. This included patient labeling reviews on 141 submissions to CDRH last year. The OHIP also issued a guidance document last year on medical device patient labeling, including a suggested sequence and content, and principles on the appearance of text and graphics.

Guidance has also been issued about when a device manufacturer may report changes or modifications to the clinical protocol in a 5-day notice to the IRB as opposed to getting formal FDA approval. It clarifies the kind of protocol changes – i.e., modification of inclusion/exclusion criteria to better define the target patient population or increasing the frequency at which data are gathered – appropriate for the 5-day notice provision. Other types of changes, such as to indication or type of study control, require prior approval.

The FDA has also posted for comment a proposed regulatory change that would require sponsors and investigators to disclose to an IRB any prior IRB review of a proposed study. In the device world companies do IRB shopping since the IRB makes the determination if the device poses significant or non-significant risk.

Device manufacturers share with pharmaceutical companies the headache of complying with the Health Insurance Portability and Accountability Act (HIPAA). In terms of sponsor access to source data, there must be statement of when authorization expires, such as until the PMA is approved or when the product is on the market. There should be a description of how far back in time the patient's medical records will need to be searched. The consent process should also include a statement that treatment, payment, and insurance reimbursement are not conditioned on signing. The document should specifically indicate information that will not be disclosed to the sponsor. And there should be a statement of when, and if, study data will be made available to study subjects. Even though the sponsor pays for a lab test, it becomes part of the patient's medical record. Patients have a right to see it unless they sign away that right during the consent process.

Under HIPAA, doctors will no longer have the right to look at the medical records of referred patients, even those within the same practice group. Investigators will need to go to the IRB to ask for a "waiver of authorization." That will add another 2–3 months to the timeline. The IRB must also get educated.

The Review Speed Problem

Device manufacturers have been pressuring the FDA to accelerate the review and approval cycle time. The average useful life span of a medical device is 18 months. It's not a question of the patent expiring. Within 18 months, the product may be obsolete. A competitor has a new bell or whistle that makes its product more desirable than yours.

In terms of review speed, FDAMA has clearly done more to benefit pharmaceutical companies than device firms. With breakthrough technology, the FDA has "a tendency to request information for 'educational purposes' that is not directly pertinent to determine the safety and effectiveness of the device in question," Weagraff explained. Timeliness and responsiveness could be improved.

A central problem at the FDA is a lack of resources and appropriately trained resources to review the mandatory, more complicated studies. "A growing number of premarket submissions are for medical technologies that pose novel review issues, like tissue-engineered products, hybrid technologies... and nanotechnology," according to the industry trade group AdvaMed.

Last year, the FDA received 70 PMA applications, the highest number in 10 years. The CDRH alone reviews some 17,000 device submissions and inspects 15,000 manufacturers a year. Though a proposed $10 million budget increase for the agency was awarded in 2003, none of these funds were earmarked for device review. "The FDA device program budget has remained essentially flat over the last 10 years, and has declined in real dollars after accounting for inflation," according to the AdvaMed report. "In addition, staffing levels have declined 8% since 1995." Limited resources have also prevented the FDA from offering up more device-specific guidance documents.

The FDA claims to be focusing on erasing holdups on PMA combination product reviews that often involve the expertise of "a drug person, a materials person and an engineer," according to one CDRH official. "The experts are all in-house, they're just not all in our center. And what's a priority for us is not necessarily a priority for anyone else." In the past, the FDA has taken as long as 13 months simply to decide which agency – CDRH, the Center for Drug Evaluation and Research, or the Center for Biologics Evaluation and Research – should perform the review. In February, the FDA also established a combination products program to help deal with the delays. Legislation is pending to create a formal combination products office to assign products to the appropriate component of the FDA.

Mark Kramer, director of the program housed in the FDA's Office of the Ombudsman, said, "Currently, we don't have an exact count on the number of combination products. And it's difficult to make a guess because a lot of these products don't require inter-center coordination and are reviewed entirely within one center that, over time, has developed certain expertise in that product area. Standard operating procedures are now under review by different centers within the FDA to make intra-agency reviews occur in a more organized and documented fashion."

"The regulatory clock on the request for a designation process used to determine which agency will review a combination product is 60 days," added Kramer. "But at times submissions need to be supplemented with additional information, or companies request a meeting during the review period because they want to provide additional information. That can cause the total elapsed time to be over 60 days. However, we generally have an agreement with the sponsor to extend the review clock."

Some FDA critics, meanwhile, believe approval times have become too short since FDAMA, and they fear that some manufacturers exacerbate the problem by doing as little testing as possible or by "fudging" clinical data. A scathing July 29 article by *U.S. News & World Report* highlighted past regulatory violations of both Boston Scientific and Medtronic, including withholding important information and details on known adverse events from the FDA. It also pointed out dangers inherent in the 510(k) process and underfunding an overburdened safety-monitoring agency. The FDA's Office of the Inspector General found that, between 1994 and 1999, regulatory violations were far from rare. Device trials were twice as likely as trials for drugs and biologics to violate FDA rules, with such violations including but not limited to missing data, poor data collection, and falsification of data.

Several FDA information sheets have also been put out to offer a needed reminder to investigators and IRBs about the difference between "significant risk" (SR) and "nonsignificant risk" (NSR) device studies – i.e., extended wear contact lenses versus daily wear lenses. NSR device studies have fewer regulatory controls and don't require submission of an IDE application to the FDA. "The IRB is supposed to make that [SR or NSR] determination," said Stark, "but they've been known to forget." FDA staff was given internal guidance in this area last fall.

Small device firms look for guidance and are respectful of clinical trial expertise once they find it. They're often idea driven rather than market potential driven. The entire organization may consist of an engineer, head of regulatory and clinical affairs, and a receptionist. Many folks in the medical device business are naïve and have little relevant experience.

Unless and until something is done to increase FDA resources, the number of required review days on some of the most medically important devices will likely continue to rise. Congress is reportedly looking at an FDA reform package that would give the agency more money to implement process improvements. A program similar to the Prescription Drug User Fee Act is now being implemented for medical devices.

Like pharmaceuticals, there are multiple steps involved in developing a new medical device. Because the product life cycle is much shorter for devices, the time lines for these steps need to be compressed.

The phases can be considered to include:

- Prototype design
- Vendor (to provide materials) selection and verification
- Biocompatability and physical chemical evaluation
- Clinical evaluation
- Regulatory filing and approval

Through the networks of contractors (CROs) to support these steps is less extensive than that for pharmaceuticals, there are still a wide variety of available sources, and the management issues remain similar.

References

ASTM. (1990). Standardization in Europe: A success story. *ASTM Standardiz. News*, p. 38.

CDRH. (1992). *Regulatory requirements for medical devices: A workshop manual. HHS publication FDA 92-4165*. Rockville: Center for Device and Radiological Health.

FAO. (1991, March 18–27). *Report of the FAO/WHO conference on food standards, chemical in food and food trade (in cooperation with GATT)* (Vol. 1). Rome: Secretariat, Joint FAO/WHO Food Standards Programme, FAO.

Gad S. C., Gad-McDonald, S. E. (2016). *Biomaterials, medical devices and combination products biocompatibility test and safety Assessmenet*. Boca Raton, FL: CRC Press.

Kahan, J. S. (2000). *Medical device development: A regulatory overview*. Waltham: Parexel.

MAPI. (1992). *The European Community's new approach to regulation of product standards and quality assurance (ISO 9000): What it means for U.S. manufacturers* (MAPI Economic Report ER-218).

MDDI. (2000, December). Industry snapshot. *Medical Device and Diagnostics Industry*, 47–56.

Nugent, T. N. (1994). *Health care products and services basic analysis*. New York: Standard & Poor's Industry Surveys.

O'Grady, J. (1990). Interview with Charles M. Ludolph. *ASTM Standardiz. News*, p. 26.

Spizizen, G. (1992). The ISO 9000 standards: Creating a level playing field for international quality. *National Productivity Review, 11*(Summer), 331–346.

USP. (2020). *The United States Pharmacopoeia, USP43 § NF-38*. Rockville: U.S. Pharmacopoeial Convention.

The Wilkerson Group. (1999). *Forces reshaping the performance and contribution of the U.S. medical device industry*. Washington, DC: Health Industry Manufacturers Association.

Functions and Types of Contract Support Organizations (Including CROs, CMDOs, Packagers, and Contract Formulators)

5

As discussed in a separate chapter, since the 1930s, the entire contract research/ development and production industry to support new drug and device development and testing into the marketplace has evolved into a major industry in its own right. The critical shortage of new drugs in the pipeline has forced a number of major pharmaceutical companies to form strategic partnerships with companies capable of bringing in resources not currently available in their own organizations, due to especially a lack of investment or downsizing. The limited number of new chemical entities (especially arising from small "start-up" companies) and the pricing pressure from the managed care organizations and the state and federal governments have made every pharmaceutical company evaluate the costs of developing a new drug and its commercial manufacturing. Additionally, most new drugs arise from small organizations which have very limited (if any) internal development capabilities. At the same time, the limits of internal resources and increased regulatory requirements for bringing new products to market powers the same needs for the medical device industry. In the midst of the process, the role of non-employee (gig-economy) clients with technical and regulatory skills to take the process increased.

There are two fundamental drivers for outsourcing in the pharmaceutical and medical device industries. The first is the need for access to sources of information, essential for the long-term success of any company. This has resulted in pharmaceutical companies buying up small innovative drug deliv-

© Springer Nature Switzerland AG 2020
S. C. Gad et al., *Contract Research and Development Organizations-Their History, Selection, and Utilization*, https://doi.org/10.1007/978-3-030-43073-3_5

ery and biotech companies, as their own laboratories run out of new drug leads and molecules. There are a variety of reasons for the lack of innovative ideas in large pharmaceutical companies, but those are beyond the scope of this book. The second major driver for outsourcing is the imperative to reduce the excessive costs and time involved in development that have developed within these companies and not having to support the necessary resources except when they are needed. The push to reduce the costs and exploit the synergies that may come with partnerships has further led to an unprecedented rate of acquisitions and mergers within these industries since the early 1990s. This has continuously accelerated.

Pharmaceutical companies have always supported a thriving service sector, partly due to the broad range of skills and technologies required to discover, develop, and manufacture a drug for the market. This has aided in the positioning of these outsourcing organizations in the role of strategic partners. Table 5.1 provides an organized index to the principal types of these CROs and their primary services.

Hole in the Virtual Model: General Contractor

The virtual companies that now predominate drug and device development have come to be as a way to reduce development costs and to facilitate the entrepreneurial drive by innovators. A major (perhaps the major) problem with the virtual company pharmaceutical development model is that the proper placement of monitoring and conduct along with the coordination of such efforts is complex and requires a level and breadth of skills which are rarely present in the virtual organization let alone in specific service providers. A single individual or organization is needed to be able to act as a "general contractor" for such activities. And such a service provider is all the better if they are experienced and able to provide some of the required key services on their own. As an example of the complexity of outsourcing operations, the task of contract formulation development should be considered.

The pharmaceutical industry is challenged by competitive pressures to shorten the new product development process. CROs have clearly demonstrated their ability to accelerate the pace of development in the clinical arena, where there are now myriad companies offering services in statistical analysis, clinical trials management, report writing, project management, and bioanalytical testing (Parikh 2001).

Table 5.1 Types of CROs

	Appendix
Nonclinical biological testing	
Pharmacology	B
Biocompatibility (devices)	A
In vitro screening	A, B
Toxicology	A
Metabolism	A, B
Pharmacokinetic modeling	B
Chemistry	
Medicinal chemistry	D
Synthesis (active pharmaceutical ingredient (API) manufacture)	D
Radiolabeled synthesis	C
Analytical method development/analysis	C
Bioanalytical method development/analysis	D
Biological product manufacturers	
Engineering	
Machine shops	B
Physical testing	B
Clinical	
Phase I centers	G
Clinical monitors	G
Statistical analysis	G
Site management organizations (SMOs)	G
Report writing services	G
Data management	G
Dosage forms	
Formulation development	E
Clinical test material (CTM) packagers	F
Labeling	F
Patient kit preparations	F
Pharmacy services	F
Contract sterilization	B
Regulatory	
IND preparation	H
NDA preparation	H
Annual update preparation	H
Regulatory advisors	H

There is a growing trend in the industry to outsource product development, including such processes as formulation development, stability testing, manufacture of clinical trial supplies, and the preparation of chemistry, manufacture and controls (CMC documents).

Formulation development is a key area (and most often overlooked) of product development patentability, lifecycle, and ultimately the success of a new product. Formulation development encompasses a very wide range of activities. Traditionally, formulation covers such functions as preformulation, including analytical assay development and characterization, excipient screening to stabilize or enhance the solubility of the product, and dosage form development, whether it involves a solid, liquid, topical aerosol, or other dosage forms. Formulation development may also include assessing delivery options.

As advances in preclinical technology have generated a massive number of putative potential drug candidates, contract formulation development has become the only way for the industry to keep pace. There are essentially three reasons for companies of all sizes to choose to outsource their formulation development functions:

(a) To compress a timeline, i.e., reduce time to market
(b) To access a particular expertise, technology, facility, or skill
(c) To offset the true costs involved with the risks of product failure

The following issues must be considered in detail for the outsourcing of any activity in general and formulations development in particular:

1. Determination of specifically what needs to be outsourced
2. Defining and establishing the scope of the project
3. Identification and selection of an outsource partner
4. Protection of the intellectual property
5. Management of the project

Determining Outsourcing Needs

The need to consider outsourcing formulation development is driven by various and unique internal factors within each company. These could include lack of skilled staff, lack of access or timely access to suitable equipment, time constraints, and a general lack of technological know-how. In short, the sponsor must decide if outsourcing is being considered for tactical reasons (contracting the project out because of time or manpower constraints) or strategic reasons (the sponsor does not have the technical resources in-house and has no intention of making the investment and taking the time to build them in-house).

The former situation is quite common among major pharmaceutical companies, where the number of projects far exceeds the available suitably skilled and experienced manpower or the time allotted. The latter scenario tends to be found among virtual companies or small firms, where resources are at a distinct premium.

Nevertheless, the determination to outsource formulation development must be made with one clear understanding: the *initial* cost of going out-of-house will always be higher than doing the same project in-house. This fact always surprises companies when they consider outsourcing for the first time. This is understandable; for a number of companies, the true cost of developing the product is hidden by the complicated way the accounting function calculates the allocation of overhead costs. An offsetting advantage is that careful selection of consultants and vendors may provide better quality at lower actual prices.

Establishing the Scope of the Project

An integral objective of formulation development is defining the ultimate clinical dosage form. In early development the dosage form is undefined. The decision often comes down to what is feasible, what is marketable, and what is cost-effective for a particular drug. A clear understanding of the ultimate goal of the project will refine the selection criteria for identifying and selecting an outsourcing organization. Formulation development projects to be outsourced span a wide range of needs. An outsourced project may range from preformulation studies to clinical supply manufacturing or it may comprise a very limited subset of the development project.

A clearly defined written list of essential activities, expectations, and responsibilities must be unambiguously established. The outsource organizations must receive such information and key objectives as a budget, a schedule of critical project milestones, and deliverables in order to supply a request for proposal (RFP) at the start and identify and visualize to participants critical path tasks and responsibilities.

The scope of the project can be subdivided into preformulation development and formulation development. Normally some of the preliminary information may be available with the originating company and can be shared with the outsourcing organization. In most cases, the preformulation and formulation development is outsourced as a single project.

The requirements for different dosage forms are obviously different and must be identified. Some of the considerations are listed in the two tables below. Some of the considerations are listed in Tables 5.2 and 5.3.

Table 5.2 Preformulation development research

1. Active pharmaceutical ingredient (API) characterization:
   - Stability indicating assay
   - Purity (IR)
   - Crystallization solvent
   - Melting point
   - % volatiles
   - Probable decay products
   - Solubility profile, pKa
   - Physical properties (i.e., LOD, dentistry, flow, particle size distribution, shape, surface area, etc.)
   - Crystal properties and polymorphism
   - Log P determination
   - Identity (chromatographic)
   - Dissolution study, x-ray diffraction, IR analysis, thermal analysis, hot-stage microscopy
   - Porosity (BET, mercury, etc.)
   - Hygroscopicity
   - Intrinsic dissolution
   - Species and route specific tolerance levels (Gad et al. 2016)
2. Compatibility testing (i.e., excipients, components)
3. Dosage form types
4. API bulk stability
5. Preformulation summary report

Table 5.3 Formulation development scope

1. Preformulation development report-review
2. Chemical/physical stability
3. Dissolution profile (if applicable)
4. Bioavailability
5. Formulation optimization
6. Clinical evaluation

Selecting an Outsource Partner

As presented in Chap. 1, just as the pharmaceutical industry landscape is always changing with mergers, acquisitions, and companies starting up or folding, so it is with the outsource service industry. The listings at the end of this book are certainly not globally complete and will be out of date by the time they appear in print in this reference (as, by the way, even some magazine advertisements for such are!!), but we hope to have provided an excellent starting place for the selection process.

After the first round of selection, one should contact the remaining organizations under consideration and conduct the following actions:

(a) Initiate Confidentiality Disclosure Agreements (CDAs).
(b) Study the printed literature and website for each outsourcer's literature.
(c) Ask each outsource organization to fill out a "Pre-Visit Questionnaire" to gain a more complete understanding of the organization, its response time, and the degree of understanding that it may have about the type of project the sponsor wants to undertake. Some of the information to request in a pre-visit questionnaire could include company name location, facility description, equipment list, history, organizational chart, mission statement, financial report (for a public company), parent company information (if applicable), regulatory audit history, references, floorplan, total number of employees (broken down by department and educational level), whether the workforce is union or non-union, industrial health and safety records, holding of any licenses (e.g., NRC), AALAC accreditation history (if applicable), complete listing of SOPs, description of project management system, description of any data capture system, description of the flow of communication, technical capabilities, and a list of the company officers clearly showing the flow of authority and ultimate responsibility. Have each organization clearly identify the individual who is to be the prime contact for your project.
(d) Once the prescreening process is complete, a quality audit needs to be initiated to further observe all the capabilities and meet the people who will be managing the project. For the best possible outcome, this activity should be conducted by someone who is familiar with CROs and that has a sound grasp of the project at hand. Find out what the workload on the formulation development staff is, how soon the project can be undertaken,

and whether the company can provide a tentative schedule for completion of certain milestones. Answers to these questions will provide a good indication of the organization's technical and project management capabilities. A reputable organization will not be unwilling to put promises of adherence to timed milestones in writing and have their lack of achievement associated with financial penalties.

(e) Discussing the reputation of the company with industry colleagues is another way of performing due diligence. Particularly in these times of change, such meticulous checks can present one actively on a now false history. These discussions can revolve around the quality of work, the meeting of promised deadlines, reaction and plan of action of the outsourcing organization when unexpected results were obtained, time between the completion of the project and the written reports, and the existence of any surprises in the final invoice for the services rendered. Make sure that the information garnered is specific, replete with adequate supporting detail, and objective. Keep in mind that the site or facility visit is the most important step in selecting an outsourcing company. If the scope of the project is beyond the formulation development, such as process development, clinical supplies, or manufacturing, it is advisable to include in the evaluation of the organization these additional anticipated outsourcing areas. If there is a remote possibility that you will need the outsource organization beyond the formulation development stage, you should consider the following:

- Experience in pharmaceutical development and manufacturing.
- Financial stability and liquidity.
- Past performance in hitting deadlines.
- Production capacity at different levels.
- Current capacity utilization.
- How do they normally sign the commercial contracts? A normal commercial contract can be signed in several different ways:

  1. A "cost plus" contract could require the contract manufacturer to reveal all of the operating costs and profits (open book) to the sponsor (not too many contractors are willing to do this).
  2. Another type of contract could be based on the "spot price," which will mean that, when you want to manufacture your product, *if* the outsource organization has the time and capacity, they will entertain

your business (this is not desirable if you want to have the assurance that the product will be available when you want it in the marketplace).

3. The third type of contract is called "take or pay," which guarantees the outsource organization a certain level of yearly production volume and, in return, the sponsor reserves a specific level of capacity to make sure product will be available to sell. There may be other creative ways commercial contracts can be signed.

- How many commercial products are being manufactured at the current location? Are any of these antibiotics especially toxic?

(f) Financial (price) and agreement reviews by the legal department for terms and conditions including the liabilities. It is advisable that you allow more than adequate time for the legal review, because it will always take considerably longer than both parties estimate.

(g) Clear responsibilities of each organization must be spelled out in the services agreement. For example, if the preformulation work is done in your own or another organization's laboratory and the development report indicates that the excipients are compatible, the outsourcing organization will complete the formulation development project based on that information. If that formulation shows a stability problem related to the compatibilities of the ingredients, the outsourcing organization should not be held responsible for any delays. There are a number of similarly unforeseen issues that may come up during the life of the project; each organization should have enough confidence in each other's professionalism that they can be resolved without too much problem. You will never be able to put every unexpected event in a contract, because that is just how drug development works. You will waste valuable time trying to do this, and only the attorneys will make money and you will lose valuable time. Rather it is important to do one's homework completely and thoroughly up front so that one knows that they are dealing with a sufficiently reputable and ethical organization and that one will be treated fairly when potential problems develop. Relationships are key in this business, so place your business where you know you will be treated well. At the same time, take reasonable steps to verify the actions of others. Drug substances and products manufactured elsewhere, particularly outside of your home country, should be verified as to identify and purify.

Protecting Intellectual Property

When you are considering outsourcing, protecting your proprietary information is critical. Signing of the secrecy agreement alone should not be considered sufficient protection. Unless you are going to license specific technology for your product from the outsourcing organization, your agreement should specifically discuss who owns the outcome of the research especially if it involves some unique process or formulation technique, or the work yields unexpected positive results, product, etc.

Managing the Project

Managing the project requires clear, facile, timely, responsive, and open communication between the parties. Because formulation development is a relatively short-term project, the sponsor company can have a member of its staff, if possible, work alongside the outsourcing organization team at the critical juncture of the project.

Typically, detailed timelines and milestones are established early. The construction of a check list may be advisable with clear responsibilities delineated. The criteria for success are defined at the beginning of the project. This makes it easier to maintain focus and to control and monitor the activities at the outsourcing organization. Monitoring such a project will give the sponsor a good understanding of the outsourcing organization's capabilities, people, and business practices. This is a valuable assessment that will be beneficial down the line, if the sponsor company ever wants to consider the outsourcing organization for the next step in the project, such as process development or commercial manufacturing of the product, and if the outsourcing organization has those capabilities.

Pharmaceutical companies are in need of a method to grow their product pipelines in order to accelerate drug development and reach revenue demands. Outsourcing formulation development can provide new technology not available in-house, besides compressing the time to market for a new drug. The processes of identifying the right outsourcing organization for a project may be streamlined by asking a series of questions internally, before seeking an outsourcing company.

A definitive project plan in terms of scope, timelines, and deliverables will help the outsource organization select a provider with appropriate cost estimates and time commitments. The proper level of due diligence after the selection of the organization must be carried out to avoid disappointments. Monitoring the project with clear milestones and proper supervision and monitoring is of paramount importance for the success of the project.

References

Gad, S. C., Spainhour, C. B., Shoemake, C., Stackhouse Pallman, D. R., Stricker-Krongrad, A., Downing, P. A., Seals, R. E., Eagle, L. A., Polhamus, K., & Daly, J. (2016). Tolerable levels of nonclinical vehicles and formulations used in studies by multiple routes in multiple species with notes on methods to improve utility. *International Journal of Toxicology, 35*(2), 95–178.

Parikh, D. (2001, October). Formulation development. *Contract Pharma*, 60–64.

CROs in China, India, and Elsewhere in the Broader World: Outsourcing Science Gone Global

6

It remains the case that most contract nonclinical pharmaceutical and device testing is performed in the United States, Western Europe, Canada, and Japan. Here we will look at CRO elsewhere and their status, strengths, and weaknesses. Considerations behind seeking such services, other than the convenience of being local, are cost, timeliness, quality, and the suitability by the range of series offered.

There was previously (going back to the 1970s) a frequent desire to perform most first in human testing in Europe, largely driven by the fact that it was possible to get into human trials outside the United States. Thus, there were a number of phase 1 trial CROs operating to offer this possibility. However, in recent years (since the implementation of the EU Clinical Trial Directive), the speed to human trials advantage for Europe has disappeared. Recently, the preferred soonest to initiate FIM trials location has become Australia, bolstered by a significant tax credit.

Starting in the second half of the first decade of the twenty-first century, CROs have been appearing worldwide. These organizations operate in almost all the areas of development support, with (currently) varying degrees of success. The major areas of operation included:

- API (active pharmaceutical ingredient) synthesis.
- Toxicology.
- Nonclinical pharmacokinetics.

© Springer Nature Switzerland AG 2020
S. C. Gad et al., *Contract Research and Development Organizations-Their History, Selection, and Utilization*, https://doi.org/10.1007/978-3-030-43073-3_6

- Drug product production.
- Phase 1 clinical studies.
- Phase 2 clinical studies.
- Phase 3 clinical studies.

The development of these CROs reflects (1) improved technology, infrastructure, and capabilities in the various countries, (2) a desire to enter the healthcare R&D business sector, (3) a response to demand for both lower costs and (in the case of clinical trials) decreased costs and a larger pool of patients, and (4) economic and financial opportunity.

For US and European companies, the factors behind going to CROs in these new countries have been somewhat different (Berens and McCoy 2005; Snyder 2010):

- Better (lower) pricing.
- For nonclinical animal work, fewer animal rights complications.
- To provide leverage to capture work in host countries that are also large economies (particularly China and India), supporting expansion of national drug development infrastructure.
- Access to larger or new pools of patients or subjects for clinical trials with these Potential advantages, however, have exposed a number of real or perceived problems:

  - Security/protection of intellectual property.
  - Regulatory (GLP, GMP, GCP) compliance.
  - Acceptance of data and goods by European and US regulators.
  - Quality of work.
  - Logistics of monitoring work (level required, costs, etc.)
  - Documentation of work and data.
  - Uneven levels of technical capabilities.
  - For clinical studies, unclear adherence to patient protection procedures.

China

Accelerating investment and growth of CROs in China builds in momentum as multinational clients look to sell more medicines in the world's most populous country and at the same time cut development costs (Ng 2009; Anon 2010). Most of the world's largest drugmakers and some of the smaller ones have turned to local Chinese drug contractors with niche specialties and a cheaper pool of scientists to deliver less costly drug trials and to gain access to China's large pool of patients. CROs in China that specialize in late stages of research, including clinical trials, have an annual revenue of about $200million, or less than 3 percent of the global CRO market. They are expected to expand at a rate of approximately 18 percent annually, with forecasts predicting an amount of $360 million by 2020. Hence, multinational CROs, including US-based Covance Inc. (CVD.N) and Charles River Laboratories International Inc. (CRL.N), are aiming to be far bigger players in this country. China, India, and other emerging markets are expected to help offset tepid CRO growth in other parts of the world. However, Brazil is now seen as another emerging potent market.

China's CROs largely came into being after the country joined the World Trade Organization in 2001 and developed a drug regulation system under China's State Food Drug Administration (SFDA). This increasingly competitive sector has at a minimum 138 CROs, 67 of which are (as of November of 2019) certified as being GLP by the Chinese government.

Beyond Chemistry to Toxicology

Over the years, Chinese CROs have focused on relatively inexpensive areas such as biology and chemistry – including screenings of chemicals to identify single entities and combinations with potential as medicines. They have also performed a significant amount of work in the manufacturing active pharmaceutical ingredients for generic drugs. Experts said an increasing number of CROs in China, local and foreign-based, are moving into more lucrative stages of the drug development chain. They include preclinical studies, such as toxicology and other animal research, as well as human studies. China's annual market for toxicology – studies that typically use animals and are designed to root out serious side effects of drugs early in the game – is worth about $180 million. With an abundant supply of nonhuman primates, and little animal rights advocacy, China has become a favorable destination for animal testing. To sell existing drugs to China, multinational drugmakers are required to conduct additional testing to obtain local approvals.

Why NOT Use a Chinese CRO? The #1 Response

"We think utilizing a Chinese CRO will put our program/project/compound at too big of a risk" (Bush 2010). This is the number one reason that Western companies cite for reluctance in leveraging resources in China for their GLP toxicology work. Most often the concern is that the FDA or EMEA will reject a GLP toxicology study from China because it does not meet global regulatory expectations, thus forcing a repeat of the study at additional direct costs and significant delays. While there is significant evidence of risk in defending on data from a number of Chinese toxicology CROs, this is not the case with the top-quality facilities. Some Western regulators do expect more careful and documented external auditing and differentiate between CROs in China as to quality.

Track Record
- GLP toxicology data from Chinese CROs have been successfully used to support multiple INDs and a few NDAs since 2006.

Points to Consider
- Due to frequent national holidays, testing programs conducted in Chinese CROs tend to take longer to complete.
- Chinese CFDA requirements (in their NMPA guidelines, currently unavailable in English) include the conduct of acute toxicity studies on all new drug candidates and anaphylaxis studies on all parenteral drugs and strongly recommend the conduct of free-standing nonclinical pharmacokinetic studies rather than toxicokinetic components being required and sufficient components of 28-day GLP studies to open clinical trials in humans.

Audits in China
- In 2002, staff from the US FDA (which has now opened permanent offices in China) audited all the CROs that have submitted GLP toxicology studies in support of INDs and NDAs. These were audits of specific GLP studies and of facilities. No studies in any of the audits were disqualified for any reason, including compliance, and only minor findings were reported in the 483 s issued (some facilities did not have a single 483 issued).

Chinese Versus Western Technicians
- How do Chinese technicians rank in comparison with their Western counterparts? Chinese animal technicians at the major CROs are top quality; they are unusually well educated, highly trained, and very committed to their jobs. To us they represent a major strength of the Chinese CRO system.

One recurrent issue has been outbreaks of flu among Chinese sourced pigs in swine studies, leading to studies having to be terminated and then restarted with new healthy animals. This became even more severe with the COVID-19 pandemic, which initiated in China and has both limited access and slowed operations.

Good Laboratory Practice

In drug development, GLP provides the framework within which laboratory (regardless of location) studies are planned, performed, monitored, recorded, reported, and archived. In 1981 the Organisation for Economic Co-operation and Development (OECD) finalized its Principles of Good Laboratory Practice (GLP). The OECD and EC (EC Directive 1999) require the establishment of national compliance monitoring programs based on laboratory inspections and study audits and recommend the use of the OECD Guides for Compliance Monitoring Procedures for Good Laboratory Practice and the Guidance for the Conduct of Laboratory Inspections and Study Audits. The harmonized ICH safety guidelines define the circumstances, duration, and types of toxicity studies on new medicinal products. These recommendations take into account the known risk factors as well as the intended indications and duration of exposure. An organization is either GLP (International) compliant or not; there is no in between. International GLP compliance and a history of it should provide at least some confidence in the organization performing the work, regardless of location

India

GLP in India

India has recently joined the OECD GLP Committee as an observer and has set up a national GLP compliance authority under DST (the Department of Science and Technology). India should move to full membership of the OECD GLP and ICH and amend its law to require GLP compliance and inspection of its testing laboratories as a condition of approvals of all medicinal products. Many Indian laboratories have obtained certification and inspection by the Indian National Accreditation Board for Testing and Calibration Laboratories (NABL), which provides a certificate valid for 3 years after inspection. Currently 48 CROs in India are certified as being GLP compliant by the Indian government.

The 2004 amendment to the law allowing toxicology testing with NCE/NME discovered abroad and the importation of standard animal models has served to attract ethical companies to contract out animal studies and cast favor of investment in toxicology labs working to attain international GLP standards.

Indian Preclinical Contract Research Organizations

The Indian pharmaceutical services industry has been attracting decent but muted attention from global pharmaceutical companies (Maggon 2004; Kumaravel and Murugan 2009). In spite of overall economy, the pharma industry has not made great strides in India in attracting foreign capital, and no major collaborations have happened except the recent acquisition of Advinus by Eurofins in 2017 which is miniscule in the context of global scale. The latter acquisition has not yielded the synergy that was expected from Eurofins, as most of Eurofins labs stand as islands of their own with no internal connectivity.

Animal Welfare and Institutional Review of Toxicology Study

Protocols

In 1960, the government of India passed a Prevention of Cruelty to Animals Act and established a Committee for the Purpose of Control and Supervision of Experiments on Animals (CPCSEA). The CPCSEA issues guidelines for laboratory animal facilities (CPCSEA 2003). The goal of these guidelines was to promote the humane care of animals used in biomedical and behavioral research and testing; the guidelines are similar to US and European guidelines. Indian pharmaceutical companies and CROs have extensive experience in handling and managing rodents and only limited experience in handling dogs. Indian pharmaceutical companies or CROs have little or no experience in conducting nonhuman primate studies. The source stock of research animals varies widely in India, and it is always important to establish where an institution is obtaining research animals. European and American stocks are often used in breeding facilities in India, but breeding strategies and general husbandry practices vary widely and should be scrutinized. It is possible to import rodent source animals from other countries in the region, and some institutions use quality facilities in Western countries, but that adds cost of transportation to studies in addition to stress on animals due to time zones.

Animal welfare movement is relatively strong through the Committee for the Purpose of Control and Supervision of Experiments on Animals (CPCSEA). The CPCSEA has a provision of Institutional Animal Ethics Committee (IAEC) which is equivalent to IACUC in the United States. Most often the CROs have learnt to manage the issues through personal tactics, rather than through thorough scientific discussion of study protocols. All non-rodent toxicology study protocols require central (federal) government approval by a committee which meets once every 2 months; also this committee does not have any strong scientific background to make sound judgment on the use of animals. In order to start a dog toxicology study, one has to have a lead time of about 4 months or more to seek central government approval. However, most labs have found alternative personal ways to get by, which is really not meeting strict government regulations. There is absolutely no CRO in India which has the capability or the competence to conduct monkey studies, and there is also no possibility of developing such facilities in the foreseeable future. However, there is no formal restriction by the government of India to conduct monkey studies. Rather, it is just the inability of Indian CRO, to breach customs or obtain the capital commitment for undertaking such endeavors.

GLP Status in India

In the Organisation for Economic Co-operation and Development (OECD 2011), India has been recognized India as a "full-adherent" country for mutual acceptance of data (GLP) from safety studies of pesticides, biocides, manufactured nanomaterials, chemicals, chemical products, and products of modern biotechnology. With new patent law, changes in regulations, and now a recognition by OECD, Indian companies are developing rapidly with many integrating full drug development capability (e.g., GCP processes, GLP/quality assurance [QA]/animal welfare compliance with regulations, toxicology/ absorption and drug metabolism [ADME]/safety pharmacology studies that meet global regulatory submission, bioanalytical development, and efficacy pharmacology and biology). However, gaps remain in adapting global International Conference on Harmonization (ICH) of Technical Requirements for Registration of Pharmaceuticals for Human Use guidance documents. Although Indian pharmaceutical companies have strengths and experience in product chemistry and custom synthesis, custom manufacturing, and bioavailability and bioequivalence studies, alliances between large, established pharmaceutical companies from the United States and Europe are critical to continue the trend in India to learn the process and, eventually, fully independently develop new drugs.

The Indian Good laboratory Practice (GLP) which is managed by one permanent official in the central government. However, for routine GLP inspections of CROs, the Indian government uses scientists working in various government institutes on a part-time basis, which is not the ideal system. According to the OECD process, the government of India does inspection of CROs using part-time government scientists and issues GLP certificate, which is valid for 3 years, which specifies as to what studies a particular CRO has competence to perform. Hence, there are very few CROs who can conduct full complement of all types of toxicology studies needed from drug development for IND and NDA.

CROs in India

There are numerous Indian pharmaceutical companies and drug development contract research organizations (CROs) involved in toxicology intended for product (drug) development. Recent sweeping regulatory improvements and restructuring of both a 1970 patent law and the Indian Drugs and Cosmetics Act of 1940 have enhanced global confidence in the drug research environment in India. In the past, the preclinical CROs offer the global pharmaceutical industry marginal opportunities in preclinical contract research. In the areas of drug discovery – which include lead optimization, medicinal chemistry research, process research and development, preclinical pharmacokinetics, and toxicology – Indian companies do not possess strong enough skills in rational drug design and optimization. However, there are only a few CROs that can conduct longer-duration studies, including 6-month or 1-year rat and dog studies and carcinogenicity studies under Good Laboratory Practices (GLPs). Western sponsors have conducted preclinical packages in the past on Investigational New Drug registration compounds that have progressed into human clinical trials. However, due to the lack of large species (dogs and monkeys), there is a definite pause in Western CROs coming to India for integrated IND drug development.

As of September 2019, there are approximately 40 GLP certified labs in India, bulk of them testing for toxicology along with few of them carrying on specifically for analytical GLP services. http://dst.gov.in/sites/default/files/Certified-Test-Facilities-with-IIBAT-26082016.pdf

Scientific Manpower

Although India has the largest number of universities and colleges, the education system lacks the Western rigor, and bulk of candidates coming out of Indian universities, these days, need lots of on-the-job training before they can manage preclinical GLP studies.

In the last decade, Dr. K.S. Rao of United States has brought the Diplomate of American Board of Toxicology (DABT) exam to India which has resulted in over 100 candidates passing the DABT exam from India. This has to some extent relieved the pressure on qualified toxicologists.

Bulk of pathologists in Indian CRO come from veterinary background who have not been well ground in laboratory animal pathology and lesions observed in control animals. In general, clinical pathology is underemphasized compared to anatomic pathology in veterinary pathology training, and clinical pathologists are underrepresented in the cadre of veterinary pathologists. Clinical pathology interpretation in drug discovery and toxicology studies is usually performed and reported by the study director/toxicologist, who may or may not be a veterinarian and who may lack training and depth of experience. This is an area of concern and should be addressed as an issue in the standards of practice for toxicologic pathology in India.

However, lack of board certification in pathology is a stumbling block for foreign labs to use Indian preclinical CROs.

Lack of formal training in toxicology in Indian universities is a stumbling block in getting qualified candidates for conducting regulatory toxicology studies. Hence, most professional level employees in toxicology labs come from general biology training with absolutely no understanding of basics of toxicology and dose response. On average, it takes a new entrant in toxicology about 3 years before they can become study directors; even then they can conduct studies where no complex issues arise in a study.

Online Capture of Data

Very few labs have any computer system for automatic collection of data (e.g., Instem or Pristina). The lack of such computer facilities inevitably can lead to suspicion of creating clean data when something does go wrong in a study, in particular where quality assurance is not independent or in bed with the study personnel, which is not uncommon in India.

General Competence of Indian CROs

Most Indian preclinical CROs can conduct rodent toxicology studies by oral and parenteral routes, and some of them have developed minimal competence in continuous intravenous infusion and have not reached the stage of global standards of continuous intravenous infusion for longer periods. Repeat dose inhalation capability in India is nonexistent to meet Western standards. Only one or two labs can conduct reproduction and teratology studies with confidence for proper interpretation with historical control data, that too the capacity is rather too small for global companies to use it on a sustained basis.

The biggest issue foreign companies would face in India is determining what studies to do for a project, which many labs do not have the competence to suggest to clients. Also, it is important to note that if a problem does arise in a study, they would be stuck with getting outside (usually foreign) consultants to solve the problem. Even though India has very good statisticians, but not many have specialized in preclinical areas to solve complex issues, in particular for handling carcinogenicity data and difficult to solve reproductive studies where anomalies may occur in selected litters.

Bioanalysis and Toxicokinetics

Bulk of the CROs in India would have only one or no more than two LC-MSs, typically of lower sensitivity. Many of the analytical scientists who manage the bioanalysis labs do not have sufficient experience in developing GLP methods for meeting with US FDA standards. In addition, even if the bioanalysis data are acceptable, very few study directors have the knowledge to interpret the kinetic parameters and related those to toxicologic findings.

In Vitro and Mechanistic Studies

Recently, few of the Indian CROs are trying to develop in vitro capability, but they do not have full complement of regulatory in vitro testing capability under GLP. Many labs can conduct few in vitro tests including mutagenicity, but they would be hard-pressed to interpret the data if there is a problem with a compound. Very few toxicologists have knowledge and understanding of biochemistry or molecular biology. Hence, it is too much to expect any CRO study the mechanism of toxicity when a problem arises.

Experience with Large Molecules

Very few Indian CROs have the working experience with novel large molecules. In the past few years, some efforts are being made to work with biosimilars; however, due to lack of knowledge and technology, compounds showing immunogenicity can be very challenging to work with due to lack of scientific talent both in analytical rigor for large molecules and the ability to understand data and interpret immunogenicity appropriately.

Communications

Very good English is spoken by most scientists, although written English is not as good as it is expected.

Report Quality

In general, if the compound does not produce any startling effects, the reports generated by the Indian CROs should be straightforward. However, when a compound does product effects in multiple parameters and organs, some study directors may find it difficult to interpret and come up with a credible NOAEL. In such cases, the client or the monitoring scientist may have to spend considerable time to polish the report and offer some constructive suggestions to the CRO and to the study director. Many of the Indian CRO may not have the in-house capability to generate SEND tables which can pose issues to the client.

Cost-Effectiveness of Indian CROs

Major CROs who have conducted IND enabling preclinical toxicology studies are on average 30% lower than US or European CROs. One factor that must be kept in mind is the Indian government requires Indian CROs to charge clients (Indian and foreign) a tax called Goods and Services Tax (GST) which comes out to be 18% as of this time. Then the client must add at least two or three trips by the client or the consultant to Indian CRO for monitoring studies during the completion of a project. When you add the GST plus travel cost to India for monitoring studies, the net savings is barely perceptible. There remains the uncertainty of something going wrong and periodic teleconferences and mentoring staff, and it consumes a lot of time of either the client or the consultant monitoring the study. There will be some Indian CRO who are very aggressive in pricing cost to the tune of only 25 to 40% of Western CRO, which should be viewed with suspicion by the client.

How to Qualify CRO in India

Based on initial inspection, a sponsor would select one or two CROs for conduct of preclinical toxicology studies. If the CRO has previously established credibility in conducting and submitting GLP studies to global regulatory authorities, then the sponsor would place a study starting with a non-GLP or shorter-duration study. However, if a CRO has not worked with global pharmaceutical companies, then there is a need to take an alternate approach to estab-lish reasonable credibility. In these cases, the decision should be made to validate these facilities using a compound with which some toxicology data has been generated.

A sponsor should send scientists and QA personnel to the selected CRO laboratory to evaluate the CRO personnel, SOPs, and documentation and to identify the gaps and work on resolution. It is important to work on the CRO's standard protocols and bring them up to international standards following ICH and/or Organisation for Economic Co-operation and Development guidelines, as appropriate. It is also important to make sure these modified protocols fit into the facility SOPs and that there are the technical capabilities to conduct these studies. Once agreement is reached on the new protocols, strain of ani-mals (rodents), and animal source, a sponsor would have the CRO begin a short-duration (1 to 2 weeks) toxicology study in rodents. The sponsor would select and provide a compound for which there has already been generated short-duration toxicology/ADME data in rodents, perhaps a compound from a well-characterized class, or a terminated chemical series. The CRO conducts a rat study with limited histopathology, clinical pathology, and live-phase param-eters and determines exposure levels on the first study day and on the final day. Once the CRO generates a summary report, the sponsor can compare data to the previous data. It is possible to assess overall the quality of the study, time to completion, and costs and, most importantly, evaluate the quality of animals available to these facilities and identify any issues with the source of these animals. If there are any issues, such as parasitic infestation or lung lesions because of the type of bedding (rice husk), then the opportunity exists to dis-cuss and resolve the issues with the facilities. It is also important to check whether the CRO satisfied any QA-identified gaps.

If the sponsor is satisfied with all of the above studies, then it is recom-mended to conduct a 4-week study in the rat. Among the components of the complete IND-enabling package would be genetic toxicology, safety pharma-cology, and 1-month rodent and dog toxicology studies with toxicokinetic analysis. Also, the CRO would conduct a dose form assay, develop a bioana-lytical method, and complete final reports. In addition to conducting the study, the CRO should demonstrate project planning and should follow timelines. The sponsor representatives should visit the CRO during the live phase and monitor the study. If special techniques need to be developed (e.g., brain trim-ming), that work should be established early, and the sponsor should plan on an independent peer review by the sponsor's pathologist. Also, the sponsor should conduct a QA inspection at the end of the study (during the draft report phase), and a QA audit report with action items should be submitted to the CRO. Overall, the sponsor should be able to fully evaluate the quality of the IND-enabling package, time of generation of the IND package, and the total cost.

Summary

There is no commitment by any company for long-term investment in developing competence and capability in full complement of regulatory toxicology studies, in particular for toxicology of large species or difficult and complex long-term studies. Numerous issues stated above like lack of qualified and experienced study directors who can competently conduct and interpret data is a stumbling block in offering carte blanche full development programs. However, Indian CROs can conduct stand-alone studies, in particular rodent studies. Ability to design programs for drug development needs development and upgrading, in most CROs. Lack of credible dog and monkey facilities makes it difficult for any Western CRO to bring programs to India for full development of drugs for IND and NDA. Last but not the least of which will be a nightmare for onsite monitoring studies in India which will be an added expense to the client. The anticipated cost saving can be lost by the imposition of Indian Good and Services Tax (GST) and travel cost by client for monitoring of studies.

Most of the Indian toxicology laboratories seem to follow the OECD protocols, which is available from the public domain. However, there are toxicology laboratories in India, which can meet the GLP requirements of FDA/EMEA in the performance of toxicology studies of new drugs. Indeed, there is one good laboratory dealing mainly with agrochemicals, which claims to have performed over 80 studies for foreign clients and passed GLP inspection from some European agrochemical and environmental regulatory authorities, but does lack experience in dealing with the ascertainment of drug toxicities.

There is a lack of trained and experienced animal histopathologists to detect early signs of drug-induced toxicity like cardiotoxicity, nephrotoxicity, hepatotoxicity, neurotoxicity, and immunotoxicity. The growth of quality clinical pathology laboratories in India and approved by US-based College of

Pathologists is limited but growing. The costs of some Indian laboratories are relatively (compared to Chinese labs) high for rodent studies, and the work may be considered GLP in India but is essentially non-GLP when compared to the international standard.

There is a tendency to issue clean reports for local registration, by excluding diseased, dead, and out of range animals, leading to overestimation of safety and underestimation of toxicity. The upgrading of facilities for animal housing, feeding, and care will require major long-term investment, continuous training of personnel, and very high standards of animal care and cleanliness.

Guidelines and rules by the Committee for the Purpose of Control and Supervision of Experiments on Animals (CPCSEA) in 1998 and revised in 2000 require a central approval by CPCSEA for all experiments on large animals (dogs, monkeys, pigs). Indian laboratories need to implement a comprehensive health program with regular and routine monitoring of experimental animals for the presence of common pathogens including bacteriology, virology, parasitology, and gross pathology to detect any breaches in health or genetic integrity of animals.

The toxicology laboratories in India should pay close attention to the bioanalytical and drug assays needed to meet GLP standards. The analytical methods development for drugs in animal biological fluids and tissues and their validation is a long complex process, which requires trained and qualified staff and sophisticated instrumentation like a mass spectrometer. Most bioanalytical methods requiring the use of LC-MS/MS, IT-MS, and SPE take considerable time even for a highly trained scientist to develop and validate. Solid-phase extraction of drugs where the concentration in biological fluids is in the low ng/ml range is a highly demanding task, and there are cases where the samples from the same animal are repeated to save on the cost of solid-phase extraction cartridges.

The repeated use of items intended to be single use is still very common in India. Several analytical laboratories doing toxicology studies lack trained and experienced staff, invariably produce positive results and assay validation as routine work within a record time, and may not pass an international analytical audit. Strict certification, audit, control, and regular annual inspections of all toxicological, pharmacology, drug metabolism, and animal PK laboratories using animals for research are required.

Until recently, Indian law made it illegal for any Indian toxicology laboratory to test NCE/NME discovered abroad. However toxicology studies have been and are still being performed for foreign sponsors.

Other New Entrants

The countries that newly host GLP toxicology laboratories continue to grow, as can be seen in Appendix I.

While Brazil, Korea, Singapore, and Australia are on the list, Eastern and Central European countries are almost all now represented. Of the estimated 1100+ CROs (nonclinical and clinical – about 70% clinical) worldwide, only a few are yet existent in any of these other countries.

Problems and Solutions

As pointed out earlier, a number of problems are attributed to work performed by newly opened labs in various countries.

A number of these problems are common with new labs, pigmented by cultural differences between existing labs (and first world regulatory agencies) and new entrants to the CRO field.

The best solutions are of course to:

1. Only deal with labs which have some track record of performing studies and submitting reports to the FDA and EMA.
2. Perform extensive and thorough qualification audits
3. Secure references for previous work if possible
4. Pay careful attention to the structure of protocols and SOPs
5. Look closely at the training program
6. Scrutinize project management techniques
7. Evaluate the potential for good, effective, solid, and timely communication. So many problems and disappointments occur because expectations have not been adequately communicated on both sides.
8. Have long-term on-site oversight (monitoring) of phases of studies conducted at such facilities.

Opportunities exist if the opportunity is managed properly. Take, for example, the United States, which has been performing GLP studies for nearly 40 years. A study of public records indicates that organizations in the United States still are not perfect in GLP. So why should one expect an entity with less experience to not require guidance and time to get up to standard?

References

Anon. (2010). *Future outlook of China preclinical and toxicology outsourcing market* (188 pages). Shanghai, China: JZ Medical.

Berens, J., & McCoy, J. (2005). Offshoring in the global pharmaceutical industry: drivers and trends. *Journal of Management Studies, 42,* 675–683.

Bush, E. D. (2010). Why NOT use a Chinese CRO? The #1 Response, *China Preclinical Management Services,* 4/12/2010 Online.

Kumaravel, T. S., & Murugan, S. (2009). Preclinical CROs in India: The next in thing. *Express Pharma,* 16–31 July, 2009.

Maggon, K. (2004). Toxicology testing in India for medicinal products. *Express Pharma Pulse,* 29 July, 2004.

Ng, I.-C. (2009) CROs booming in China. *Drug Discovery & Development,* October 19, 2009.

Snyder, S. (2010) The year in review. *Contract Pharma,* January/February 2010, pp. 30–32.

Selection of CRDOs

7

The selection of service providers that outsourcing development activities require is a demanding activity. A successful development team will certainly include not just a single provider but rather a group of specialist companies, individuals, and organizations (Jackson 1985).

Despite the difficulties and new challenges this approach to R&D presents, more and more companies – large and small – are implementing outsourcing programs as part of a strategy to accelerate the discovery process, control development costs, exploit profitable niche markets, and minimize time to market. Indeed for small and midsize companies, an adequate outsourcing strategy is of paramount importance from the beginning.

The Trend Toward Outsourcing

The "contracting out" or "outsourcing" of chemical scale-up and, more particularly, bulk manufacturing has always been an integral part of pharmaceutical industry activities, but the outsourcing of biology is a more recently developed phenomenon. This is because the more mature industrial chemical industry was already using contract providers, an approach that then became acceptable to the younger pharmaceutical industry entities. The expense of investing in and maintaining a chemical plant means that its capacity must be fully utilized in order to maintain profitability; its use by a number of clients

© Springer Nature Switzerland AG 2020
S. C. Gad et al., *Contract Research and Development Organizations-Their History, Selection, and Utilization*, https://doi.org/10.1007/978-3-030-43073-3_7

has obvious cost-saving and revenue-producing elements. In the past, there existed neither the requirement nor the services necessary to consider outsourcing biological studies.

This changed in the early 1960s, when the tragedy of thalidomide revealed the importance of adverse findings in toxicology and transformed the public policy surrounding drug safety. It was furthered by the introduction in 1977 of Good Laboratory Practice (GLP). Since these two events, the pharmaceutical industry has adapted outsourcing of preclinical safety studies and their components as an integral and essential part of their overall strategy. This can be similarly applied to the clinical work that is performed to supply proof of safety and efficacy of new drugs and has been the norm for medical devices since the 1990 Safe Medical Devices Act.

Outsourcing is now an essential element in the strategy of pharmaceutical companies. Far from being solely the province of large company strategy, outsourcing is used intensively by small companies aiming to adopt modern techniques in a flexible, cost-sensitive, and competitive environment. Outsourcing can be taken to mean more than just contractual R&D and can involve both academic and industrial collaborations. In the widest sense, outsourcing can range from contract R&D to acquisition, with a wide spectrum of joint ventures and collaborative research efforts in between. Arrangements between parties can stretch from preferred provider contractual relationships, through to equity investments interlaced with research collaboration. For the purpose of this chapter, we'll narrow our definition of outsourcing to the contractual relationship between technology provider and client. This may involve a research or a development contract; however, the intellectual property in this definition remains with the sponsor, with payment based on completion of the sponsored work and not related to the ultimate success of the project.

Rapid Growth

In a recent report, outsourcing in the pharmaceutical industry was estimated at contributing to about 90% of overall R&D spending (50% for large pharmaceutical companies) and rising. Given that pharmaceutical R&D is estimated to run at more than $250 billion for the year 2008, this amounts to some $220 billion of expenditure annually. The overall outsourcing market is expected to continue to grow significantly over time, driven by the financial performance expectations of companies. In some areas such as outsourcing of chemistry-related functions, the figure has recently been rising at a compound annual rate of 40–50%. Given the huge amounts of money spent on outsourcing, it is perhaps surprising that more attention is not given to the process and procedures of selection.

This rather oligopolistic market representation should not disguise the fact that there is huge diversity among the smaller organizations that is not shown in the chart, and indeed, in the somewhat older manufacturing function, the split is much wider among a larger number of companies. In clinical and toxicological evaluation, many (though not all) of the tasks have similar skills requirements, and the generic nature of the processes involved tends to favor the agglomeration into larger business units. In chemical manufacture, there is a greater degree of specialization and a greater importance of specialized machinery and facilities required to execute different synthetic routes or manufacture different formulations. However, it is also true that this segment of the outsourcing market is less mature than chemical manufacturing; this may also be a factor in the number of companies represented.

The Buying of R&D

Management of outsourcing is a much more complex process than that of internal R&D. While the selling of R&D is a well-advanced process, the buying of it is not. Many companies incorrectly regard this as a normal extension of their in-house efforts with little training being given to those personnel who are expected to manage it. Frequently, they consider outsourcing as part of the purchasing function. The process of buying R&D can be divided into the following segments:

- The identification of potential providers
- Selection of preferred providers
- Negotiation of a contract
- Management of the work
- Receipt and utilization of the resulting product

Identification of potential partners is itself a complex process, with more than 2300 companies in the business of offering contract pharmaceutical and medical device services. While there are "for hire" directories of such organizations published (DIA 2010; FDLI 2010; Contract Pharma 2020), only these volumes cover the entire span of available resources.

Reflecting the complexity involved, a few of the larger CROs are offering a wider menu of services, in an effort to capture "one-stop-shop" outsourcing. However, the risk for the buyer in choosing such offerings is that the quality value for money and coordination between groups are not always equally high. One is far better served by selecting different companies with expertise specific to the type of service sought.

Selecting, planning, and budgeting for the use of a CRO are critical to project success. CRO use continues to increase in the United States and Europe, and yet sponsors continue to encounter difficulties in these areas. Typical problems include:

- Insufficient knowledge of available providers.
- Lack of understanding of CROs, their function, and how to select and deal with them.
- Finding the time and resources for evaluating and selecting a high-quality, experienced CRO.
- Unrealistic bid expectations.
- Poor bid specification leading to poor CRO performance.
- Difficulty comparing competing bids.
- An inability to specify rates and terms for any additional work on a basis comparable to the initial contract. This reflects the "scope creep" problem faced by both the client and the provider.

Sources of Information on CROs

Identifying Competent Laboratories

The first step is to obtain a list of laboratories engaged in the contract provider field such as toxicological testing. Although other opportunities exist for obtaining such services, for example, university laboratories, laboratories of a consortium member's company, and, in some cases, government laboratories, the vast majority of externally placed studies involve the contracting party (the "sponsor") placing a study in a "contract research organization's laboratory." Therefore, this situation will be used as the model for the rest of this chapter. The CRO (contract research organization) or CRDO (Contract Research Development Organization) industry has become truly international, as is reflected in the lists provided in this volume. Laboratories can be selected based on a range of factors, as we shall see.

Published Lists

Several lists of contract providers exist, but the most currently available list should be utilized. These lists are updated from time to time, since the contract laboratory industry is dynamic and the capabilities of an individual laboratory change over time. Also, it must be recognized that the contract research industry has become an international one, with services both provided and required by organizations in a large number of companies.

These compendia serve as basic sources of information for finding CROs capable of performing a specific task. More detailed information can be obtained by contacting (by phone, mail, or email) the individual provider organizations and requesting literature or by visiting a website.

Information Available at Meetings

A great deal of information about CROs can be obtained at various scientific and industry meetings (e.g., Society of Toxicology, American College of Toxicology, Safety Pharmacology Society, American Association of Pharmaceutical Science, etc.). Brochures which explain the types of services a CRO is capable of providing, and descriptions of facilities, staff, and price ranges for standard activities, are prominently displayed at such meetings by many contract service providers. Laboratory sales representatives (the current trend is to call these "BD" or business development personnel) attend these meetings frequently to discuss specific study needs with prospective sponsors. Sometimes actual working scientists attend these meetings and are available for discussion.

A second source of information available at meetings is the experience of professional colleagues, who may be able to provide advice on their personal preferences as to where to have certain kinds of services provided, having had similar work done previously. Of particular importance is information about where their work was done, its perceived quality, the hitting of timelines, the handling of errors, and how to avoid mistakes or misunderstandings in dealing with a particular contract laboratory.

This latter source of information needs to be taken with the proverbial "grain of salt." Almost anyone who has contracted R&D activities has had some problems; those who have contracted many projects have had at least one with a major problem; and probably every good contract provider has been inappropriately criticized for poor work at least once. A distorted evaluation is altogether possible if, for example, uncontrollable events (power shutdowns, shipping strikes, etc.) might have affected study results and the sponsor's overall impression of the provider. Remember the importance of effective and adequate communication in any work relationship. Keep in mind the essential nature of a quality business relationship. While mistakes and problems are not desired, they do occur because of human nature, and you will want to ultimately place your work at an organization or organizations where you ultimately have the confidence that you will be treated fairly and ethically. Relationships are key!

For highly specialized work, choices in providers may be very limited. The service and availability of phototoxicity testing, for example, is still a relative rarity. Reproductive and developmental toxicity evaluations, although offered by many laboratories, are tricky, demanding, and performed well by only a few. Inhalation toxicity testing is in similar circumstances. An even more complex situation involves tests requiring several kinds of relatively unusual expertise or equipment. A developmental toxicity study which requires inhalation exposure, for example, may limit laboratory selection to only a few facilities. Contract providers will usually provide information on the availability of services in specialized areas, if they are unable to provide such testing themselves. When looking at services, do not be misled by the availability of stunning new technology that a laboratory is trying to sell, in order to help pay for the investment. Rather the services sought should be well-based in regulatory requirements and/or solving a specific scientific problem that could be an issue in the drug development process at some time. Extra credit is not given by any agency for providing data using some new esoteric technique, which may not even have adequate background of historical data. Including "extra" service studies always has the potential of causing problems downstream.

"Freedom of Information" Requests

Copies of reports of laboratory inspections conducted by federal agencies are available under the Freedom of Information (FOI) Act and online at the FDA website (www.fda.gov). These reports generally follow the format of the laboratory inspection guidance given to Food and Drug Administration (FDA) investigators and provide a great deal of information of varying utilities. Since they are purged of references to proprietary activities, trademarks, specific sponsorship of studies, and much other information, it is sometimes difficult to understand the intent of the report. In addition, they present the opinions of individual investigators concerning isolated activities and events and therefore may not be truly representative of a laboratory's usual practices. Although this information is at least theoretically intended to be objective in nature, sometimes it is not. Effort must be made to truly understand the nature, relevance, and importance of any citations. All points noted on an audit report are not equal in severity, and sometimes points are of no consequences at all. The analysis, interpretation, and advice of a good consultant can help a lot here.

On the other hand, since the laboratory inspection procedures used by a particular agency are usually consistent, the FOI reports permit some comparison among laboratories. This information, coupled with other inputs, is therefore valuable and should not be ignored.

FOI requests should be made to the specific agency which conducted the inspection. Since the FDA's inspection program has been in existence for some time, they are the logical first agency to call in seeking inspection reports on a particular laboratory.

Having developed a list of laboratories able to do the study in question, the most critical part of getting a good job done is in selecting *the* laboratory at which to place the study. The rest of this chapter will be spent reviewing selection criteria in detail.

This volume, of course, is intended to meet several unmet needs. A number of organizations provide an interface between the provider and the client. These intermediaries provide a range of services, from information databases to consulting services, and in some cases even conducting studies themselves, acting as a sort of general contractor CRO.

Such companies can offer more extensive information on CROs than pharma or biopharma companies tend to have in-house, which allows a savings of time and contract costs by facilitating charge comparison and the negotiation of better CRO selection, thereby reducing the risk of selecting a poorly qualified CROs. Mistakes in selection can be very costly both in terms of increased time to completion, project costs, and poor performance, particularly where there may become a need for additional studies to make up for poorly conducted contracts. Lost time is lost market opportunity. There are a number of independent consultants who also act as "one-stop" CROs, arranging and coordinating all required activities for development. These can each, however, usually handle only a few projects at a time (see, e.g., www.toxconsultants.com or www.chemconsultants.com).

DataEdge (www.dataedge.com) has collaborated with 30 larger pharmaceutical companies to define benchmarks and divide unit costs into 20 common budget categories, ranging from pretrial regulatory filing to manuscript preparation. They prepared a unified process for CRO selection, which the company claims makes the preparation and evaluation of requirements for proposal a much more facile and rapid task. The CRO responds to a proposal involving detailed tasks described in familiar terminology. This all-inclusive proposal reduces initial and add-on costs by eliminating double charges. Preferred provider rate can be readily compared to industry rates paid by other companies and comparisons with other means of carrying out the work, such as using internal resources.

Similarly, Arachnova (www.arachnova.com) offers services in project leadership and outsourced project management, providing a database (the Technology Web) with more than 1000 companies specifically in the CRO industry. Limited searching of the database is freely available via the BioPortfolio web portal at www.bioportfolio.com, but a CD-ROM version is available at a commercial rate.

Technomark (www.technomark.com) has provided a register of CROs since its conception in 1988. Initially focused on toxicology and clinical outsourcing, an addendum has recently been published which identifies contract pharmaceutical manufacturers and chemical synthesis companies. The information provided by the Technomark registers has also recently been enhanced by an online version of the database. As well as basic contact information, there are details on the finances and the number of staff in an individual CRO. This information is not provided for all CROs and is particularly lacking from the small, often private entities, which make up the bulk (in number) of the service providers. While it is often said that it is the smaller private provider that is more financially exposed, the recent failures of Oread and Azopharma exemplify the wide range of this business risk. It is interesting to compare the failed strategy of Oread which was to become a fully fledged multidisciplinary development service provider with that of Albany Molecular Research, which, while expanding its offerings, has nevertheless remained focused on chemical service provision.

A smaller version of the Technomark database is provided by InPharm (www.inpharm.com) in the FlexiPages part of the website. The information, which is given more in a directory format than a database, provides contact details for a wide range of agencies and suppliers serving the pharmaceutical and healthcare industries. The information is accessible for free on the web and can be searched by keyword or browsed by category. There is little information on many of the featured companies, but some have a profile with more information. Although the total number of companies is around 1000, few are specifically in the contract pharmaceutical R&D field. From a business perspective, this data is funded by organizations paying for a profile to be included on the website. This has the advantage of being free to the user, but the disadvantages of being partial in scope and biased toward those that do pay for a profile. This is not the case with the information provided in the appendices of this volume.

The Middle Tier

As with the client pharmaceutical and medical device companies themselves, the merger trends of recent years in pharmaceutical outsourcing could be seen as suggesting a future with ever fewer, ever larger providers. While there has remained room for niche CROs, there is a trend to provide a wide range of pharmaceutical development resources to optimize the drug development services within a single organization. The real business challenge from such reorganization is to use this very large development resource to optimize the drug development process for the benefit of the pharmaceutical industry. As in any industry sector, integrating the activities of a large CRO organization, particularly one that has recently merged, has been a substantial internal challenge.

This trend has now been countered by the emergence of a new tier of company intercalating itself between the sponsor and the CRO, with the outsourced management of clinical trials through site management organizations (SMOs) as an example. SMOs provide CROs with physicians and coordinators to enable clinical research coordination and monitoring of phase I, II, III, and IV clinical trials. The SMO often has a number of therapeutic specialties and access to a large and diverse patient population for inclusion in the proposed research. In addition, SMOs usually employ full-time certified clinical research personnel for trial documentation and case report form completion. SMOs are judged by their ability to enroll patients in studies and start and complete a clinical drug trial in a timely manner. In essence, therefore, SMOs aim to streamline the functions of CROs and operate between the CRO and the investigator.

Unless and until the cost-savings and efficiencies promised by the continuing round of CRO mergers can be realized, there will remain room for such intermediate-size organizations, which can operate in a highly flexible sense to add value to the outsourcing process in pharmaceutical R&D.

The CRO business is highly competitive, and in this respect it is similar to the product-based industry it serves. However, there is a major difference in the way the two industries compete for business. The pharmaceutical industry can hope to very clearly differentiate its products based on hard data obtained from efficacy, safety, and pharmacoeconomic studies. Even in today's new healthcare environment, the market place is less price sensitive when clear clinical evidence for product advantage can be shown. This is in marked contrast to the CRO industry, which has an ever-shrinking number of large well-founded mature customers and a vast and expanding pool of young and small and venture capital-hungry customers. Differentiating and selling technical services to senior R&D management is very different from marketing products to doctors and healthcare providers. Claims that work can be completed faster, error-free, and reported to agreed timelines are simply generally not credible to customers: because all CROs make these claims. A highly placed big pharma executive once said "…all CROs are the same, they promise you the world and then fail to deliver. One does not truly find out what he or she has until something goes wrong. The way that the situation is handled and the client is treated is the key to success." This is also the key to the development of business relationships. As stated previously, relationships are key, and work should be placed with organizations, management, and study directors that one can trust.

The real added value that an individual company might bring in its service offerings needs to be more carefully considered. Given that the facilities, GLP/GMP/GCP status, and technical competence and the like are mostly undifferentiating for the successful CRO, the simple answer has to be the knowledge and experience that an organization has, that is, of the technical and scientific complexity of the pharmaceutical and medical device development process. CROs that can capture this knowledge by employing professionally experienced leaders who can then cultivate the scientific culture of pharmaceutical development into their organization will be the winners of the fight to capture increased market share in a generally mature or shrinking market. Such people-based elements last only as long as these individuals are employed by the organization. Knowing the good and bad elements comes from experience of working relationships; expertise in one area does not imply equal or similar talent in all areas. In some cases, specific technologies might add a further element of uniqueness, for example, inhalation technology, continuous infusion technology, telemetry, and transgenics.

There is increasing recognition that specialist companies can add value to the outsourcing process, and many now see the role of an intermediary organization as beneficial to serving the research-based pharmaceutical sector. Indeed we should not be surprised. The word "entrepreneur" literally means "to take between": in all industries, as they mature and become more integrated, companies often become more specialist in their offerings, and opportunities can open up for new commercial intermediaries. A useful comparator here is the computer manufacturing industry, which is highly fragmented and based on outsourced networks. A final validation of this concept comes from the large CROs themselves, which, in order to offer the one-stop shop from which they can benefit substantially as a provider, often resort themselves to subcontracting. It will be interesting to see how this trend develops in the next few years, in an age when the business of pharmaceutical development is still growing, becoming ever more international in scope, more competitive, and more complex.

Outsourcing is no doubt a trend that will continue to expand, and, in order to improve it efficiency, the ways in which it is managed are likely to see dramatic evolve.

Key Considerations in Selecting a Lab

Dependability Far and away of greatest importance should be confidence that the contractor will perform as agreed to (on time, on budget, honestly, and delivering the agreed product in the quality anticipated) and will inform the client or their agent of any problems and issues as they arise in a timely fashion. For longer projects, such unexpected occurrences will occur and are most likely and easily solved or addressed if attended to early.

Experience (activity or study type specific) Unless a study or activity is very unusual, any CRO selected to perform it should be able to demonstrate having previously performed the desired type of work in a successful manner. If the lab has not performed the work previously, keep in mind that everybody at some time has to be the first. To that end, fair and due consideration should be given to an organization that presents a plan that provides a detailed description of the important aspects of the study in such a fashion as to provide sufficient confidence in the proper execution of the project. It is not whether or not one is the first or the 99th, but rather is the organization adequately prepared with sufficient resources to perform the work. If the desired work is unique or of an unusual nature, the CROs wishing to provide the service should provide a plan for "refresher" training or performing a "pilot study" (at no charge to the client) so as to maximize the chances of success.

Does the laboratory employ personnel trained in the needed specialty? What about ancillary expertise (clinical pathology, special services, ophthalmology, cardiology, pathology, statistics, pharmacokinetics)? If not directly employed by the laboratory, are trained specialists available on a consulting basis? For example, if the major emphasis of a study is the determination of the inhalation toxicity of a test agent, but a minor component concerns teratogenic effects, the selected laboratory should require the presence of skilled, experienced inhalation toxicologists on staff. The laboratory does not necessarily have to employ its own teratologists, however, since coverage of these evaluations may reasonably be conducted by consultants in this specialty.

A skilled, competent staff will be necessary to the conduct of the work. Prospective laboratories' personnel environments should be scrutinized for signs of frequent or rapid staff turnover, difficulties in recruiting and retaining new staff, lack of career pathways for staff currently employed, and good wholesome interaction between employees. When visiting a laboratory, observe how the employees interact. Do they work well together? If they work well together, they can probably work with you.

Many laboratories rely on independent organization certification to demonstrate a standard of achievement and competence on the part of their technical and scientific staff. For example, both the American Board of Toxicology and the American College of Toxicology have certification programs for toxicologists. Likewise, the American Association of Laboratory Animal Sciences (AALAS) has three stages for certification of laboratory animal technical staff (ALAT, LAT, LATG). Other specialties have similar certification programs based on some combination of experience and achievement demonstrated by written and practical testing (e.g., quality assurance, pathology, laboratory animal medicine).

Hand in hand with personnel availability is the selection criterion of technical expertise. Many different specialties are brought to bear on a particular study. The more complex the study, the greater the difficulty in finding a contract laboratory with all the necessary expertise.

In attempting to evaluate the qualifications of contract laboratory staff, organizational charts, training records, job descriptions, and curriculum vitae should be obtained. These documents are standard tools, which are used by contract laboratories as marketing aids. FDA's Good Laboratory Practice (GLP) regulations require laboratories to maintain documentation of the training, experience, and job descriptions of personnel. This is usually done by means of compilations of curricula vitae.

Another important point in evaluating staff capabilities is the number of people employed by the laboratory. The proposed study staff should be sufficient to perform all the work required. Attention should be directed to the laboratory's overall workload relative to available staff. While this is difficult to specifically assess, an open and frank discussion between the CRO and the client should take place. Do not fall into the trap of calculation of various staff to study ratios, which will not be applicable in a cost-effective organization where there is a substantial degree of cross-training and cross-departmental sharing of technical resources based upon workload.

Equipment Are all of the required instruments, tools, supplies, reagents, computers, and such in place, operational, properly maintained, calibrated, validated (if necessary), and labeled (check records)? Are the knowledge and skills of senior scientific staff suitable to the required works? Do they have prior experience performing such works? Are the actual technicians who will be performing the day-to-day works suitable? What is the turnover rate for the staff at the facility?

Cost As a general rule, all contract research and development should be put out for bid by several CROs (but not too many because such bids take work and time to prepare, and it is unfair to ask for such a proposal if there is not a good chance that a contract will be awarded). Three or possibly four bids are common, but requests in excess of a half-dozen are unprofessional. Care should be exercised to provide sufficient information and detail to the potential bidders to ensure that all participants end up rendering bids on the same scope of work.

Facilities Are the facilities (buildings, rooms, and environmental support services such as water, heat, air, and power) sound, well maintained, suitably monitored, sufficient to the tasks, and clean? Particularly if living organisms are involved, it is essential that provisions for any power failures (i.e., backup generators) be present.

Laboratory animal care facilities may be accredited by the American Association for Accreditation of Laboratory Animal Care (AAALAC). This is a voluntary organization which accredits laboratories based on its own standards as supplemented and reinforced by those of other organizations (academic and industrial). Accreditation is based on elements of several major activities, programs, or capabilities of the individual laboratory, such as veterinary resources, physical resources, administrative matters, pain management policy, animal enrichment program, and the presence and activity of an effective animal care and use (animal welfare) committee. AAALAC accreditation is frequently the only objective symbol of the general compliance of the laboratory with standards of good practice in animal use and care, veterinary, physical plant, and administrative areas. Although this provides no guarantee that the laboratory does good testing, AAALAC accreditation represents a worthwhile first step toward excellence in the care, handling, and management of animals and a sound level of assurance that one's study will not be featured on the 6 o'clock news for violations of animal welfare.

Regulatory history Regulatory agencies remember both good and bad performances by regulated contractors. They regularly audit such, and the results of such audits are public records which should be provided upon request by the contractor and which are available online from FDA.

A large portion of the initial visit to prospective contract laboratories can usefully be spent in reviewing standard operating procedures (SOPs). These should be written for all routinely performed activities.

GLPs require that SOPs be established in the following general areas: animal room preparation, animal care pain management, test and control substance management, test system (animal) observations, laboratory tests, management of on-study dead or moribund animals, necropsy, specimen collection and identification, histopathology, data management, equipment maintenance and calibration, identification of animals, the IACUC, and quality assurance. Although not specifically required by GLP regulations, the laboratory should also have SOPs for archiving activities. In each of these areas, numerous individual SOPs should be in place. For example, in the area of histopathology, SOPs should be available to describe tissue selection, preparation, processing, staining, and coverslipping; slide labeling and packaging; and storage and retention of wet tissues, blocks, and slides. Similarly, SOPs should be available for maintenance and calibration of all equipment and instrumentation which requires these activities.

The laboratory's SOPs should be clear, understandable, and sufficiently detailed to permit a technically experienced person to perform them. They should be up to date, and the method for keeping them current should be described. They should have the sanction of facility management, usually provided by signature of the person responsible for the pertinent laboratory activity. The SOPs should be simply written and in a level of detail that provides confidence in the task being done repeatedly well, but not so much detail that it is impossible to be in compliance with the SOP. SOPs should be written by the people performing the work and not by management, so look closely at the signatures on each SOP.

To be effective, SOPs should be readily available to those who need them. For example, animal care SOPs should be available to vivarium workers, as analytical and clinical chemistry SOPs should be available in these laboratories. Compendia of SOPs which sit pristinely on shelves in offices may not reflect what is actually occurring in the laboratories and animal quarters. Likewise, SOPs which have not been reviewed or revised in several years should be viewed with suspicion. Improvements in actual methods occur frequently and should be reflected in the written procedures.

If the laboratory has contracts with other laboratories, SOPs should be available for the secondary laboratories as well. Both the SOPs and these contracts should be reviewed in the same way. Subcontractors used by the CRO should be audited on a regulator basis.

Computerization The days when all but a minority of data and records were recorded, captured, and manipulated by hand are gone. The degree and quality of automation and computer resources of a potential contractor must be assessed as should the overall integration of such systems and plans and progress toward GLP compliance section 2.

Financial Soundness In Chap. 1, a listing of extinct laboratories was provided. Several of these ceased operations with studies in progress and without notifying sponsors in advance due to financial failure. To avoid this, one needs to assess the financial ability of a contract organization to continue operations and complete works. For many contractors, Dun and Bradstreet can provide such information. However, such information is difficult to secure from privately held companies. However, in these cases, do not be afraid to sit down and talk with the president of the company and/or its owner about financial performance.

Location Much is sometimes made (frequently by competitors in a negative way) as to the importance of location of facilities. While there are some factors which are related to location which should be considered (ease of trend and perhaps trend cost, stability, and availability of technical staff and security come to mind), the authors' belief is that this is near the bottom of the list in terms of priority.

A consideration in selection of contract laboratories is the sponsor's ease of monitoring the study, which is largely a function of distance between the sponsor and the laboratory. In some studies, this may be a major consideration, in others, not worthy of mention. If the study is complex and requires frequent oversight, a trade-off may need to be made between the best laboratory relative to the previously mentioned selection criteria and monitoring ease.

On the other hand, sponsors do not plan complex studies unless they anticipate substantial product safety evaluation concerns and, therefore, considerable potential profit. If this is the case, the relatively small additional sum spent in the increased cost of frequent or distant monitoring may be minuscule in the eyes of those selecting the laboratory.

Site Visits of Prospective Contract Laboratories

In scheduling site visits with contract laboratories, the objectives should be clearly defined up front. Meeting those people who will be directing and contributing importantly to the study provides an opportunity to evaluate their understanding of the nature of the questions or problems which may arise. Ancillary contributors (pathologists, statisticians) should be interviewed carefully as well, since their contributions can be of fundamental significance to the quality and outcome of the study.

The facilities should be toured, looking for appropriate size, construction, spacing, and design. GLP regulations as promulgated under the Food, Drug, and Cosmetic Act, the Toxic Substances Control Act, or the Federal Insecticide, Fungicide, and Rodenticide Act provide guidance as to the general facility, equipment, and operational requirements of laboratories.

Storage areas for extra racks and cages, feed and bedding, and so forth are frequently inadequate in laboratories (cost issue), but these facilities should be inspected and evaluated anyway. One's evaluation of a facility should be against a reasonable standard of functionality and not against some prior experience with a multi-billion dollar year operation that had no limits to spending.

The FDA provides their field investigators who conduct laboratory inspections for compliance with GLPs with "Compliance Guidance Manuals." These are comprehensive documents which use a checklist approach to inspecting a laboratory for adherence to all the elements of GLP regulations. They can be obtained from the agencies and can be used as guidance for study sponsors in evaluating prospective laboratories. An advantage of using this approach is that the sponsor will not omit an important element in inspecting a prospective laboratory. However, the sponsor should not get so bogged down in reviewing checklist items that actual observation of the laboratory is abbreviated.

Once an initial review of potential service providers has been conducted, some organizations will be eliminated from consideration, but those that remain in consideration (no more than three is a suggested limit) should be visited for on-site qualification. Table 7.1 (with CV's provided) provides a sample agenda for such a visit.

Cost

A key factor in the selection of a laboratory for most sponsors is the cost of the study. This single element can largely affect the quality of a study. "Caveat emptor" applies equally to the toxicologist as to the home consumer. Many of the negotiable elements of a carefully defined study will not be performed in a similarly titled study at a different laboratory for a lower cost. Conversely, some of the extras offered for a higher-priced study should not be included for

Table 7.1 Sample agenda for a qualification visit to a CRO

Global presentation by the CRO/vendor
  Range of services offered
  Company history
  Organizational chart of the company
  Presentation of potential study team
  Previous experience and references
  Number and type of ongoing/future projects
  Previous audits

Presentation by and specific to the business of the company placing the work
Tour of the facility
Project management
  Discuss interfaces/coordination with CRO and sponsor, project team structure and reporting processes (including review of staffing estimate, CVs, training plan/records, job descriptions)
  Discuss logistics/process review and project team coordination (including data flow, data transmission capabilities, reconciliation with other databases, management of committees, samples of timelines, quality controls, problem identification, and resolution processes)

Data management
  Demonstration of the data management system (data entry, data query system, tracking of CRFs, tracking of queries, process flowchart, standard metrics, e.g., time from the last subject out to database lock)
  Demonstration of the central randomization system
  Review drug distribution capabilities and interface with the central randomization system
  Review data management and central randomization system validation documentation
  Review procedures for reconciliation with other databases
  Review manual vs. automated processes and validations
  Discuss ability to use sponsor coding dictionaries

Quality assurance
  Review CRO organizational structure (organizational charts, mission/quality statement, training records, training policy)
  Review QA department activities, reporting relationships, quality manual, quality records, and QA SOPs/standards
  Review reference files management (regulatory documentation/guidelines)
  Review SOPs
  Review quality controls and audits
  Review equipment inventory

(continued)

Table 7.1 (continued)

Wrap-up/summary of findings (sponsor)

Present and discuss any finding from SOPs or other departmental review

Determine need for additional qualification data or visits by additional sponsor personnel

Establish plan for CRO to provide any missing data identified during visit

Schedule a mutually acceptable time for presentation of the formal report of the sponsor's findings. During this meeting the CRO will need to be ready to create a plan to address and "deficiencies" found during the visit

The written audit report should in NO way be a surprise to the CRO and should be entirely consistent with discussions held during the exit interview

extra cost if they are neither scientifically or regulatorily necessary nor desirable. The objective in considering the cost of a study is to select the laboratory which offers all of the same essential study elements at the lowest cost consistent with good quality. Good quality in turn relies on the other criteria previously discussed. When a laboratory is found which can perform all desired elements of the study, does high-quality work, and offers a lower price for the study than its competitors or highly competitive price with its competitors, then this is probably the laboratory to choose to perform the study. Pricing of studies from competitors should be clustered together (within 10% of each other). Organizations providing extremely high prices (fliers) or low prices (sinkers) should be eliminated from consideration, unless a rebid process is desirable for some reason due to bid requirement confusion. The former typically tells you that the laboratory is full and they are only willing to perform the work at an extremely high margin. Similarly an extremely low price tells you that the laboratory is hurting for business.

It is so very important to compare bids carefully to make sure that the prices are for the same work. Unfortunately it is not an uncommon event to see prices for studies quoted at a very low amount, because some essential study components have not been included (ECG, ECG analysis, ophthalmic exams, limited histopathology, etc.). The strategy in this case is to provide a very low bid to secure the business and once the business is secured to raise the study price with all the "necessary" additions. In the end, the actual true price tends to be very similar to that of others. The strategy usually works as clients tend for a variety of reasons to not walk away, as they should.

Remember the golden triangle, quality, cost, and timing. You can only get two of the three parameters at any one time. So, for example, if one wants it fast, the cost will not be cheap, and the quality may be marginal. Similarly if one wants very high-quality work with a lot of detail, the price will not be cheap, and it will take longer to execute.

In discussing costs, the sponsor should attempt to determine whether the laboratory will be able to add elements to the study if this appears desirable as the study progresses. The laboratory should have the capability to expand the original study design. Sponsor and laboratory should attempt to foresee how the cost of such additions would be determined.

Reputation

The reputation held by particular contract laboratories is clearly a guide in laboratory selection. Although not an absolutely reliable indicator of the worth of a contract laboratory's efforts, by and large laboratories earn their reputations over a long period of time. Again, beware of laboratories which submit extremely low bids for studies and either cut corners to stay within their quoted cost or include add-ons, at the sponsor's expense, through the course of the study. Study additions can significantly increase the actual cost if the contract requires the sponsor to pay for them.

Other laboratories try to foresee likely additional aspects of the study, which may increase the quoted cost but yield a much better product. A good CRO will at least discuss with a potential client possible future extensions of cost. Producing the study at the price quoted is only one part of a contract laboratory's reputation. Quality, professional qualifications of staff, activity in scientific professional societies, accreditation, regulatory performance, and many other issues are important as well.

Protection of Client Confidentiality

Most contract laboratories expend considerable effort in trying to maintain confidentiality on behalf of their clients. In walking through a laboratory, clients should not be able to see proprietary labels on test material containers, or cage labels which state company names. A contract laboratory concerned about client confidentiality will be careful not to allow visible evidence to be seen by other potential clients. Confidentiality is usually of significant concern and should be discussed with laboratory management. The laboratory's master schedule should maintain client confidentiality as well.

Prior Experience

Prior experience with specific contract laboratories highly simplifies the task of selecting a laboratory. Establishing a continuing relationship with one or several laboratories in the case of routine testing provides an opportunity to fine-tune study protocols. This will be discussed in greater detail in section "The Study Protocol".

Scheduling

Undoubtedly, starting the study as soon as possible is important. The ability of the laboratory to begin the study soon may well determine where the study is performed. Most of the larger contract houses can start all but very large studies within 4–6 weeks. Some studies may be able to be initiated on even shorter notice. Certainly for shorter studies, less complicated protocols are needed, and generally less lead time is required to begin the study. The converse is equally true, so if the study is large, long-term, or complicated, a fairly long time before study initiation will be needed to get the details of the study worked out with the laboratory. As a result, a laboratory which is willing to start a lengthy or complex study before the details have been settled should generally be avoided. Again, most contract research organizations can start studies relatively quickly, unless they are very complicated. However, the biggest delays in getting studies started are the supply of test article, adequate formulation for the test article, availability of an adequate bioanalytical method, and a signed protocol.

Special Capabilities

As the science of toxicology and the questions society, regulatory agencies, and companies seek to answer become more complex, technical skills and equipment which are not widely available become more in demand. Such special capabilities are frequently resident in smaller or university laboratories where procedures, documentation, and adherence to regulatory standards may not be as rigorous as either one's own corporation or larger contract laboratories. One may even have to help investigators develop protocols, standard operating procedures, and record keeping systems.

Evaluating technical competency for specialized procedures is obviously difficult, as one is usually dependent on others to initially identify such specialists and they may have to also get outside help to evaluate the appropriateness and quality of the results. A not uncommon case of special capabilities is when human testing (such as repeat insult patch testing or RIPT) must be performed.

Here one must understand the special regulatory, legal, and ethical constraints on work with human subjects and generally deal with an IRB (institutional review board) which must review, approve, and oversee any such human studies from the perspective of subject protection and ethics.

The Contract

General terms of the contract should address such aspects as timeliness, proprietary rights, confidentiality, adherence to regulatory requirements (in the research effort and in the laboratory's practices in waste disposal, workers' protection, safety, etc.), type and frequency of reports, communications between parties, conditions under which the study may be aborted and restarted, timing and method of payment, insurance, and the like. Such a contract "… should be negotiated by a team of lawyers and scientists who have a thorough understanding of the problems to be investigated, including both the scientific issues and the potential business implications. Armed with this understanding, the lawyers can then proceed to develop a contract that is appropriate to the situation. Much of the language will be routine or 'boiler plate', the type commonly found in agreements of various kinds."

The contract should specify who does what in the furtherance of the study. For example, if analysis is necessary, the sponsor may wish to retain the responsibility to analyze the test material as a means of keeping its identify confidential. The derivative concern about documentation of the analysis is presumably also retained by the sponsor, but the contract should be clear on the responsibilities of both parties.

When discussing study personnel, various degrees of authority are vested in contract laboratory study staff by the sponsor. The study contract should define as clearly as possible the degree of authority vested in the contract laboratory staff and at what point the sponsor would be consulted for a decision when unforeseen situations arise. In general terms, then, the contract should define the rights and responsibilities of both parties.

The contract should also address financial matters, such as the cost of the study and the method and timing of payment. Certain unanticipated activities not directly related to the study may increase the cost to the laboratory; the contract should attempt to anticipate these events and establish reasonable incremental costs to the sponsor to deal with them. For example, study-specific inspections by agencies authorized to review a study (FDA or EPA) may add to the cost to the laboratory for additional staff time to accompany inspectors, copy documents, and otherwise field the inspections. If the sponsor wishes to be present at such inspections, additional direct costs will be incurred. Although many readers would view this simply as part of the laboratory's cost of doing business, the contract should anticipate how each party is expected to respond financially if the inspection becomes very time-consuming or onerous.

Likewise, post-study activities and responsibilities should be defined in the contract. Who will archive tissue and other samples and specimens? For how long? If statistical analysis is to be performed, of what does it consist? Who decides? If further analysis appears desirable after evaluation of the data, will the sponsor incur extra costs? If a failure should occur, the details of how this is to be handled with regard to timing and cost responsibility need to be addressed in the contract.

The Study Protocol

The study protocol is not a contract and items that are to be placed in the contract have no basis to be in a scientific document such as a study protocol. The most important part of site visits to laboratories will be the discussion of the specifics of the study and establishment of the protocol. Extensive prior experience of the sponsor in conducting the contemplated study is very helpful although many elements may still have to be negotiated. If the sponsor has limited experience, the importance of the protocol increases, since it contains the specific language of the scientific and regulatory contract between sponsor and laboratory which governs the conduct of the study.

To write a protocol with little flexibility may preclude the study director's judgment and may actually compromise the quality of the study. Each party must feel comfortable that the study protocol provides sufficient detail to specify what is to be done, when it is to be done, and under what conditions it is to be done. However, the protocol must not be so rigid that the study director is hampered in responding to changing conditions and events as they occur during the course of the conduct of the study. Since unanticipated events almost always occur, the objective is to provide a protocol which permits the study to be conducted as closely as possible to the original study plan, to answer all the important study questions and yet provide sufficient flexibility for the study director to adequately manage the study and not create a quality assurance and regulatory nightmare.

Other Terms

Authorship

The question of authorship of publications resulting from the proposed study should be covered in the contract and not the study protocol. Not all work is worthy of publication nor do contract laboratory staff often get an opportunity to author papers. But if the laboratory has contributed significantly to the work, and a publication is contemplated, help in writing portions of the manuscript should be solicited from members of the study staff, for which co-authorship is a deserved award.

Reports

The contract again and not the study protocol should specify the nature and frequency of reports which the laboratory will make to the sponsor. For example, a short-term study (2 weeks or less) may require only telephone confirmation of study start, status of the animals at the halfway point, confirmation of termination, and the usual draft and final report.

For a longer study, the sponsor may request written status reports at regular intervals. In the case of chronic studies, the sponsor may wish to have formal interim reports prepared by the laboratory. The contract should clearly specify the expectations of both parties concerning reports.

Inspections by the Sponsor

Most contract laboratories do not like the thought of unscheduled site visits by study sponsors, for understandable reasons. Under ordinary circumstances, a large amount of staff time is spent escorting visitors through the laboratory. Unscheduled visitors therefore place an additional burden on already stretched resources.

Nevertheless, the right to monitor a study's progress at any reasonable time should be explicitly affirmed in the contract. This right, although perhaps never exercised by the sponsor, should not be relinquished. As a practical matter, unscheduled monitoring visits almost never occur, since the sponsor must recognize that the study staff may be unavailable at the time of the visit, making the trip a wasted one.

Likewise, the contract should explicitly grant the sponsor access to the laboratory's quality assurance (QA) inspection reports of the study. These reports are ordinarily *not* available to government investigators, and some contract laboratories prefer not to share them. However, a sponsor should ensure that the contract grants access to the QA reports.

References

Contract Pharma (2020). Contract Services Directory.

DIA. (2010). *Contract service organization directory*. Fort Washington, PA: Drug Information Association.

FDLI. (2010). *Directory of lawyers and consultants*. Washington, D.C.: FDLI.

Jackson, E. M. (1985). How to choose a contract laboratory: Utilizing a laboratory clearance procedure. *Journal of Toxicology: Cutaneous and Ocular Toxicology, 3*, 83–92.

Study Directors and PIs

8

Christopher Papagiannis

Prologue

Let it not be lost among the very busy days or occasional frustrations that the research for which we are responsible is critical in the development of new drugs for the treatment, or cure, of many diseases, or to allow for hazard and risk assessment associated with exposure to chemicals in the environment. Our work is providing a tremendous benefit to our society and the world and, even perhaps more closely, to our own friends and families or ourselves. This chapter is dedicated to the efforts of those who have been fortunate enough to serve in the role of study director during their careers and who have given back and mentored others in a collaborative scientific spirit that has always engaged, inspired, and motivated the next generation of study directors in the wonderful journey that is scientific research.

In optimally explaining the study director role and all it entails, portions of this chapter sample relevant sections of various training matrix modules that have been utilized as orientation and instructional material for newly hired (internal or external) study directors at the Mattawan site of Charles River

C. Papagiannis
Senior Director, Safety Evaluation/Principal Reserach Scientist,
Charles River (CR-MWN), Mattawan, MI, USA
e-mail: Christopher.Papagiannis@crl.com

© Springer Nature Switzerland AG 2020
S. C. Gad et al., *Contract Research and Development Organizations-Their History, Selection, and Utilization*, https://doi.org/10.1007/978-3-030-43073-3_8

Laboratories, Inc. A very special acknowledgment goes to Dr. Theodore Baird, Dr. Christopher Stewart, and the late Dr. Paul Newton for their efforts in creating some of this key and valuable explanatory content that sets the stage for the detailed overview provided in this chapter. In addition, a heartfelt thank you goes to my mentor, Dr. David Serota, who saw potential abilities and talents in me before I ever had the confidence to envision them in myself and who always put in the time necessary to optimally cultivate them and create teachable moments for me.

The Study Director

As a sponsor, your interactions and working relationship with your study director(s) are one of the most important elements in the conduct of a successful study or package of studies for your program. A large part of the trust that a study will be scientifically sound involves the performance of the study director.

The role of the study director is defined as the single point of control, which includes various GLP compliance responsibilities (from FDA 21 CFR Part 58 Subpart B and EPA 40 CFR Parts 160 and 792). (FDA, n.d.; EPA, n.d.-a, n.d.-b)

> The study director has overall responsibility for the technical conduct of the study, as well as for the interpretation, analysis, documentation, and reporting of results, and represents the single point of study control.

The study director is also required to assure the following:

1. *The protocol and any changes are approved and followed; test systems are as specified in the protocol.*
2. *Experimental data, including unanticipated observations, are accurately recorded and verified.*
3. *Unforeseen circumstances which may affect study quality and integrity are properly noted, and appropriate corrective actions are taken and documented.*
4. *All applicable GLP regulations are followed.*
5. *Raw data, documentation, protocols, specimens, and final reports are transferred to the archives.*

6. *Prompt and accurate communication of significant or unusual observations, particularly those that may require changes in study design or conduct.*

In the context of a matrix-style organization, while the study director may not routinely operate "hands-on" in the performance of protocol-required functions, they must play an effective organizational, consultative, and oversight role to ensure that protocol requirements are achieved.

GLP regulations also require that the study director ensure technical staff is appropriately trained to complete protocol requirements and, as such, play a vital role in the translation of procedural/testing requirements to effective practice among technical staff. Due to the intrinsic leadership nature of the study director role, it is understood that the study director may often be the source of initial translation, training, and implementation of a wide variety of study procedures. The technical nature of some procedures may require the conduct of pilot studies, whereas other procedures are more readily transferred without such in-depth qualifying efforts. Generally, a sampling of the kinds of interactions/roles that a study director must master may include:

Technical/Scientific

- Creation of a study plan/protocol design.
- Translation of procedures from relevant literature to technical staff (training).
- Oversight of data collection, interpretation, analysis, documentation, and reporting of results.
- Interaction with peers in the form of contributing scientists or principal investigators (PIs) that may be responsible for specific protocol requirements (e.g., electrocardiographic (ECG) interpretation, bioanalytical, specialized biomarker assessment, etc.)
- Scientific peer interactions and participation in professional career activities.
- Coordination/communication with any off-site study activities (usually through their PIs) if a multiple site study.

Business/Administrative

* Business development, initiating and maintaining sponsor relationships, and identifying opportunities to cross-sell services.
* Overseeing the study budget.

Compliance

* Ongoing regulatory compliance (GLPs, Animal Welfare Act, etc.).
* Protocol/report compliance.
* Properly recorded unanticipated events/observations and quality corrective action/preventive action (CAPA) events are captured and reported as required.

Practically speaking, the study director is the main conduit and reconciler of sponsor feedback and expectations. The study director must understand the various capacities of the laboratory areas, appreciate possibilities to stretch capabilities outside of traditional routine, appreciate when and how to become involved in facilitating necessary functions, know implicitly the logistical and organizational realities of internal departments, and know how company resources may be responsibly leveraged to provide value to the sponsor, which promotes effective and sustainable working relationships.

In most preclinical contract research organizations (CROs), the typical study director does not often have direct responsibility for the personnel and other resources required for their study; thus, there are optimal skills that the proficient study director utilizes to manage the multifaceted demands of the role and to appropriately delegate where applicable. These involve a number of traits that as a sponsor you want to see your study director consistently and deftly exhibit when conducting studies, which allows them to successfully maximize their ultimate responsibility for the overall scientific conduct of the study. For all of these, dependability in performance is essential.

First and Foremost Are Communication and Relationship Building Skills

The study director should be an effective and timely internal and external communicator, with a supreme focus on two-way communication and asking the right questions. This includes a consistent listening mind-set and both verbal and written communication skills, be it by phone, by email, by study documents, or in person. Whether the study director is an introvert or extrovert is immaterial to the development and enhancement of these skills (many scientists are by nature introverts), as internal and external relationship building is a soft skill that can be mastered and developed for the prototypical needs and expectations of the study director position and utilized to achieve study compliance and a quality outcome. Some of the needed qualities may be innate, while others are learned or developed through practical experience. For you as a sponsor, your study director can and should become your advocate within their organization, one who can navigate and marshal the resources of the CRO for your benefit and foster productive and proactive two-way communication that builds long-term trust and a relationship of respect between your organizations. Similarly, the relationship between the study director and study personnel from the numerous internal departmental areas of technical expertise involved in any study within a CRO is just as important. All should feel comfortable approaching the study director to report any issues in real time, ask questions if they are at all unsure of protocol intent or how to handle a particular situation, or provide any ideas, suggestions, or alternatives to a process for the study director to consider or champion on their behalf.

The responsibility and role of the sponsor in these matters of quality communication is also of paramount importance to both study director and study success and cannot be understated. A non-responsive sponsor, who *does not* answer questions or consider options, provide necessary details and deliverables in line with CRO deadlines, discuss their specific expectations and preferences, or engage the study director or CRO as a true partner or teammate in the project, can lead to less than desired outcomes, increased chances for error, or, ultimately, dissatisfaction in study performance. Do your best to help your study director (and CRO) help you.

Also of Optimal Importance Are Technical and Troubleshooting Skills

The study director is the person everyone looks to on a study when something happens, either good or bad, both in terms of the guidance they provide and how they react as events or situations unfold. When CRO staff or a sponsor sees a study director who panics or appears overwhelmed or defeated by challenging situations, they may by nature tend to panic as well. It is important to realistically note that no one is perfect and that no CRO is error-free. When a significant error occurs, how it is handled is of utmost importance, both internally and externally, and the study director is the point person who can either make or break a situation or relationship with colleagues/coworkers or with the sponsor. The study director should communicate any salient errors to the sponsor immediately so that they are not blindsided after the fact, even before the full breadth and depth of applicable investigative work has begun or any root cause analyses and CAPA is conducted/determined. As the investigative work progresses, the ongoing study director communication with the sponsor should then involve key items such what happened, why and how it happened, what is being done to fix it, and what new plans or processes are being put in place to ensure it does not happen again. The study director should take a prominent and positive role in formal investigations when they are needed. It is paramount for the study director to assist in troubleshooting and providing possible solutions while continuing to keep the sponsor in the loop. The study director should never merely deliver bad news to the sponsor and ask them what they want to do or merely toss the ball into their court, but rather should provide various options and their associated pros and cons to the sponsor for discussion and consideration ahead of a viable decision that can be justified prospectively.

As a sponsor, you obviously never want to see a significant error happen on your study and neither does the study director. The study director and CRO will typically want to do everything they can to make things right for you, and depending on the seriousness of what has happened, this may even involve an offer to restart the study for you at their cost and expedite the report to minimize any overall program delays. However, in most situations the study can be viably continued with applicable corrective actions in place and with no effect on the overall integrity of the study or on an ultimately successful regulatory submission outcome. How the study director and/or CRO come through for you in such a situation is indicative of the importance they place on their relationship with you and your organization and is a key indicator of their organizational and customer service philosophies. In fact, their sometimes heroic efforts or an above and beyond response in such a situation can turn a negative into a positive and further cement the relationship and level of trust going forward.

Scientific Interpretation and Results Writing Skills

The report is the ultimate product that the CRO generates. In fact, the CRO product you are purchasing is a promise to produce a scientifically sound report that is delivered on time and meets all of the requirements and expectations of the sponsor. In that regard, the sponsor cannot see what they are buying on the front end. Part of the trust that the report will be scientifically sound involves the reputation and ability of the study director, who should make every effort to stay current by reading scientific journals, publishing study results whenever possible, and visibly participating in scientific meetings and continuing education courses. The study director must display the ability to optimally tell the story of the study when writing the results/discussion/conclusion and to do so in a manner that presents a cohesive and integrated text for the reader. This is most especially enhanced and evident when the study director also leads applicable prewriting integration meetings with the key contributing scientists (including the clinical pathologist, anatomical pathologist, and toxicokineticist) to assure optimal correlation of findings across sections. The following is a recommended listing of the types of considerations a study director should keep top of mind when interpreting the data for a study report and composing their text and that a sponsor should consider when reviewing a report.

The first study results section should be a summary of the analytical results because the actual test article formulation used is critical to the study and interpretation of the results. This is what the animals were dosed with, and it is crucial to know that the test article formulation was homogeneous and stable for the appropriate time and what the achieved dose levels were. The section following it should include a discussion of the toxicokinetic data as further documentation of the relationship among the dose levels and what the animals were actually dosed with. This is especially critical if the target dose levels weren't achieved or some untoward event happened. In-text tables with summaries of the results are very helpful and may be used as applicable so that the reader does not have to go digging to find the data.

The sections following the analytical and toxicokinetic results sections then present detailed discussions on the data for each of the endpoints evaluated. The same format or style should be used for each section to make the report user-friendly. A more complete overview on how the study director should determine and discuss test article relationships is presented later in this section.

Conclusion

For the conclusion, bottom line what did the study director conclude about the results of the study? This should be the take-home message. "Under the conditions of this study, where…." The message may be as simple as the test article "…was not a carcinogen."

Because the regulatory agencies use "no-observed-effect level" (NOEL) or "no-observed-adverse-effect level" (NOAEL) in their risk assessment, stating what the NOEL or NOAEL is can be very useful. There can also be more than one NOEL. In the case of a dermal study, one may have a NOEL for the site of dermal application and an additional NOEL for systemic toxicity.

The Spin

- Focus on severity at lower doses.
- When in doubt, err on the side of safety.
- Transient? Reversible? No degenerative changes? Species-specific?
- It is OK to be uncertain.
- Present the good news last.

The Perspective

- Never underestimate the importance of proper data interpretation and presentation.
- Don't forget that the FDA (or other agencies) is the ultimate "customer" and reader.

Discussion Style or Format

It has been said that the best teachers use the following technique. "Tell them what you are going to tell them, tell them, and then tell them what you told them." This approach may be used when discussing the data results. Start off with a summary statement that states either "Test article-related effects were seen in…" or "No test article related effects were seen in…." These test article-related effects can then be discussed, followed by any changes that were of uncertain relationship, followed by unrelated or spurious non-test article-related changes.

Again, in-text tables (and perhaps figures) can be very useful to help support the conclusion and help the flow of the discussion. The study director has had the opportunity to pore over the study data and know it well, but they must now spoon-feed these results in a logical manner to first-time readers in such a way as to allow them to follow their reasoning and understand their conclusions. Using this style consistently in each section will also greatly help the readers.

If the changes are test article related, they should be referred to as "effects." If the changes are not test article related, then they should be referred to as "changes" not "effects."

Other Perspectives

- Attention to detail is essential.
- Every sentence counts.
- Use simple sentence structure where possible and strive for clarity that can withstand translation into multiple languages and the perhaps limited attention of an overloaded agency reviewer.
- Subdivide sections or use bullets as necessary for clarity.
- Cross-reference where appropriate.
- Cite literature when appropriate.

Data Interpretation

Data interpretation is a three-step process.

Step 1: Identify changes.
Step 2: Determine relationship to test article.
Step 3: Assess biological significance.

Identify Changes

Relative to concurrent control group (or historical control).
Time-dependent (versus pretest data).

Determine Relationship to Test Article

- Dose response? (If all treated groups are similarly different from control, maybe the control group values changed. Check relative to historical control.)
- Both sexes?
- Group effect or individual animals?
- Magnitude? (mean, range).
- Time course? e.g., onset, maximum response, persistence, and recovery.
- Biologically meaningful or relevant time frame?
- Within normal variability (inter-animal and over time)?
- Statistically significant?
- Consistent with known pharmacologic activity?
- Previous experience in same species? e.g., the propensity of dogs to vomit.
- Effects of related drugs or chemicals?
- Expected effect? i.e., seen in previous studies or with related test articles.
- Related to other changes? e.g., increased AST and ALT, increased liver weight, and microscopic hepatotoxicity.
- Numerous other effects at the same or lower doses?

Other Considerations

- Preexisting condition?
- Procedural related? e.g., stress-induced neutrophilia in monkeys.
- Possible sampling bias?
- Caused by vehicle?
- Secondary to moribundity?
- Caused by anesthetic agent or other ancillary treatments?
- Spurious measurements?

Qualifying Language: Suitable Terminology to Utilize

- Related, unrelated, uncertain.
- Clearly, most likely, probably, suggestive, possibly, doubtful, unlikely, definitely not.

- "...could not be attributed to the test article with certainty."
- "...could not be clearly distinguished from normal variability."

Assess Biological Significance

- Incidence/severity/magnitude relative to untreated animals (control, pretest, historical).
- Magnitude relative to maximum response.
- Dose levels affected; species/sex specificity.
- Other associated alterations, e.g., vomiting, can produce a decrease in potassium.
- Reversibility.
- Nature of response, e.g., degenerative (necrosis) vs. compensatory (hypertrophy).
- Exaggerated pharmacologic action?
- Unique species sensitivity.

A test article-related effect is not necessarily biologically significant if the mean of the treated group(s) is outside the historical control range; nor is the converse always true. A 50% increase in AST and ALT is outside the normal range, but that magnitude of increase isn't that great. Conversely, a small change in bilirubin may be biologically significant.

As a sponsor, you and/or others in your organization will be reviewing the report and providing comments (or perhaps you will contract with a consultant to do so), but your role in the outcome of sound scientific interpretation starts much earlier than that. In fact, prior to the start of the study, it is important for sponsors to share details of the test article such as indication, clinical plan/status, mechanism of action, expected pharmacological effects, and previous findings seen in other studies (if conducted in a sponsor vivarium or another CRO) with the study director. While many years ago, some sponsors were concerned that such detailed sharing of information might cause subconscious bias toward potential calls/findings, the advantages far outweigh that questionable and frankly unrealistic concern. Not only does such transparency give the technical staff (who are the life blood of any study) an increased sense of ownership of the study, but it allows veterinary/clinical medicine staff to be on standby for anticipated or potential outcomes or to assist in developing a pre-study plan of ameliorative treatment options so as to be optimally prepared and proactive rather than reactive. It is also important to note that this type of detail is now increasingly required by many institutional animal care and use committees (IACUC) as part of their protocol review/approval processes. This is important both for the scientific quality of the study and the welfare/health status of the animals on study, as such positive planning and strategies can preempt unforeseen or undesirable issues on a study, thus allowing for a report that does not get bogged down in extraneous noise in explaining such issues and their potential impact(s) on the integrity of the study. Study directors at CROs typically preside over a pre-initiation or pre-study meeting with the operational/departmental areas that will be involved in conducting the study in order to discuss the protocol and address any potential concerns or issues that may be articulated. It is helpful for sponsors to participate in those meetings (even if by phone) to share the above-discussed information in more personal detail and to be readily available to assist in answering questions that may arise or in vetting any alternative process or methodology suggestions that may be made.

As you review the draft report and provide comments to your study director and CRO, it is important to be specific and clear as to what you are asking of them. Tracked changes in a document that provide alternate wording suggestions that you may prefer or an explanatory background of why you are requesting a particular interpretational change are helpful, while a stream of consciousness commentary in the margins that does elucidate a definitive point or desired path forward is much less so. Comments should be collaborative, businesslike, and professional, without disparaging or denigrating the author(s), or in any suggesting any type of business repercussions if a specific change in interpretation is not made. Any hint of undue influence exerted by sponsors is a primary focus of regulatory authorities, and care should be taken when working through any differences in interpretational opinion to make sure the communications and back and forth across what can sometimes be multiple rounds of comments and revised draft reports reflect sound and pragmatic scientific analysis and decision-making. The study director and the contributing scientists from a CRO will work very closely with you to discuss and address your comments, offer compromise wording that is amenable to both parties, and do their best to fine-tune the report as needed as you work together toward a signed finalized report.

What Should the Experience Level, Training, or Background of Your Study Director Be?

CRO study directors have historically come from varied backgrounds and experiences, rather than any particular "one-size-fits-all" standard educational or career path. Many CROs have an abundant mixture of homegrown or externally hired study directors of differing degree levels. Homegrown/internally hired study directors may come from almost any departmental area of the CRO, while externally hired study directors may come from industry (including sponsors), academia, or other CROs. All, regardless of their background, should go through an applicable study director training program within that CRO and be provided a mentor or mentors to guide them on an ongoing basis and be there to provide support in the areas of problem-solving and managerial skills. Some of the most important instruction and oversight toward the development of an effective study director is guided by ongoing mentorship involving the mentee and more senior staff. Individual mentee needs will vary, depending on their relative qualifications (experience factors such as education, applied practice, etc.). For example, the mentoring involvement for an individual with more limited academic and/or practical applied experience will typically be more extensive than for an individual with advanced training/certification and/or practical application. Accordingly, it should be recognized that due to the background/experience and ongoing mentoring relationships, the qualifications of a specific trainee at any given point in time are not determined by any rigid set of competencies, as might be devised for the training/qualification of technical/operational staff.

As a sponsor, you may perhaps ask the CRO to provide the curriculum vitae (CV) for a number of potential study directors for your consideration or request that your study director have certain credentials as a prerequisite. You might also seek out recommendations from colleagues in the industry who swear by the capabilities of a particular study director at that CRO. The toxicology community is a relatively small one, and word gets around, both good and bad. However, the definitive tried and true assessment is how an individual performs on your study or studies and if the developing relationship exhibits the foundation and bonding indicative of two-way respect and trust and shows potential for the future (someone you want to work with long-term and that provides a level of customer service that meets your needs). You would also ideally like to see your study director to be looked upon as a leader in the field by publishing articles, opinion pieces, or study results and attending and participating in scientific meetings and their related symposiums, roundtables, and continuing education courses. While younger or newer professionals in the role may not have had the opportunities to accumulate a wide variety of such accomplishments just yet, they should not be dismissed out of hand, as their future potential needs to be considered. Someone of comparatively little overall experience (when compared with others of more veteran ilk) may already be on the way to becoming the next superstar study director that sponsors will swear by and clamor for and that you can establish a productive long-term relationship with from the get-go.

Be Cognizant of and Maximally Utilize the Abilities of the Study Director's Team and Colleagues

Although you will be working most closely with your assigned study director in terms of day-to-day interactions and discussions, do not miss the opportunity to also get to know and interact with the members of his or her direct team. Study directors will often have a study coordinator or scientific coordinator (the title varies among CROs) that serves as their administrative right hand, a report coordinator that works on methods and tables and keeps all aspects of the report on track, and an alternate contact (typically a study director colleague who is available to assist as needed if the study director is briefly indisposed or unavailable). These individuals can be valuable and additional go-to people for you within your CRO, most especially when your study director is unable to readily respond (if they are observing study functions in an animal room or other parts of the laboratory, giving a presentation, participating in an internal meeting, etc.) and you perhaps need something urgently. In addition, many CROs have a study director staff that in totality may reflect literally hundreds of years of overall industry experience. The larger group (and its senior management) can be tapped by your study director on your behalf for any unique study situations or questions that may arise, as typically someone on such a staff is likely to have run into a similar or exact situation at some point in their career and can provide counsel or advice as needed. In short, CROs and CRO study directors have seen and experienced an impressive breadth and depth of situations across all types of compound and indication platforms, what has worked and what hasn't, what processes the agency has perhaps recently frowned on or recommended against, etc. While the CRO or study director cannot typically present themselves as a bona fide regulatory consultant, the range of anecdotal knowledge is often impressive and is a valuable source of information that should be tapped for decision tree purposes and in weighing the relative merits or pros and cons of particular paths forward. This is also true of contributing scientists within the CRO, such as clinical pathologists, anatomical pathologists, toxicokineticists, veterinary cardiologists, as well as other professionals such as staff veterinarians, veterinary ophthalmologists, etc. that your study director can put you in direct contact with or pose questions to on your behalf.

The Principal Investigator Role and Its Relation to the Study Director

Multi-site studies are becoming increasingly more common place in the industry, which often creates situations where the study director is geographically remote from portions of the actual experimental work that are conducted at another site (a test site) and cannot affect immediate supervision. In those instances, the Organisation for Economic Co-operation and Development (OECD) Principles of Good Laboratory Practice give the study director permission to delegate specified responsibility (a particular or defined phase of the study) to a person serving as principal investigator(OECD, n.d.). However, this does not countermand the study director's overall responsibility for the conduct of the study (as single point of control), which cannot be delegated. Thus, clear lines of communication and optimal quality of communication between the study director and principal investigator are of paramount importance and should particularly focus on any study issues or problems, standard operating procedure (SOP) and protocol deviations, and study updates. In fact, the key skills and attributes of a study director as discussed in this chapter also apply to the principal investigator and how they should ideally approach their portion of the study, since some of the duties of the study director (minus the ultimate responsibility) are delegated to the principal investigator in these instances. In a similar fashion, expectations should be discussed up front between the study director, principal investigator, and sponsor so that all are on the same page and the work can proceed in a seamless manner without any confusion or surprises. Ultimate determination of the impact on study of any issues that arise at a test site remains the responsibility of the study director.

While CROs may subcontract a phase of the study to a test site within their organization or outside their organization (and which has typically been vetted and/or qualified by them), it is often sponsors who directly choose and contract with a specific "sponsor-designated laboratory" other than the CRO for a particular portion of the study (or perhaps choose to conduct it within their own internal sponsor facility/laboratory). In the instance of a specific sponsor-designated laboratory, it is critical that the sponsor is confident of their scientific and technical abilities, the robustness of their quality programs and regulatory philosophies, and the reliability of the timing of their deliverables within the overall reporting timeline that the study director and CRO are working with. In addition, setting the communication expectations for the principal investigator on the front end is of utmost importance so that communication from the principal investigator is timely and detailed, flows seamlessly, and includes both the study director and the sponsor so that there are no information gaps. If you as a sponsor notice that the principal investigator from your selected sponsor-designated laboratory is communicating key items (data updates study issues, SOP and protocol deviations, etc.) to you as the sponsor, but is not including the study director, do make it clear that the study director must be included. The study director can and will make their expectations clear if they are excluded, but since you are paying for the services of the sponsor-designated laboratory, your attention to these details can provide additional positive reinforcement for such things to be handled in an optimal manner for the study.

Chapter Epilogue

While this chapter was generally written from the perspective of a sponsor in regard to working with a study director at a CRO and maximizing the effectiveness of that relationship, let us now conclude by providing an overall summary of helpful hints for all our study director colleagues throughout the industry (of which I am one), as I am sure they are also among the readers.

How to Be a Highly Effective Study Director

1. Invest the time to understand the capabilities of the laboratory and operate within those boundaries.
2. Learn the preferences of each department for the conduct of their portion of the study.
3. Expect the laboratory to perform to the level of their capabilities; trust the laboratory to do their best.
4. Understand the intent of each section of the protocol from an operational perspective.
5. Help the sponsor to understand the capabilities of the laboratory (the can do's and can't do's).
6. Ensure (through peer and operational review) that you properly and accurately capture the sponsor's intent in the protocol.
7. Share background information of the test article with the laboratory (including any personal protective equipment (PPE) requirements).
8. Maintain a level of presence in laboratory areas (to interact with technical staff and see animals/functions firsthand).
9. If you have been informed of animal health status issues from clinical observations or veterinary consultations/observations, observe the animals firsthand so that you can speak from a personal view and perspective when updating the sponsor and describing the effects to them.
10. Keep your alternate contact(s) informed about salient issues should they need to act in your stead/on your behalf.
11. Commit to timely review and approval/signing of study documents and respond promptly to quality assurance observations; issue all internal/external documents and protocol amendments in a timely manner.
12. Communicate study progress with the sponsor according to their expectations. Conduct real-time review of data to spot early results trends or any unexpected issues. While operations staff will let you know of major issues/findings, they should not be used to replace your eyes and ears on a study. Do your best to keep sponsors continually updated in real time, so there are no surprises for them. Quickly inform them of mortality, important findings, and key deviations. Frequency of data updates depends not only on the sponsor's preference but on how "busy" the study is in terms of critical issues/findings.
13. Communicate changes to the sponsor and laboratory in a timely manner. Keep laboratory personnel informed of any potential design changes that

are being discussed with the sponsor during the study, even if a decision has not yet been made. The more lead time to digest and plan for possible changes, the better, and the more smoothly they can be enacted. Avoid lag time in capturing any price/cost revisions resulting from design changes.

14. Freely share knowledge/experiences with and accept counsel from other study directors and from sponsors.

15. Justify all decisions prospectively; determine acceptable pros and cons before a decision is made.

16. Accept the quality assurance unit as an ally.

17. When errors happen, never place blame; do identify the cause and lead or assist in problem-solving where possible. Take a prominent/positive role in formal investigations when they are needed. Assist in troubleshooting and providing possible solutions while keeping the sponsor in the loop. Make suggestions to the sponsor about such study issues or errors and provide options. Do not toss bad news at them and let the ball sit in their court to come up with a plan of action. Be an active partner and extension of their laboratory and fully engage with them by presenting you and your CRO's ideas.

References

FDA. FDA 21 CFR Part 58, Good Laboratory Practice for Non-Clinical Laboratory Studies.

EPA. EPA (FIFRA) 40 CFR Part 160, Good Laboratory Practice Standards.

EPA. EPA (TSCA) 40 CFR Part 792, Good Laboratory Practice Standards.

OECD. OECD Series on Principles of GLP and Compliance Monitoring Number 8 (Revised); Consensus Document, The Role and Responsibilities of the Study Director in GLP Studies.

The Inner CRO: Laws, Regulations, and Guidelines for Animal Care and Use in Research

9

Charles B. Spainhour and Shayne C. Gad

Introduction

An individual was once quoted as stating "It is harder to perform research in animals than it is in humans." This is probably the same thought that many of us have also had at least at one time or another. What he was referring to were the multiple and varied requirements, rules, and regulations that had to be put in place and closely followed when setting up an animal care and use program. And these efforts all had to be completed prior to actually procuring and then using animals in research projects. Many countries have a specific doctrine on the use of animals in research, some of which involve a plethora of rules and regulations that require a great deal of administrative time and effort, while others have very basic requirements. The requirements for the use of animals in research range from laws that must be followed and are enforced. If these laws are not followed, there are serious repercussions ranging from significant monetary fines to incarceration. However, some guidelines are voluntary. These voluntary guidelines provide facilities with the standards and information necessary on how to attain what is considered to be the "gold standard of

C. B. Spainhour
Scott Technology Park, Calvert Laboratories, Scott Township, PA, USA

S. Gad
Gad Consulting, Cary, NC, USA
e-mail: scgad@gadconsulting.com

© Springer Nature Switzerland AG 2020
S. C. Gad et al., *Contract Research and Development Organizations-Their History, Selection, and Utilization*, https://doi.org/10.1007/978-3-030-43073-3_9

animal care and use." This chapter will provide the reader with an overview of the laws, regulations, and guidelines for the care and use of animals in a research setting as well as resources that will provide more in-depth information to the reader.

History and Background

Animals have been used in research thousands of years, and often the procedures performed on animals when they were first used to gain an understanding of how living systems functioned were essentially brutal and inhumane. The Greeks studied anatomy and physiology by using the dead as well as living animals. In order to determine how the body functioned, surgical procedures were performed on fully awake animals to see how blood flowed, how the heart beats, etc. Of course early man did not have access to anesthetics, and many did not feel that animals perceived pain as we do because they were assumed to be inferior creatures. Experimentation on live animals was justified as a "path to the truth" (Brewer 1999). To put things in perspective, one must also remember that surgical procedures at this time were also being performed on humans without anesthesia and that learning anatomy and physiology from animals helped early healers to better understand how to help humans and understand physiologic processes and diseases. The development of anesthesia occurred in the middle of the nineteenth century as well as an evolution out of the dark ages that led to an era of inquiring minds wanting to know and with it came an increase in the use of animals in biomedical research. Initially animals were being used by researchers that had no idea of how to properly care for animals or the complications that various disease entities could have on their research. Proper animal care began to evolve from researchers hiring "animal caretakers" who genuinely cared about the animals and their health. These individuals were the predecessors to our modern animal care technicians.

With the realization of the progress and knowledge that could be gained from the study of animals in relationship to human conditions and diseases, the use of animals in research became popular which in turn led to an increase in the number of animal colonies that was being established for research purposes. Researchers began to realize that in addition to choosing the correct animal models for the type of research they were performing, they also needed healthy subjects. As the use of animals in research became widespread and animal facilities at prestigious institutions such as the Royal Prussian Institute for Experimental Therapy, Harvard, Johns Hopkins, and the Mayo Clinic were being established, the development of the proper husbandry for the specific species being housed as well as the importance of disease control and elimination of disease in animal colonies was advancing (Brewer 1999). Institutions began hiring veterinarians, who often were already involved in various research projects at the institution, to manage their animal colonies. The desire to properly care for and humanely use research animals basically began with veterinarians, animals caretakers, and researchers. This is the group that started the first organization for the humane care and use of research animals, the Animal Care Panel (ACP). The ACP was founded in 1950, and its first meeting was also in 1950 and would later become the American Association for Laboratory Animal Science (AALAS). The ACP prepared numerous publications on the proper care and use of laboratory animal species. The first publication, *Standards for the Care of the Dog Used in Medical Research*, was published in 1952, and many more publications followed including the first *Guide for Laboratory Animal Facilities and Care, 1963* (Mulder 1999). The ACP also implemented training courses for animal care technicians. The Association for Assessment and Accreditation of Laboratory Animal Care (AAALAC) also evolved out of the ACP in 1965 and encouraged institutions to voluntarily become accredited in order to promote the establishment and development of high-quality animal care programs. In addition to these organizations, others such as the Institute of Laboratory Animal Resources (ILAR) (Wolfle 1999) and the American College of Laboratory Animal Medicine (ACLAM) (Middleton 1999) were established in the 1950s to also promote the proper care and use of laboratory animals. Other programs that involved training, the development of new and improved husbandry techniques in support of developing improved laboratory animal care, and dissemination of that information were also being established in the late 1950s and early 1960s but are beyond the scope of this chapter to discuss in further detail.

It was not until 1966 that the United States developed federal regulations to "protect" research animals. Advocates against the use of animals in research often use the media to fuel their campaigns as was the case in 1966. In response to the public outcry ignited by an article published in a 1966 issue of *LIFE Magazine* on the inhumane care of dogs by dealers selling them for research, legislature for the protection of animals that were to be used in research was enacted (Schwindaman 1999). The US Department of Agriculture (USDA) was charged with the oversight and enforcement of the Laboratory Animal Welfare Act (LAWA). The USDA had to develop minimum standards for the care and management of laboratory animals. The USDA consulted with a multitude of various groups to establish the minimum standards of animal care. The initial LAWA only required those facilities that were using dogs and cats for research and received federal funds to register with the US Department of Agriculture (USDA). Furthermore, only dealers that bought and sold dogs and cats, conducting business over state lines, were required to be registered. The LAWA was amended in 1970, changing the name to the Animal Welfare Act (AWA), 1979 and 1985. Each amendment broadened the scope of items, species, and groups that were covered by the AWA as well as the regulatory and enforcement responsibilities of the USDA. The 1985 amendments brought the greatest changes and accountability to research facilities in the United States. These amendments required the conduct of a search for alternatives to the performance of any research procedure that had the potential to cause more than the presence of momentary pain or distress to research animals, The establishment of an Institutional Animal Care and Use Committee required the definition of a program for the use of pain- and stress-relieving measures as necessary, identified the Institutional Official (IO) as having the accountability and responsibility for meeting the AWA requirements, established the importance of exercise programs for dogs, required environmental enrichment programs for nonhuman primates, and put in place a program where USDA inspectors mandatorily visit facilities unannounced at intervals of a minimum of once each year. The compilation of a list of criteria that an IACUC must use to evaluate protocols, the training procedures for personnel working with animals and establishment of the Animal Welfare Information Center (AWIC) (Schwindaman 1999). Since 1985 there has not been much new formal legislative activity concerning the AWA other than the Pet Theft Act of 1990 which requires animal shelters to hold dogs and cats for at least 5 days prior to selling them to dealers and the recent January 30, 2013, amendment on Handling of Animals; Contingency Plans (Federal Register 2012). Dealers must provide to any research facility to which they sell the dog or cat the source and origin of the dog or the cat, and a contingency plan on possible disasters that may affect a facility must be formulated and written, and employee training on the plan must be implemented. Other legislative bills that are being considered include the Pet Safety and Protection Act of 2011 (H.R. 2256 2011) and the Great Ape Protection and Cost Savings Act of 2011 (S. 810 2011). The Pet Safety and

Protection Act of 2011 proposes the elimination of dog and cat dealers that obtain dogs and cats from random sources such as private breeders, pounds, individuals relinquishing pets, etc. The USDA has classified dealers who market random source dogs and cats as class B dealers. This bill would virtually eliminate the use of random source dogs and cats by research facilities. Currently the majority of large breed dogs often used in cardiovascular and orthopedic research are obtained from class B dealers as there are very few dealers who breed animals specifically for research also known as class A dealers who can provide these animals in any quantity. Also the pool of class A cat breeders is currently severely limited considering there is only one major breeder remaining. Unfortunately this bill has been introduced into the legislature every year since 1996 and fortunately still has not passed. The Great Ape Protection and Cost Savings Act of 2011 has come very close to becoming law. It prohibits the use of chimpanzees in "invasive" research since these are the only great apes currently used in laboratory research settings. The definition of invasive outlined in this Act precludes the use of chimpanzees in any type of biomedical research. If this bill becomes law, it will impede research on conditions and diseases for which chimpanzees are judged to be the closest model for the condition or disease in humans such as in infectious disease research involving entities such as Hepatitis B, Hepatitis C, AIDs, etc. (Committee on Long-Term Care of Chimpanzees 1997). The National Institute of Health (NIH) is currently providing testimony to Congress on the need for chimpanzees in biomedical research albeit on a limited basis. The NIH is attempting to reach a compromise that will alter the stringent wording in the current Act that will only allow the use of chimpanzees in research on a very specific as-needed basis requiring a very strong scientific justification for the use of the animals. These are the main acts that are being presented to the federal government that currently affect biomedical research using animals, but there are countless legislative bills at various levels of government (state and local) that are being considered or passed that deal with animal welfare and rights (National Association for Biomedical Research, Animal Law 2012; Pennsylvania Veterinary Medical Association, Veterinary Laws and Regulations 2012). Many of these potential bills are being presented and advocated by animal rights groups such as the Humane Society of the United States (HSUS), People for the Ethical Treatment of Animals (PETA), Physicians Committee on Responsible Medicine (PCRM), and many others.

Laws, regulations, and enforcement agencies that govern animal welfare have been established worldwide. In Europe, animal welfare laws are set by the European Union (EU) (The European Parliament and the Council of the European Union. Directive 2010/63/EU 2010). The EU is made up of various countries in Europe, and each country can have its own animal welfare laws, regulations, and enforcement agencies, but they are expected at a minimum to comply with the regulations established by the EU. For example, Italy is advocating some legislative actions that are much more restrictive than the EU requirements. The Italian government is proposing a ban on the breeding of dogs, cats, and nonhuman primates for research purposes, prohibiting the performance of any experiments that may cause pain without using anesthesia, and stricter government oversight on the use of transgenic animals (Nosengo 2012) The EU has banned the use of great apes in research and the testing of cosmetics in or on animals (Commission of the European Communities 2004). In Canada, animal welfare guidelines are established by the Canadian Council on Animal Care (CCAC) (CCAC Guide to the Care and Use of Experimental Animals, Vol 1 1980 and Vol 2 1984; Guidelines on: choosing an appropriate endpoint in experiments using animals for research, teaching and testing 1998; Guidelines on: euthanasia of animals used in science 2010). Japan's animal welfare requirements can be found in the Law for the Humane Treatment and Management of Animals and Standards Relating to the Care and Management of Experimental Animals. These are a few examples of the animal welfare requirements of various countries. As the laws, regulations, and guidelines of various countries are reviewed, one can appreciate the range of animal welfare advocacy and anticipate that the further protection of animals is accelerating at a rapid pace.

US Animal Laws and Regulations

Animal Welfare Act (AWA)

The Animal Welfare Act contains the details of the federally mandated laws and regulations governing animal welfare in the United States. The US Department of Agriculture (USDA) is the government agency that was chosen by Congress to formulate the regulations for compliance with the AWA and the enforcement of these regulations (Schwindaman 1999). Under the AWA, research facilities are required to register with the USDA if they use any AWA-covered species in research, tests, teaching, or experiments. Research facilities are required to renew their registration status every 3 years. Species that are not covered by the AWA are birds, mice (genus *Mus*), and rats (genus *Rattus*) bred for use in research; horses not used for research purposes; farm animals, including livestock and poultry, used or intended for use as food or fiber or in agricultural research; fish; and invertebrates (crustaceans, insects) (United States Department of Agriculture, The Animal Welfare Act: An Overview 2006). The latest version of the Animal Welfare Act and Animal Welfare Regulations (AWA) was published in August 2002 by the USDA, Animal and Plant Health Inspection Service (APHIS) (United States Department of Agriculture, Animal Welfare Act and Animal Welfare Regulations 2002). This document contains the requirements of the AWA as well as the regulations followed by the USDA to ensure sound animal welfare. Additional documents used by the USDA for guidance on how to interpret and carry out the AWA and its regulations are The Animal Care Resource Guide Policies (United States Department of Agriculture, Animal Care Resource Guide Policies 2011) and the consolidated inspection guide (United States Department of Agriculture, Animal Care Inspection Guide 2012). The species specifically covered in the Animal Welfare Regulations include dogs, cats, rabbits, guinea pigs, hamsters, nonhuman primates, marine mammals, and then a general category of all other warm-blooded animals. The subsections for each species include Facilities and Operating Standards, Animal Health and Husbandry Standards, and Transportation Standards. Minimum requirements for cage size can be found in the Facilities and Operating Standards section for each species and in Table 9.1.

In addition to the space requirements for the various species covered in the Animal Welfare Regulations, temperature, lighting, ventilation, facility structural requirements, waste disposal, feeding, bedding/caging surfaces, sanitization, watering, housing (single vs. group), etc. are covered for each species. Facilities are now also required to have a disaster plan in place as well as an employee training program on how disasters should be handled as stipulated in the facility disaster plan. The items covered in the Regulations are mandatory and not elective requirements. Transportation requirements for each species are comprehensively covered including how many animals may be transported in the same container (e.g., no more than 15 rabbits in one primary container), container ventilation requirements, structure of the transport container, how often animals need to be fed and watered on a trip, how often animals need to be observed while in transit, and handling of the transport containers when they hold animals, etc.

Table 9.1 AWA requirements for minimum space of primary enclosures (August 2002)

Species	Weight	Floor area/animal	Cage height[a]	Comments
Dog	NA	$$\frac{\left(\text{dog length}\left(\text{in.}\right)+6\right)^2}{144}$$	6" above head of tallest dog in the enclosure	Bitches with nursing puppies must be provided with additional floor space. Generally each puppy should get a minimum of 5% of the minimum floor space requirement of the bitch
Cat	≤4.0 kg	3.0 ft² (0.28 m²)	24" (60.96 cm)	Queens with nursing kittens must be provided with additional floor space. Generally each kitten should get a minimum of 5% of the minimum floor space requirement of the queen
	> 4.0 kg	4.0 ft² (0.37 m²)	24" (60.96 cm)	
Guinea pig	<350 g	60 in² (387.12 cm²)	7.0" (17.78 cm)	
	≥350 g	101 in² (651.65 cm²)	7.0" (17.78 cm)	
	Female + litter	101 in² (651.65 cm²)	7.0" (17.78 cm)	
Hamster	<60 g	10 in² (64.52 cm²)	6.0" (15.2 cm)	
	60–80 g	13 in² (83.88 cm²)	6.0" (15.2 cm)	
	80–100 g	16 in² (103.23 cm²)	6.0" (15.2 cm)	
	>100 g	19 in² (122.59 cm²)	6.0" (15.2 cm)	
	Female + litter	121 in² (780.45 cm²)	6.0" (15.2 cm)	
Rabbit individual	<2 kg	1.5 ft² (0.14 m²)	14" (35.56 cm)	
	2–4 kg	3.0 ft² (0.28 m²)	14" (35.56 cm)	
	4–4.5 kg	4.0 ft² (0.37 m²)	14" (35.56 cm)	
	>5.4 kg	5.0 ft² (0.46 m²)	14" (35.56 cm	

(continued)

Table 9.1 (continued)

Species	Weight	Floor area/animal	Cage height[a]	Comments
Females + litters	<2 kg	4.0 ft² (0.37 m²)	14″ (35.56 cm)	
	2–4 kg	5.0 ft² (0.46 m²)	14″ (35.56 cm)	
	4–4.5 kg	6.0 ft² (0.56 m²)	14″ (35.56 cm)	
	>5.4 kg	7.5 ft² (0.70 m²)	14″ (35.56 cm)	
Nonhuman Primates[b]				
Group 1	<1 kg	1.6 ft² (0.15 m²)	20″ (50.8 cm)	
Group 2	1–3 kg	3.0 ft² (0.0.28 m²)	30″ (76.2 cm)	
Group 3	3–10 kg	4.3 ft² (0.40 m²)	30″ (76.2 cm)	
Group 4	10–15 kg	6.0 ft² (0.56 m²)	32″ (81.28 cm)	
Group 5	15–25 kg	8.0 ft² (0.74 m²)	36″ (91.44 cm)	
Group 6	>25 kg	25.1 ft² (2.33 m²)	84″ (213.36 cm)	

[a]From cage floor to cage top
[b]The different species of nonhuman primates are divided into six weight groups for determining minimum space requirements, except that all brachiating species of any weight are grouped together since they require additional space to engage in species-typical behavior. Examples of types of nonhuman primates in each group: Group 1 – Marmosets, tamarins, and infants (less than 6 months of age) of various species
Group 2 – Capuchins, squirrel monkeys and similar size species, and juveniles (6 months to 3 years of various species
Group 3 – Macaques and African species
Group 4 – Male macaques and large African species
Group 5 – Baboons and nonbrachiating species larger than 15 kg
Group 6 – Great apes over 25 kg

In addition to the basic care and handling of the species covered by the USDA two laboratory species that have additional requirements. Along with the mandatory minimum floor space requirement, the dog must be given the opportunity to exercise. This exercise cannot be forced such as putting the dog on a treadmill; rather the dog must be given additional floor space to exercise and play. The methods and frequency of the opportunity to exercise are delegated by the facility. The facility along with the attending veterinarian must draw up a plan to provide the dogs with the opportunity to exercise. When exercising, the available floor space must be twice the floor space of the minimum required floor space. Many facilities have various methods for providing dogs with the opportunity to exercise, and some of these methods include walking on a leash, allowing dogs to run around on the floor of an animal room for a set amount of time, pair housing in caging that at a minimum meets the floor space requirement of each dog, thereby doubling the floor space when the dogs are together (e.g., having a sliding door between two primary enclosures and opening the doors to allow the dogs to comingle), indoor or outdoor pens, etc. If dogs are group housed and the enclosure floor space equals the floor space required for each dog or an individually housed dog has double the required minimum floor space, additional opportunity to exercise is not required. Dogs can be exempted from exercise by order of the attending veterinarian for reasonable medical or behavioral reasons. If the animal is exempt from exercise, the attending veterinarian needs to re-evaluate the animal every 30 days to see if exercise can be reinstated. If the attending veterinarian determines that the animal has a permanent condition that is not conducive of exercise, this needs to be completely and thoroughly documented, and the opportunity to exercise will not be required. Dogs may also be exempt from exercise based on an IACUC-approved scientific protocol that has *adequate* scientific justification for the exemption. Records for any exemptions must be maintained and reported on the USDA annual report.

The second common laboratory animal species that have special requirements are nonhuman primates. An environmental enrichment/enhancement program must be in place to promote the psychological well-being of nonhuman primates, and it is essential that this be developed by the individual research facility. Facilities that house nonhuman primates are advised to consult publications and organizations that provide information on the needs of various species of nonhuman primates and tested and tried methods of providing environmental enrichment/enhancement to meet these needs as the basis of their programs (Committee on Well-Being of Nonhuman Primates 1998). Social housing is considered one of the mainstays of psychological enrichment in nonhuman primates and is now strongly advocated by the USDA. In the past, individual housing of nonhuman primates in research facilities was common practice, for reasons such as food consumption measurements, odd number of animals in dose groups, transfer of test article between animals, injury potential to both the animals and staff when social housing animals, etc. were considered acceptable. In 2010 these reasons were no longer considered acceptable. Dose groups with odd numbers of animals should be housed in triplicate or greater with one strategy being using tunnels on the front of the cages to allow bottom animals to also use top cages and vice versa. The Food and Drug Administration accepts group housing data such as group observations of fecal and urine output and group food consumption and does not seem concerned with potential test article transfer as long as animals from the same dose group are housed together. Animals can be separated for dosing procedures by closing off individual cages or using innovatively designed dosing cages where the nonhuman primates are trained to enter a dosing cage, removed from the common pen, dosed, and returned to the common area. There are some exceptions to the rules of group housing, and some of these include the presence of an overly aggressive or vicious animal or a debilitated animal. For animals that are overly aggressive, extensive documentation needs to be available to support and verify that there have been multiple attempts that failed to work before an animal can be labeled in such a manner. Other exceptions include animals presenting with signs of a contagious disease unless the whole group has it then they could be group housed if they are not debilitated or are noncompatible. Nonhuman primates also are required to have environmental enrichment. The enclosure environment must be enriched by providing a means for the nonhuman primate to express species-specific behaviors. Many items are being used by a variety of facilities in order to provide enrichment to nonhuman primates. Some of these items such as foraging boards, perches, mirrors, toys, televisions, treats, etc. are available commercially. There are even more items that innovative facilities have invented on their own, and many of these items and ideas are shared at various laboratory animal meetings and on websites or list servers. Similar to the exemption of exercise in dogs, exemptions from participation in environmental enhancement for nonhuman primates are allowed. Veterinary exemptions can be made, must be documented, and must be reviewed every 30 days. Permanent exemptions can be made with an appropriate level of detailed documentation. Exemptions can be protocol driven with appropriate scientific justification and IACUC approval. Exemptions due to research requirements must be reported yearly on the annual report. Nonhuman primates do not have to be exempt from all aspects of the environmental enrichment program. For example, a nonhuman primate that cannot be group housed can still be allowed access to activities that permit enrichment of their environment and actually be exposed to more types of enrichment or complex enrichment in an attempt to make up for the lack of social housing.

In addition to animal care standards, the Animal Welfare Regulations require research facilities that are subject to the AWA to establish an IACUC. Institutional Animal Care and Use Committee requirements as stipulated by the regulations will be covered in the section of this chapter on IACUCs. Other requirements for research facilities include the proper training of employees that care for, handle, and/or use animals in research, a program for the provision of adequate veterinary care, detailed record keeping requirements and maintenance (records must be maintained for 3 years), the mandatory completion and submission to the USDA an annual report, and the completion or righting of deficiencies as identified and specified during the course of an inspection being conducted by a USDA inspector. Each research facility must employ an attending veterinarian. The veterinarian can be full time or part time. If the veterinarian is part time, then a written program of veterinary care must be developed between the veterinarian and the research facility. All animals must be observed at a minimum of once daily by adequately trained personnel in order to assess their health and well-being. There must be a mechanism for the direct and timely communication with the attending veterinarian if animal health issues develop. Each research facility is required to fill out an annual report on the use or intended use of AWA-covered species. The time frame for the annual reporting period for the USDA is from October 1 to September 30 of the following year, and the report is due by December 1. The annual report includes statements that assure that animals are being properly used in research. The number of animals being housed and used at the research facility between the dates stated above must be documented in the annual report. Animals are placed in one of four categories. Category B should include animals that are being held for research, teaching, testing, etc. but on which no procedures have been conducted. Animals placed in Category C have been used for procedures that cause no more than momentary pain or distress such as blood collection, routine injections, etc. Category D should contain animals that have had procedures performed on them that would cause more than momentary pain or distress but were administered the appropriate anesthetics, analgesics, or tranquilizing drugs (e.g., surgical models). Animals placed in Category E had procedures performed on them that caused more than momentary pain or distress but had appropriate anesthetics, analgesics, or tranquilizing drugs withheld as the administration of these substances would interfere with the procedure being performed, the results, or the interpretation of the data. Examples of such studies are experiments that use pain models, models of inflammation, chronic disease models, etc. If a research facility has animals that are in pain Category E, a detailed explanation of why the alleviation of pain or distress could not be provided needs to be attached to the annual report. Exemptions of dogs from exercise and nonhuman primates from the environmental enrichment program that are required by IACUC-approved protocols must also be included on the annual report.

The USDA is required to inspect all registered research facilities to be in compliance with the AWA and its regulations at a minimum of once a year if not more frequently. These unannounced inspections are conducted by veterinary medical officers (VMOs) or other trained personnel such as veterinary technicians who are designated as animal care inspectors. The inspector will conduct a detailed walk through the facility to assure that animal care is in compliance with the regulations, that the structural aspects of the facility (i.e., caging, equipment, walls, flooring, doors, walls, etc.) are in satisfactory condition, and that all paperwork is thorough and complete and has been performed in a timely fashion. If they are inspecting a research facility, the Institutional Animal Care and Use Committee (IACUC) minutes, membership, attendance, deliberations, etc. are closely scrutinized for compliance. Research facilities must furnish the inspector in a timely fashion with any information or records requested that the facility is required by the AWA and its regulations to maintain. The inspector has the authority to make copies of these records and take photographs of any areas of noncompliance. Regardless of any SOPs that a facility may have in place with regard to the use of cameras, the USDA inspector is permitted because of his or her authority to take such pictures for documentation. However, the facility should completely understand why the picture is being taken, make sure that the inspector takes a photograph of the item of concern only and not just a broad photograph, and finally request a copy of all photographs taken. At the end of the inspection, the inspector will write up an inspection report. Any noncompliant items (NCI) will be enumerated in the report. The section and subsection of the Animal Welfare Act and Animal Welfare Regulations will be cited along with the pertinent NCI on the inspection form. The report is signed by the inspector and the responsible member or suitable designate of the research facility. If the responsible party of the facility does not agree with the inspector's findings, there is an appeals process that can be followed. If a facility wins the appeal, an amended USDA inspection will be filed by the USDA. All inspection reports are posted to the web and available for anyone to read and study.

The year 2010 was declared the "Age of Enforcement" by the Deputy Secretary of the Department of Agriculture, and along with this declaration was a substantial increase in the monetary value of fines to be assessed as well as the "two strikes" and you're out rule (Bennett 2012). If a facility has two NCI items that are classified under the same section of the AWA, the facility may now be considered to be in violation of the AWA. This in turn can lead to the levy of significant fines. It is important to recognize that recurrent findings do not have to be consecutive nor do they have to occur in the same area of the facility or the same administrative function. It is imperative that research facilities have a well-managed animal care program, facilities, and inspection management program and have the support of the facility administration up to the highest levels of management to provide the necessary resources to avoid the discovery and citations of NCIs and potential fines.

Office of Laboratory Animal Welfare (OLAW)

The Office of Laboratory Animal Welfare (OLAW) is the division of the Public Health Service (PHS) that reviews an institution's proposed program of animal care and use in PHS-conducted or supported activities (Office of Laboratory Animal Welfare 2002). If the proposed program of animal care and use meets PHS requirements OLAW will issue the institution an Assurance number. The Public Health Service is the parent organization of the National Institutes of Health (NIH), which is the branch to which researchers typically submit their grant applications in order to secure funds for their research. If an institution does not have an OLAW Assurance number, no NIH grant-supported research can be conducted at the facility. In order to obtain an Assurance number from OLAW, the institution must submit its proposed Institutional Program for Animal Care and Use. The institution's animal care and use program must use the most recent version of the *Guide for the Care and Use of Laboratory Animals (Guide)* (Committee for the Update of the Guide for the Care and Use of Laboratory Animals 2011) that has been approved by OLAW for the basis of developing and implementing an institutional program for activities involving animals (United States Department of Health and Human Services, OLAW, Position Statements: OLAW Responds to Concerns Regarding Adoption of the Guide for the Care and Use of Laboratory Animals, Eighth Edition 2012). The Program Description requirements can be found in the *Public Health Service Policy on Humane Care and Use of Laboratory Animals.*

Institutions are placed by OLAW into one of two categories, which then determines the documentation that will be required by OLAW for obtaining an Assurance and Assurance Number. Category 1 institutions are those who are currently accredited by the Association for the Assessment and Accreditation of Laboratory Animal Care International (AAALAC). These institutions do not have to submit their most recent semi-annual IACUC evaluation reports with the Assurance application. Category 2 institutions are not AAALAC accredited and can rely only on their IACUC to evaluate their animal care and use program. These institutions are required to send the most recent semi-annual report into OLAW with the Assurance application. OLAW can also perform special reviews and/or a site visit in order to further assess the facility's compliance with the requirements of the PHS Policy.

Once an Assurance number has been obtained, facilities are required to keep records of items such as copies of the approved Assurance, IACUC minutes, proposed projects and subsequent IACUC deliberations on research proposals, minority opinions on research to be conducted, semi-annual IACUC reports, and any records of accrediting body inspections. All records must be maintained for a period of at least 3 years. Records for ongoing approved proposals must be maintained until the activities on the proposal are completed plus 3 years beyond that date. Assured facilities must submit an annual report to OLAW in writing through the Institutional Official (IO), and the report must include any changes in the AAALAC accreditation status (or any other acceptable accreditation), any changes in the institution's program for animal care and use, any changes in IACUC membership, and disclosure of any and all dates that facility inspections and program reviews were performed by the IACUC. If there are no changes in any of these points, this must be stated in writing by the IO to OLAW. If there are any serious or continuing noncompliance issues with the PHS Policy, serious deviations from the *Guide*, or suspension of an activity by the IACUC, they must be reported to OLAW. Minority opinions expressed by IACUC members must be disclosed and filed also.

Applications for grant monies from the NIH must be submitted through OLAW if animal use is involved. The applications must contain a section describing the care and use of the species that are being proposed for use. The required information includes the identification of the species and the numbers of animals for the program, a statement on the rationale for the selection and use of the animals as well as statements on the appropriateness and relevance of the species chosen and numbers of animals requested, a complete detailed description of the proposed use of the animals, a detailed description of procedures to be used to minimize pain and distress if it occurs, and methods of euthanasia. The proposal must have IACUC approval. The IACUC is expected to review and assess the protocol taking into consideration the requirements of the US Government Principles which can be found in the PHS Policy manual, August 2002 and Table 9.2. IACUC approval can be filed anytime prior to the grant, and approval is good for 3 years. If IACUC approval is subsequent to the submission of the proposal, any modifications required by the IACUC must be verified. The verification of IACUC approval must be signed by an individual authorized by the institution. Grant awards will not be released until IACUC approval is verified.

Table 9.2 US government principles for the utilization and care of vertebrate animals used in testing, research, and training

The PHS Policy implements 9 US Government Principles that are the foundation for humane care and use of laboratory animals in this country. These principles were developed by the Interagency Research Animal Committee and adopted in 1985 by the Office of Science and Technology Policy. The principles are:

I. The transportation, care, and use of animals should be in accordance with the Animal Welfare Act (7 U.S.C. 2131 et. seq.) and other applicable federal laws, guidelines, and policies*

II. Procedures involving animals should be designed and performed with due consideration of their relevance to human or animal health, the advancement of knowledge, or the good of society

III. The animals selected for a procedure should be of an appropriate species and quality and the minimum number required to obtain valid results. Methods such as mathematical models, computer simulation, and in vitro biological systems should be considered

IV. Proper use of animals, including the avoidance or minimization of discomfort, distress, and pain when consistent with sound scientific practices, is imperative. Unless the contrary is established, investigators should consider that procedures that cause pain or distress in human beings may cause pain or distress in other animals

V. Procedures with animals that may cause more than momentary or slight pain or distress should be performed with appropriate sedation, analgesia, or anesthesia. Surgical or other painful procedures should not be performed on unanesthetized animals paralyzed by chemical agents

VI. Animals that would otherwise suffer severe or chronic pain or distress that cannot be relieved should be painlessly killed at the end of the procedure or, if appropriate, during the procedure

VII. The living conditions of animals should be appropriate for their species and contribute to their health and comfort. Normally, the housing, feeding, and care of all animals used for biomedical purposes must be directed by a veterinarian or other scientist trained and experienced in the proper care, handling, and use of the species being maintained or studied. In any case, veterinary care shall be provided as indicated

VIII. Investigators and other personnel shall be appropriately qualified and experienced for conducting procedures on living animals. Adequate arrangements shall be made for their in-service training, including the proper and humane care and use of laboratory animals

IX. Where exceptions are required in relation to the provisions of these principles, the decisions should not rest with the investigators directly concerned but should be made, with due regard to Principle II, by an appropriate review group such as an institutional animal care and use committee. Such exceptions should not be made solely for the purposes of teaching or demonstration

State and Local Regulations

In addition to the federal regulations governing animal welfare and research facility operations, one must also be aware of the variety of state and local statutes that must be followed. State and local laws can in some cases be more stringent than the federal laws. A facility must follow federal regulations, but if the state and local regulations have requirements that exceed the federal requirements, a facility must also comply with these laws. Many of the state and local laws make an attempt to exempt research facilities from their oversight such as the Pennsylvania dog law. Pennsylvania passed a revised version of their dog law in 2008 that expanded the sections on the requirements to house dogs in a kennel. The housing requirements were directed at improving the conditions of dogs maintained in "puppy mill"-type operations. Pennsylvania's new kennel housing requirements were not directed at research facilities as it was well-known that they were inspected annually by the USDA; the state of Pennsylvania exempted research facilities from further inspections by Pennsylvania dog wardens. However, research facilities in Pennsylvania are required to submit their USDA inspection reports to the state once a year. Some states require specific permits to house exotic animals such as nonhuman primates. Therefore, research facilities in these states are required to obtain permits from the state to possess and house such animals. Some states have laws pertaining to the use of animals in consumer product safety testing. New Jersey has a state law that requires alternatives to be used, if they are available. In addition to the Drug Enforcement Agency (DEA) requirements of obtaining, handling, and record keeping of controlled substances, there are additional state and possibly local laws regarding controlled substances. State and local control of veterinary practices also exist. In some municipalities in California, declawing of cats is prohibited. Many states have laws against ventriculocordectomy in dogs. States also have "sunshine" laws that require documents and records at public institutions such as universities to be made available to the public. These laws can lead to public requests of research records from academic institutions. These requests have sometimes led to court proceedings to determine exactly what type of information can be considered proprietary and not open to the public. Disclosure laws are something to consider when performing research or testing at academic institutions. These are just a few examples of the myriad of state and local laws that can and do affect the care and use of animals in research facilities as well as the actual research and testing that is being conducted. The National Association for Biomedical Research (www. nabr.org) is an excellent resource for keeping up to date with state and local legislation (National Association for Biomedical Research 2012). In addition to the NABR, state veterinary associations are also good sources of state laws and regulations affecting the local practice of veterinary medicine that may in turn influence the legality of procedures performed on laboratory animals (Pennsylvania Veterinary Medical Association 2012).

International Laws and Regulations

European Union (EU) Laws and Regulations

The European Union issues directives that members of the union are required to follow. This is the minimum that constituents of the union are expected to meet (such as ETS 123). If they choose they can go above and beyond these directives. The new directive, *Directive 2010/63/EU of the European Parliament and of the Council of 22 September 2010 on the protection of animals used for scientific purposes* ((The European Parliament and the Council of the European Union. Directive 2010/63/EU 2010), covers the requirements that member countries must meet when using animals in research. Organizations or businesses that use animals for research and are either based in European countries or have branch facilities in Europe often require research facilities in non-European countries to meet these directives. One of the main differences between the EU directive and US requirements is the housing requirements for dogs and nonhuman primates. The requirements of the *Guide* will be used for comparison of housing requirements in the United States. The following are the floor space requirements for dogs: dogs <15 kg require 0.74 m^2 of floor space, dogs up to 30 kg require 1.2 m^2, and dogs over 30 kg require greater than 2.4 m^2 of floor space. The EU directive requires a minimum of 4 m^2 for dogs up to 20 kg and 8 m^2 for dogs over 20 kg. The EU floor space requirements are approximately four times the floor space required in the United States. The EU minimum floor space requirements can accommodate two dogs without additional space, and every additional dog added to the pen is required to have an additional 2–4 m^2 depending on the weight of the dog. Dogs must be socially housed and can only be separated from each other for a period of time to not exceed more than 4 hours a day. The EU floor space requirements effectively will reduce the number of animals that can typically be housed in a room especially in facilities that were designed when floor space requirements for dogs were significantly less and used cages rather than runs. Studies that may have been accommodated in two rooms essentially would need to be housed in four rooms according to this directive, which will significantly raise the cost of animal care. These costs will then be passed on to clients. In addition to dogs, nonhuman primate (NHP) EU space requirements significantly exceed US requirements. Both the EU and US require NHPs to be socially housed. The space requirements for the EU accommodate up to two animals, while the US requirements are based on the individual animal. EU requirements are based on age, while the US requirements are based on weight. In order to perform a direct comparison, cynomolgus monkeys will be used as the model. Typically a juvenile cynomolgus monkey used in a toxicology study is approximately 2 years of age and weighs less than 3 kg. For an animal of this size and age, EU space requirements are 2.0 m^2 of floor space and 1.8 m of vertical space. Space requirements for this same animal in the United States would be 0.28 m^2 of floor space and 76.2 cm of vertical space. Two animals would require 0.56 m^2 of floor space in the United States. As with dogs, the EU requirements are approximately four times the US requirements. Individual countries in the EU also have some additional requirements, which may be requested when studies are being placed by companies that are based in a particular country.

International Regulations and Resources

A listing of animal research regulations from countries around the world can be found at www.aaalac.org.

Institutional Animal Care and Use Committee Requirements and Function

The Animal Welfare Act (AWA) came into existence in 1966 to provide guidance and regulations for the care and use of animals used in research, testing, teaching, exhibition, and transportation. The original AWA did not require research facilities to form an Institutional Animal Care and Use Committee (IACUC). It was not until 1971 that the National Institutes of Health (NIH), which is a major component of the Public Health Service (PHS) of the Department of Health and Human Services, issued its first "Policy, Care, and

Treatment of Laboratory Animals" reference with which research institutions that were about to receive or were receiving NIH grant money had to comply (Gordon 1999). This directive first introduced the animal care committee as a means to ensure the proper care and use of laboratory animals. In 1985 the AWA was amended to include the requirement that research facilities institute an IACUC. The current difference between IACUC requirements for the AWA vs. OLAW (Office of Laboratory Animal Welfare which oversees NIH grant monies) is the number of members that is required to be on the committee. The AWA requires a minimum of three committee members, attending veterinarian (AV), a chairperson, and an unaffiliated community member. OLAW requires a minimum of five members (AV, chair, unaffiliated community member, non-scientist, and a scientist). Members of the committee are appointed by the Chief Executive Officer (CEO) or highest-ranking management individual within an institution or business. The committee reports to the Institutional Official (IO). The IO is the person who has the financial authority and resources to assure compliance with the requirements of the AWA and OLAW (United States Department of Health and Human Services, Institutional Administrator's Manual for Laboratory Animal Care and Use 1988). The responsibility of the IACUC chairperson is to conduct the meetings and report any issues to the IO. The attending veterinarian must be either specifically certified or possess training and experience in laboratory animal science and medicine or be highly experienced with the use of the species at the institution and must have specifically direct or delegated animal care and use program responsibility. The unaffiliated community member represents the unbiased interests of the general community. The community member cannot be in anyway affiliated with the institution and not a member of the immediate family of a person who is affiliated with the institution. It is imperative that the community member regularly attend meetings, be made aware of all committee-related activities that occur outside a regularly convened meeting, and are included in the conduct of facility inspections. Unaffiliated committee members can receive compensation for their meeting attendance but not at a rate that is considered to be adding substantially to their regular income. The two additional members required by OLAW, the scientist and non-scientist, are added to help provide a well-rounded membership to participate in discussions. The scientist must be experienced in research using animals, and the non-scientist adds a different level of understanding and perspective to the committee from a non-research perspective. Typically, the unaffiliated member and the non-scientist are often the ones whose questions in an attempt to understand the rationale for the research/ testing being performed lead to a more in-depth evaluation of the procedures being carried out on the animals which may in turn lead to protocol modifications which benefit the animals and the research. OLAW will allow some members to fit into more than one category such as the unaffiliated member can also be considered the non-scientific member as long as he or she is not a scientist, etc. OLAW also allows for alternate members of the committee. Alternates are appointed to the committee by the CEO or equivalent, and each alternate has a one-on-one designation to the category of the voting committee member they can replace (Office of Extramural Research (OER) Web Site 2008). They must receive the same training as regular committee members, and they can only vote if the regular committee member they are representing is not present. The AWA does not address the concept of alternate members but does not appear to object to the concept. Neither the AWA nor OLAW limits the number of members that may be on an IACUC committee. It is generally recommended that the number of members on a committee be an odd number to obviate the development of an impasse when voting. Other individuals that may add valuable expertise to the functioning of the committee are animal care staff, statisticians, information specialists, research technicians, etc. (Applied Research Ethics National Association 2002). One stipulation set by the AWA is that not more than three members of the IACUC may report to the same administrative unit within an organization, business, or institution.

There are a few conflicts of interest that are best to avoid. One is designating the AV as the chair, and the other is appointing the IO as a voting member of the IACUC. The attending veterinarian's role on the IACUC is one of oversight and guidance concerning animal use and welfare. If the AV is also the chair, this can be seen as basically shifting the balance of power to one person. The IO should not be a voting member of the IACUC since the committee reports to the IO, and allowing the IO to vote on IACUC issues could be construed as overly influential. Some recommend that the IO attend IACUC meetings in order to have a better understanding of the function and deliberations of the committee. The benefits of having the IO attend will need to be weighed against the impact of potential influence their presence could potentially have on the committee members and their behavior, depending on the dynamics of the relationship between the IO and the committee.

Responsibilities of the IACUC are delineated in the law (AWA amendments of 1985) and federal policy and regulations (OLAW). The mandate of the committee is to "maintain oversight of the facilities' animal care program." This is achieved by the IACUC overseeing the facility's animal care and use program, facilities inspections, and protocol reviews. The IACUC must review the institution's animal care and use program at least once every 6 months. This review provides an ongoing mechanism for ensuring that the institution maintains continued compliance with applicable animal care and use policies, guidelines, and laws. The review also serves as an opportunity for constructive interaction and education for the animal care staff, research staff, and IACUC members. The reviews also aid facilities in preparing for outside inspections and site visits. Key aspects of the review include IACUC membership adequacy, functions, and procedures of the IACUC, how protocols are reviewed by the IACUC, the facility inspection process, provisions for reviewing and investigating concerns regarding animal care and use, record keeping practices, methods employed to meet reporting requirements, occupational health and safety programs, veterinary medical program, personnel qualifications and training, and review of written institutional policies such as standard operating procedures (SOPs). The IACUC may use subcommittees comprised of a minimum of two members for required activities except for protocol review. All members need to be aware of evaluations being performed by subcommittees so they have the opportunity to participate and contribute, if they so desire.

Methods an IACUC may use when reviewing protocols include full committee review and designated member review. When a protocol is submitted to the IACUC, the following information must be included in the protocol before the review process can begin. There must be a sound rationale and purpose of the proposed use of the animals in a study. The species and number of animals that are to be used must also be thoroughly justified. Housing and husbandry details should be included especially if these conditions differ from routine or recommended procedures. For example, the Guide for the Care and Use of Laboratory Animals, 8th ed. (Guide), recommends social species be group housed and rodents be housed on solid bottom caging. If animals are single housed or housed on wire-bottom caging, there should be scientific justification as to why these animals are to be maintained and housed in this manner. The protocol must include a complete description of the proposed use of the animal including the procedures to be performed as well as any drugs that may be used for relief from pain and distress or reasons for disallowance of pain-relieving medications (Committee on Pain and Distress in Laboratory Animals 1992). If surgical manipulation of the animals is proposed, then preoperative, intraoperative and postoperative care, including the use of anesthetics, analgesics, tranquilizers, and any other medications, must be adequately addressed in detail in the protocol. Anytime multiple major survival surgeries are proposed, scientific justification must be given. Methods of and reasons for euthanasia must be indicated in the proposal. Humane endpoints must be well-defined with criteria and a process for timely intervention, treatment of the affected animals, removal of animals from study, or euthanasia if painful or stressful outcomes are anticipated. The principal investigator (PI) must document consideration of alternatives to painful procedures and provide a written narrative description of the methods and sources used to determine that alternatives were not available. Assurance that the protocol is not unnecessarily duplicative must be provided. Any deviations from the AWA regulations or the Guide if funded by the NIH must be identified and approved by the IACUC. The IACUC must be assured that the personnel conducting the procedures on the animals have been adequately trained and are qualified in the procedures being performed.

Full committee review requires that the protocol be reviewed at a convened IACUC meeting with at least a quorum of the members present. The protocol is presented to the committee members either by the principal investigator or a committee member who preferably has expertise or familiarity with the protocol design being submitted. It is advantageous to allow each committee member to have access to a copy of the protocol prior to convening the IACUC meeting. This will allow the members to review the protocol ahead of time and formulate any questions they may have allowing the meeting to run more efficiently. All deliberations on protocols presented at a full committee meeting must be included in the IACUC minutes. If the PI is a voting member of the IACUC, he or she must abstain from voting on the proposal and is not considered to be a part of the quorum required for deliberations on the proposal. This abstention from voting must be noted in the minutes. When all of this is complete, then and only then can the committee vote to approve the protocol, require protocol modifications to secure approval, withhold protocol approval, or defer or table the review for additional future discussions (rare).

A designated member review (DMR) process can also be used for protocol review. Each member of the committee is given the opportunity to review all protocols or significant protocol changes prior to review. A member can then call for a full committee review if they deem this is necessary prior to DMR review. If no member calls for a full committee review, then the protocol can go for DMR review. The designated reviewer is then designated by the chair. The designated reviewer can approve the protocol or require modifications in order to secure approval or call for a full committee review. The designated reviewer cannot withhold approval.

Any significant changes to a protocol must be approved by the IACUC before the change occurs. Significant changes include but are not limited to changes in the objective of the study, altering the proposal to switch from non-survival to survival surgery, changes in the invasiveness of the procedure, changes in key personnel, changes in the use of pain-alleviating drugs or the nonuse of these drugs, changes in the methods of euthanasia, etc.

Protocol review is required on a regular basis, and the frequency depends on the species being utilized in the protocol which dictates under which regulatory body the protocol falls. If the species being used in the protocol falls under the purview of the USDA, a yearly IACUC review of the protocol is required, and a search for alternatives for protocols containing painful or distressful procedures will be required every 3 years (United States Department of Agriculture, Animal Care Resource Guide Polices 2011). Protocols that fall under the auspices of OLAW and do not involve USDA-covered species must be reviewed by IACUC every 3 years. In addition to protocol review, post-approval monitoring (PAM) of the approved protocol-driven procedures is highly recommended (Silverman et.al. 2007). Post-approval monitoring involves ensuring that the objectives and the procedures stated in the protocol are being followed. Post-approval monitoring can be achieved in many ways such as during the facility inspections that occur every 6 months, quality assurance oversight of protocol activities, veterinary staff rounds, compliance officer inspections, etc.

Facility inspections involve the IACUC assessment of areas that house animals and their support areas. If a subcommittee is being used to evaluate the facilities, it is highly recommended that the unaffiliated member be a part of the facility inspection subcommittee. Satellite facilities where animals are housed for more than 24 hours must also be inspected. Areas where surgical manipulations are performed are evaluated. The AWA/AWR require that surgery on nonrodent species be performed in a dedicated surgical suite and surgery on rodent species be carried out in an area that is dedicated for surgery when the surgical procedure(s) are being performed. In accordance to the AWR, animal study areas that hold USDA-covered species for more than 12 hours and holding facilities also need to be assessed. Laboratories where routine work such as weighing, blood collection, dosing, etc. are performed are not required to be evaluated on the inspection, but many IACUC's evaluate these areas on a rotating basis since animal manipulations are occurring in these areas, even though the animals are not actually housed in the area for any length of time. The IACUC during the course of their inspections needs to evaluate caging, physical plant, sanitation, food and water provisions, animal identification, animal health records, controlled drugs, expired drugs, environmental controls (HVAC), lighting, watering system, occupational and health concerns, staff training, security, knowledge of applicable rules (are employees wearing appropriate PPE), disaster plan, etc. A written report of the semiannual facility inspection must be written and signed by a simple majority of the IACUC members. All deficiencies must be categorized or classified as being either significant or minor. A significant deficiency is defined as a situation that is or may be a threat to animal health or safety. Once any deficiencies are identified, a reasonable and specific plan as well as a time schedule with dates for completion of each finding must be documented. If any significant deficiencies are not remedied by the assigned completion date, the IO must inform the USDA APHIS within 15 days of the lapsed deadline. The report must be sent to the IO in a timely fashion (usually within 1 month of the completion of the inspection) for review and kept on file a minimum of 3 years (Applied Research Ethics National Association 2002).

The IACUC must have provisions for reviewing any concerns pertaining to animal welfare raised by the public or institutional employees. Procedures must be established to ensure that any concerns are effectively communicated to the IACUC. The AWR provides personnel with a "whistleblower" policy. It states that "no facility employee, committee member, or laboratory personnel shall be discriminated against or be subject to any reprisal for reporting violations of any regulation or standard under the Act" (United States Department of Agriculture, Animal Welfare Act and Animal Welfare Regulations 2002). The IACUC chair is typically responsible for ensuring that concerns are investigated, but he or she can delegate a subcommittee to handle the conduct of any investigation. Conditions that reportedly jeopardize the health and well-being of the animals must be investigated immediately. In some cases the veterinarian or a specifically designated individual can evaluate the situation and stop any procedures that do not comply with institutional policy or are perceived as not in compliance with institutional policy until the IACUC can convene and consider the matter formally. The committee needs to formally acknowledge the complaint, and if an investigation is deemed necessary, the findings must be documented as well as the details of any corrective actions, if the situation warrants such. The AWR and PHS Policy authorize the IACUC to suspend any activity after review of the matter at a convened meeting of a quorum of the members. Suspensions must be reviewed with the IO in consultation with the Committee. Appropriate corrective action is taken, and the IO must report any suspension to OLAW and the USDA depending if the grievances involved an NIH-funded study and/or a USDA-covered species.

If the facility has an OLAW Assurance number and/or AAALAC accreditation, any departure from the Guide must be documented on the semi-annual review. Departures from this course of action must be approved by the IACUC prior implementation of the departure, or the departure will be considered to be a noncompliance matter reportable to OLAW and AAALAC.

The IACUC responsibilities cover many aspects of the functionality of a facility. This committee must be able to ensure to all governing and accrediting bodies that a facility's animal care and use program meets all the standards set by the various entities. It is imperative that all facets of a facility work closely and in harmony with the IACUC, with the ultimate goal being the attainment of compliance with the governing agencies. A strong, compliant animal care and use program equals healthy and well-conditioned animals which lead to good science and ethical and moral behavior as well as a good image to the public.

Euthanasia

The word euthanasia was derived from Greek and literally means "good death." In research and testing, euthanasia is very often the final outcome for the greatest majority of the animals. One of the ultimate goals for most individual toxicology studies is the histopathological evaluation of an all-encompassing tissue list which requires that tissues be harvested from the animals. There have been some strides made where imaging techniques are being used to evaluate target tissues such as tumors over time so that animals do not have to be euthanized at each time point. By using these techniques, less animals are required for a given study, which in turn leads to less animal death, but the ultimate fate of even the imaged animals is still euthanasia at the end of a study. Culling of animals especially rats and mice in breeding colonies that do not express or harbor the desired traits or gene is commonly performed. Early termination of animals due to endpoints (tumor size, genetic diseases, toxicity, etc.) being reached is a common scenario. Since death is the ultimate outcome, every attempt must be made to make the event as painless and unstressful as possible. Euthanasia is a procedure that is commonly used in veterinary practice, because the euthanasia of animals usually for end-stage disease is considered a standard procedure in veterinary care. Euthanasia of animals unfortunately to control animal populations is also commonplace. In order to standardize and ensure that the best practices are being used to euthanize animals, the American Veterinary Medical Association (AVMA) has developed guidelines for what is considered acceptable, conditionally acceptable (if used in a research setting requires scientific justification and IACUC approval), and unacceptable euthanasia methods in animals. The document is called the AVMA Guidelines on Euthanasia, June 2007 (American Veterinary Medical Association 2007). This is the latest available edition. The AVMA periodically updates this document as more information becomes available on euthanasia methods.

Table 9.3 below indicates the methods of euthanasia that are acceptable or conditionally acceptable for euthanizing commonly used laboratory animal species. For other species, please refer to the AVMA document cited above.

The following methods are not acceptable for euthanasia: air embolism, concussive blow to the head (for most species), burning, the administration of chloral hydrate (unacceptable in dogs, cats, and small mammals), the administration of chloroform, the administration of cyanide, decompression, drowning, exsanguination alone, the administration of formalin, various household products or cleaning agents, and various solvents.

Organizations Associated with Laboratory Animal Care and Use

Association for the Assessment and Accreditation of Laboratory Animal Care International (AAALAC)

"AAALAC International is a private, nonprofit organization that promotes the humane treatment of animals in science through voluntary accreditation and assessment programs" (AAALAC:About AAALAC, What is AAALAC? 2012). AAALAC inception began with the Animal Care Panel (ACP) that held its first meeting in Chicago, IL, in 1950. Members of ACP recognized that there was a need for standards, certification, and accreditation in the use and care of laboratory animals. Over time members of ACP realized that the

Table 9.3 Agents and methods of euthanasia by species

Species	Acceptable	Conditionally acceptable
Amphibians	Barbiturates, inhalant anesthetics (in appropriate species), CO_2, CO, tricaine methanesulfonate (TMS, MS 222), benzocaine hydrochloride, double pithing	Penetrating captive bolt, gunshot, stunning and decapitation, decapitation, and pithing
Birds	Barbiturates, inhalant anesthetics, CO_2, CO, gunshot (free-ranging only)	N_2, Ar, cervical dislocation, decapitation, thoracic compression (small, free-ranging only), maceration (chicks, poults, and pipped eggs only)
Cats	Barbiturates, inhalant anesthetics, CO_2, CO, potassium chloride in conjunction with general anesthesia	N_2, Ar
Dogs	Barbiturates, inhalant anesthetics, CO_2, CO, potassium chloride in conjunction with general anesthesia	N_2, Ar, penetrating captive bolt, electrocution
Fish	Barbiturates, inhalant anesthetics (in appropriate species), CO_2, tricaine methanesulfonate (TMS, MS 222), benzocaine hydrochloride, 2-phenoxyethanol	Decapitation and pithing, stunning, and decapitation/pithing
Nonhuman primates	Barbiturates	Inhalation anesthetics, CO_2, CO, N_2, Ar
Rabbits	Barbiturates, inhalant anesthetics, CO_2, CO, potassium chloride in conjunction with general anesthesia	N_2, Ar, cervical dislocation (<1 kg), decapitation, penetrating captive bolt
Rodents and other small mammals	Barbiturates, inhalant anesthetics, CO_2, CO, potassium chloride in conjunction with general anesthesia, microwave irradiation	Methoxyflurane, ether, N_2, Ar, cervical dislocation (rats <200 g), decapitation
Ruminants	Barbiturates, potassium chloride in conjunction with general anesthesia, penetrating captive bolt	Chloral hydrate (IV, after sedation), gunshot, electrocution
Swine	Barbiturates, CO_2, chloride in conjunction with general anesthesia, penetrating captive bolt	Inhalant anesthetics, CO, chloral hydrate (IV, after sedation), gunshot, electrocution, blow to the head (<3 weeks of age)

accreditation unit should be an autonomous entity and not a part of any particular professional or scientific organization, in order to gain acceptance by the scientific community in general. AAALAC founding member organizations numbered 15, and in 1965 AAALAC became an official not-for-profit organization based in Illinois (Miller and Clark 1999). AAALAC accredits programs both domestically and internationally. Currently AAALAC has more than 850 companies, universities, government agencies, and other research institutions in 36 countries that have achieved accreditation (AAALAC:About AAALAC, What is AAALAC? 2012). AAALAC accreditation for animal care and use programs is achieved by contacting AAALAC and filling out a Program Description form. This form requires an intensive review of an institution's animal care and use program and includes all aspects of the program such as occupational health and safety, IACUC functions, animal facilities, veterinary care, standard operating procedures, etc. AAALAC has established a Council on Accreditation, whose members are responsible for reviewing Program Descriptions.

The Council bases its evaluation of programs primarily on three documents, *Guide for the Care and Use of Laboratory Animals* (Committee for the Update of the Guide for the Care and Use of Laboratory Animals 2011), the *Guide for the Care and Use of Agricultural Animals in Research and Testing* (Federation of Animal Science Societies, *Ag Guide* 2010), and the European Convention for the Protection of Vertebrate Animals Used for Experimental and Other Scientific Purposes, Council of Europe (ETS 123) (AAALAC:About AAALAC, AAALAC International Mission Statement 2012). AAALAC offers a Program Status Evaluation (PES) service to programs that are applying for AAALAC accreditation for the first time. This is a peer review assessment that allows the institution to determine if its animal care and use program meets AAALAC standards and if not how improvements can be made so that the organization can meet these standards. It also familiarizes the institution with the accreditation process. The advantages of obtaining AAALAC accreditation are that it portrays to the scientific and business communities that a facility is committed to excellence in their humane care and use of research animals (AAALAC: Accreditation, Benefits of AAALAC International Accreditation 2012). This further indicates that the facility is dedicated to providing a high-quality product in all other aspects of its operations such as preclinical testing, research results, etc.

American Association for Laboratory Animal Science (AALAS)

The American Association for Laboratory Animal Science is a membership organization of professionals from around the world who are dedicated to the humane care and use of laboratory animals (American Association for Laboratory Animal Science: About AALAS 2012). AALAS is the premier organization for education in proper laboratory animal care and use. The organization offers programs for Laboratory Animal Technician certification at three different levels, Assistant Laboratory Animal Technician (ALAT), Laboratory Animal Technician (LAT), and Laboratory Animal Technologist (LATG). Technicians achieving these certifications indicate a competence in technical knowledge that is nationally recognized. AALAS also publishes two peer-reviewed journals, *Comparative Medicine* and *the Journal of the American Association of Laboratory Animal Science* (JAALAS). These journals contain numerous articles on various topics related to laboratory animals and their use as experimental models, laboratory animal medicine, biology, husbandry, comparative medicine, etc. Other literature provided by AALAS includes the Laboratory Animal Science Professional, Tech Talk, and AALAS in Action. AALAS provides the greatest amount of training resources and continuing education in the industry. Continuing education is provided through the National AALAS meeting as well as regional and branch meetings. Regional and branch groups provide member networking and support at a local level. AALAS provides a Learning Library that is used by many training programs around the world. Laboratory animal managers can take advantage of the educational opportunities provided by the Institute for Laboratory Animal Management (ILAM). Professional and technical awards of excellence are granted each year at the National AALAS meeting. Job search resources are also provided by AALAS. The AALAS Foundation provides funding and support for programs and materials for public outreach and education on the value of biomedical research.

American College of Laboratory Animal Medicine (ACLAM)

The American College of Laboratory Animal Medicine is a specialty group founded in 1957 and recognized by the American Veterinary Medical Association (AVMA) that provides for the board certification of veterinarians working in the field of laboratory animal medicine (Middleton 1999). In order to become board-certified, a veterinarian must have graduated from an AVMA-approved or AVMA-accredited school, have a foreign equivalency certificate, or be qualified to practice in some state, province, and territory in the possession by the United States, Canada, or other countries. The veterinarian must then meet the educational and experience requirements prior to sitting for the board examination. The training required prior to sitting for the board examination currently can be achieved by two methods, a specific training program in laboratory animal medicine that is of at least 2 years duration or through 6 years of full-time experience in the field of laboratory animal medicine. The veterinarian seeking board certification must also publish at least a single paper on a relevant topic in a peer-reviewed journal accepted by ACLAM. In addition to the board certification of veterinarians, ACLAM provides continuing education to veterinarians in the field, publishes laboratory animal textbooks, and issues position statements on issues of importance in the laboratory animal medicine field that are used by other organizations and facilities for advancement of the their animal care and use programs. ACLAM also sponsors research projects that advance the scientific knowledge of laboratory animal medicine and surgery.

Other Associations and Alternative Organizations

There are many organizations (Table 9.4) dedicated to the care and use of laboratory animals as well as those that are seeking for alternatives to animal testing (Table 9.5) (American Association for Laboratory Animal Science: Links 2012). These tables are shown below.

Agencies That Provide Regulations and Guidelines on Animal Testing

The safety testing of products in animals such as pharmaceuticals, chemicals, pesticides, cosmetics, etc. is required by law in many countries. The methods of how these tests are to be carried out are dictated by a number of regulatory bodies such as the Environmental Protection Agency (EPA), Food and Drug Administration (FDA), Department of Transportation (DOT), Pharmaceutical

Table 9.4 Associations for The care and use of laboratory animals

ACLAD – American Committee on Laboratory Animal Diseases

ASLAP – American Society of Laboratory Animal Practitioners

AMP – Americans for Medical Progress

ASM – American Society of Mammalogists

ASR – Academy of Surgical Research

AWI – Animal Welfare Institute

ANZCCART – Australian and New Zealand Council for the Care of Animals in Research and Teaching

ARENA – Applied Research Ethics National Association (PRIM&R's website)

CAAT – Center for Alternatives to Animal Testing, The Johns Hopkins University

CALAS – Canadian Association for Laboratory Animal Science

FBR – Foundation for Biomedical Research

FELASA – Federation of European Laboratory Animal Science Associations

FRAME – Fund for the Replacement of Animals in Medical Experiments

ICLAS – International Council for Laboratory Animal Science

ILAR – Institute for Laboratory Animal Research

LAMA – Laboratory Animal Management Association

LASA – Laboratory Animal Science Association (UK)

LAWTE – Laboratory Animal Welfare Training Exchange

NABR – National Association for Biomedical Research

NCA – Netherlands Centre Alternatives to Animal Use

PRIM&R – Public Responsibility in Medicine and Research

Scand-LAS – Scandinavian Society for Laboratory Animal Science

SCAW – Scientists Center for Animal Welfare

UFAW – Universities Federation for Animal Welfare

Administration and Regulation in Japan, Organisation for Economic Co-operation and Development (OECD), International Committee on Harmonization (ICH), European Commission Enterprise Directorate-General Pharmaceuticals and Cosmetics, European Regulatory Commission on the Registration, Evaluation, Authorisation and Restriction of Chemical Substances (REACH), etc. The guidelines that many of these organizations provide and their regulations are in a constant state of flux, and in order to ensure compliance with the various agencies, these regulations and guidelines should be frequently consulted. When referring to agency guidelines, attention must be paid to whether the guideline or alteration of a guideline has been accepted or is merely in draft form. For example, the OECD has a number of changes in their guidelines that are still in draft form and therefore are not the guidance that has been approved and accepted. Many of the changes in the regulations and guide-

Table 9.5 Alternatives to animal testing

Alternatives Search Service – UCDavis Center for Animal Alternatives

Alternatives to Skin Irritation Testing in Animals

ALTWEB – Center for Alternatives to Animal Testing, The Johns Hopkins University

Animal Welfare Information Center

Center for Animal Welfare, University of California – Davis

Centre for the Study of Animal Welfare (CSAW), University of Guelph

European Centre for the Validation of Alternative Methods (ECVAM)

In Vivo Imaging Community – Resources For In Vivo Imaging Researchers

Information on Alternatives Databases – hosted by the Norwegian Reference Centre for Laboratory Animal Science and Alternatives

InterNICHE Alternatives Loan System (based in Europe). List of training media and devices

isogenic.info – has two sub-webs: 15 steps in the design and statistical analysis of animal experiments and information about isogenic strains

Model Organisms for Biomedical Research – Mammalian and nonmammalian; Funding Opportunities. National Institutes of Health

National Centre for the Replacement, Refinement, and Reduction of Animals in Research (NC3Rs) – NC3Rs provides a UK focus for the promotion, development, and implementation of the 3Rs in animal research and testing. NC3Rs brings together stakeholders in the 3Rs in academia, industry, government, and animal welfare organizations to facilitate the exchange of information and ideas and the translation of research findings into practice that will benefit both animals and science

Netherlands Centre Alternatives to Animal Use – coordinating research and disseminating information on alternatives to animal experiments for the Netherlands

NORINA (Norwegian Inventory of Alternatives) – a comprehensive collection of information on audiovisual aids and other alternatives to the use of animals in teaching, at all levels from junior school to university

University of California Center for Animal Alternatives

lines address the use of animals. The European directive on cosmetic testing eliminates all animal testing of cosmetics. The testing ban on finished products has been in effect since September 11, 2004, and on ingredients or a combination of ingredients since March 11, 2009 (Commission of the European Communities 2004). The marketing ban for cosmetics tested on animals for all human health effects has been in force since March 11, 2009, with the exception of repeated dose toxicity studies, reproductive studies, and toxicokinetics. The marketing ban will apply as soon as alternatives to the three studies listed are validated and adopted by EU legislation with a maximum of 10 years after entry into force of the directive. Once 10 years have passed, the marketing ban will apply whether there are validated alternatives or not. The impetus of keeping up with this regulation is that if cosmetic companies use animal testing and attempt to market their products in Europe, they will be unable to put their product on the market. This can lead to a reduction of profitability for the company. IACUCs must be well versed in the changes in the guidelines and regulations to make sure when searching for alternatives to painful or distressful procedures they are aware of acceptable alternatives that are allowed by the various regulatory agencies. These in vitro alternatives need to be seriously considered by the client. An example of an accepted alternative is the local lymph node assay (LLNA) for sensitization where a lower species, the mouse, replaces a higher species, the guinea pig. This assay also reduces the number of animals used on a given study. Organizations such as the Interagency Coordinating Committee on the Validation of Alternative Methods (ICCVAM) and the European Centre for the Validation of Alternative Methods (ECVAM) are working diligently to validate alternative testing methods that use less animals, lower-level species, and ultimately do not even use animals. Both of these agencies also present their data to the regulatory agencies in order to obtain their acceptance of the alternative test methods.

The Food and Drug Administration has taken the position that they no longer require Draize testing (acute ocular or dermal irritation studies) or the performance of LD50 determinations. They also want species justification to ensure that the proper species is being used in the safety evaluation of a compound (Schofield 2011). The FDA has indicated that the nonhuman primate should only be used if absolutely necessary which will require that a suitable justification for their use be provided. In addition to the efficacy of a compound in a particular species, the availability as well as the feasibility of performing the required techniques in a particular species also needs to be taken into consideration. For example, the daily intravenous administration or blood withdrawal in guinea pigs is not feasible unless cannulated animals are used. Once animals are modified, cost as well as the development of complications induced by these modifications must be taken into consideration when planning a study and the interpretation of results. The OECD has modified the LD50 for chemical testing to an up-down procedure which uses fewer animals but still provides the necessary data. In the past, animals had to die on an LD50 study, but now the OECD has established endpoints that may be used to determine if an animal is moribund in order to humanely euthanize rather than allowing it to die on its own (Organisation for Economic Co-operation and Development 2000). Again, one needs to stay abreast of the changes in the guidelines and regulatory requirements in order to ensure compliance with the regulatory agencies and ensure the marketability of a product as well as to use the least amount of the proper species of animals humanely.

Facilities – An Overview

Proper Care and Use of Animals

How a facility that uses animals is managed should be based on the requirements of the animals being housed. Documents that provide guidance on the proper care and use of laboratory animals are *Guide for the Care and Use of Laboratory Animals* (Committee for the Update of the Guide for the Care and Use of Laboratory Animals 2011, the *Guide for the Care and Use of Agricultural Animals in Research and Teaching* (Federation of Animal Science Societies, *Ag Guide* 2010) and the European Convention for the Protection of Vertebrate Animals Used for Experimental and Other Scientific Purposes, Council of Europe (ETS 123) as well as other guidances depending on the country of residence or the organizations for which research is being conducted. Various departments of the US Government have their own guidelines in addition to the Guides (Guide, NRC 2011; Ag Guide, FASS 2012) and the Animal Welfare Act/Regulations on the use of animals in research or testing that must also be followed when research or testing is performed or funded by the departments. Examples include the Department of Defense (DoD) (Department of Defense 2012), Department of Veterans Affairs (Department of Veterans Affairs 2011), and the National Institutes of Mental Health (National Institutes of Mental Health 2002). In addition to general and agency/department guidelines, guidelines have been formulated for the care and use of animals used in particular types of research such as behavioral research (Committee on Guidelines for the Use of Animals in Neuroscience and Behavioral Research 2003). Recommendations based on species can also be found throughout the literature (Committee on Dogs 1994). Regulatory bodies such as OECD also have recommendations on the proper care and use of animals for testing that can be found in their testing guidelines. The use of animals in research is a privilege and not a right. To this effect, animals used for research must be treated humanely and with respect as they are living entities with very similar perceptions and reactions to their environment and manipulations that humans have. With this in mind, the *US Government Principles for Utilization and Care of*

Vertebrate Animals Used in Testing, Research, and Training should be accepted and endorsed (see Table 9.2) by all facilities and organizations that promote and support research and testing such as the Society of Toxicology (Society of Toxicology 2008) In order to best follow these principles, it is very important to always take into consideration the 3R's (Replacement, Reduction, and Refinement) (Russell and Burch 1959). Whenever a proposal to use animals is made, it should be carefully scrutinized to ensure that the 3R's have been applied. Are the proper numbers of animals being used? Through the use of pilot studies and statistical power analysis, the minimal number of animals to use on the study can be determined rather than just picking an arbitrary number of animals that is not based on any type of scientific data or method. Carefully evaluating animal numbers is very important since choosing the number of animals in an attempt to reduce the use of animals may not always be in the best interest of the study and the information needed. Not enough animals may cause the study to fail which may in turn require the use of more animals as the entire study may have to be repeated rather than conducting the first study with more animals that would allow for proper data collection and interpretation. Reducing animal numbers without good justification can actually lead to an increase in the number of animals used rather than a "reduction." Refinements can often be made to study proposals such as using whole body imaging over time rather than sacrificing animals at each time point. This is not only a refinement, it is a reduction in animal numbers. Nursing care for ill animals that can occur with various research models such as nerve injury models, specific disease models, etc. is considered a refinement as the discomfort of animals is being alleviated. Complete replacement of animals in testing and research is the ultimate goal when searching for alternatives, but often this is not possible, but it may be possible to use a lower species such as substituting a fish for a rat or rabbit in developmental studies. There are currently a number of assays that have been developed and are being developed to replace the use of animals especially in the field of skin and eye irritation studies that historically have used the rabbit.

Training Personnel

Animal care and research staff training is an important aspect for the success of an animal care and use program as well as the successful collection of scientific data for the benefit of man and animals. Training can be accomplished through various mechanisms such as hands-on training, professional society meetings with training seminars, online training courses, in-house seminars, etc. Documentation of training should be implemented, which will allow an accurate assessment of an employee's abilities. Training documentation is also required by many agencies such as FDA, EPA, USDA, AAALAC, etc. Employee proficiency at a specific task should always be assessed at a timely point prior to the employee actually performing the task in order to ensure that proper animal care and use is being performed. This safeguards the animals as well as the employee from injury and ensures that animals are being taken care of and manipulated in an acceptable manner. The IACUC is also responsible for assuring that personnel working with animals from principal investigators (PI) to animal care staff are properly trained. Proper training is often assessed when post-approval monitoring (PAM) is performed by the IACUC. During PAM the proficiency of investigators and technical staff can be evaluated as study records and actual performance of the technique(s) can be reviewed. The veterinary staff is also responsible for training and determining proficiency of personnel involved in projects, animal husbandry techniques, handling techniques, dosing techniques, and sample collection techniques. Any deficiencies identified must be immediately addressed, and retraining of individuals needs to be implemented immediately. Recertification of staff should also be considered especially for techniques that are not routinely performed and to help curb drift from proper standard procedure. In addition to animal care and research staff training, IACUC members require training to ensure they have the proper knowledge and understanding of their responsibilities as an IACUC member.

Occupational Health and Safety Program

An occupational health and safety program (OH&S) should be established by each institution. If the institution is governed by regulatory bodies (USDA, OLAW) or accredited by AAALAC, an OH&S program is required. The OH&S program should ensure that the facility complies with all federal (OSHA), state (DEP), and local regulations and establish safety practices that safeguard employee health. The presence of a safety committee is highly recommended and in some cases required by regulatory agencies to oversee ongoing evaluations of health and safety, conduct facility inspections, facilitate communication, and promote occupational health and safety at the facility. The OH&S program must conduct a risk assessment evaluation of the various procedures carried out at the facility as well as an evaluation of potential exposure to hazardous substances such as chemicals, biologic agents, radiation, physical hazards, and exposure to animals. Based upon a risk assessment, appropriate precautions to guard personnel against potential hazards must be instituted (Committee on Occupational Safety and Health in Research Animal Facilities 1997). Appropriate precautions include the proper and effective use of personal protective equipment (PPE). Appropriate PPE must be made available to all personnel working in an area that contains a hazard that requires the use of PPE. Proper PPE will be determined based on the hazards present in a given area. Personnel must receive the proper training on how to use the required PPE, and this training should be documented. Standard operating procedures (SOP) should be written covering when and how PPE should be used. If respirators are part of the required PPE, personnel must receive respirator fit testing yearly as well as periodic medical evaluations to ensure that individuals are physically and physiologically competent to wear a respirator.

Medical evaluations of personnel working with animals should be conducted pre-employment and then on a routine basis to assess the development of any physical impairments that could potentially preclude an individual from performing their duties or that may require modifications of an individual's work environment in order to allow them to continue in their current position. An example would be the development of allergies. Latex allergies may require the facility to provide alternate glove material. Animal allergies may require the facility to offer medical treatment for the allergies such as hyposensitization treatment, limitations in the types of species the individual can work with, and/or PPE that provides a higher degree of protection from the presence of airborne allergens. There are cases where some individuals will no longer be able to work with animals, and the facility may need to provide them with alternate job requirements. Proper immunization programs should be established as necessary. Personnel working with animals should be current with their tetanus immunization status. If it has been determined that personnel have a risk of rabies exposure such as those working with wildlife, bats and raccoons, with the rabies virus on research projects, rabies prophylactic vaccination should be provided. Personnel working with human-based materials should be provided with the opportunity for hepatitis B immunization. Other immunizations may be offered based on risk assessment. The training and screening for the presence of zoonotic disease should be instituted based on potential exposure to these entities. Personnel working with nonhuman primates should be screened at least yearly for tuberculosis. The measles status of personnel is also important since measles can be contracted from nonhuman primates or alternatively; personnel with an active measles infection can in turn infect nonhuman primates. Since diseases can be spread from people to animals, policies should be in place to address the proper precautions that should be taken by personnel when they are ill. Polices should also be in place to address personnel with special needs such as those that are immunocompromised, pregnant, etc. All medical information obtained must meet the confidentiality requirements as well as other medical and legal factors that are required by federal, state, and local laws.

Personnel training on safety in the workplace is absolutely essential in the animal testing and research environment. Policies and SOPs must be in place to address the proper precautions that must be taken when working in a laboratory setting. Eating, drinking, using tobacco products, applying cosmetics, and handling contacts in laboratories and animal rooms should be strictly forbidden. Proper personnel hygiene should be reviewed such as frequent handwashing, changing into appropriate uniforms and dedicated facility shoes, showering procedures, etc. Proper facility and equipment safeguards should be in place as appropriate for the hazard being addressed and functioning properly. Policies on facility security should be in place and strictly enforced. Excellent sources of information when developing an OH&S program include *Occupational Health and Safety in the Care and Use of Laboratory Animals* (Committee on Occupational Safety and Health in Research Animal Facilities 1997), OSHA regulations, and the *Biosafety in Microbiological and Biomedical Laboratories* (United States Department of Health and Human Services 2009).

Husbandry

Facilities that utilize animals for research and testing must provide the species housed with the proper environmental conditions, housing, and husbandry requirements. The equipment needed will depend upon the species that is or area to be housed. It can be as simple as the purchase of filtered polycarbonate shoebox cages on a shelf in an environmentally controlled room to house mice to as complicated as the group housing of nonhuman primates with extensive environmental enrichment devices along with ancillary equipment to separate out the animals when manipulations are required. In the laboratory setting, the temperature, humidity, lighting, and ventilation are controlled to keep the animals healthy as well as to reduce variables in testing and research projects. Parameters for these environmental factors can be found in the *Guide for the Care and Use of Laboratory Animals* (Committee for the Update of the Guide for the Care and Use of Laboratory Animals 2011). Caging must be adequate for the species that is to be housed and to allow for species-specific behaviors. There are many different types of caging that are available, from wire-bottomed or grate-type stainless steel cages to solid bottom plastic cages. Solid bottom caging is now being advocated as the standard for the housing of rodents. It is felt that rodents are more comfortable in solid bottom cages with bedding and the development and incidence of foot lesions that have been associated with long-term housing on wire-bottom cages are avoided. Wire-bottom cages have been the standard in toxicology testing for many years and still confer the benefits of being able to evaluate the changes in fecal output, fecal consistency, urine amount and color, and the presence or absence of food crumbling. All of these observations can provide a significant amount of information of the effect of a compound on a rodent. Some of these changes may eventually be observed in a rodent on bedding, but the observation is picked up in a more timely fashion when the cage paper under a wire-bottomed cage is observed on a daily basis. This can also aid in the more timely assessment of an animal's health since changes in the characteristics of urine and feces can be one of the first signs that an animal may be having health issues. There is some evidence in the literature that rats do not necessarily prefer solid bottom caging over wire-bottom caging (Rock et al. 2000).

Animals also need to be provided with food and water (generally ad libitum) on a daily basis. Animals must be fed diets that provide them with adequate nutrition, and in some cases where studies are to be conducted under Good Laboratory Practice (GLP), animals are fed certified diets. Certified diets come with a contamination profile, so there is evidence that the level of substances considered to be contaminants is below levels that are set by agencies such as EPA and FDA. Diets can also be autoclavable or irradiated to ensure they are sterile when fed to animals that may be immunocompromised or to animals in barrier facilities to prevent contamination of the barrier by an organism or organisms contained in the diet. As mentioned previously, many species are fed ad libitum, but animals that are housed long term are often limit fed to prevent the development of obesity. All animals must be provided with potable water, and this is usually supplied through an automatic watering system or a manual system such as water bottles/sacks, bowls, etc. Water is treated in many ways (reverse osmosis, acidified, autoclaved, etc.) depending on the requirements of the facility and the work they are doing. Cages must be cleaned and sanitized according to a set schedule. How frequently this is done depends on a number of factors. The USDA has specific cleaning and sanitization requirements depending on the species. The *Guide* is more opened-ended and performance-based in the recommended requirements, and the frequency of cleaning is based on "the maintenance of environmental conditions conducive to health and well-being" of the animals (Committee for the Update of the Guide for the Care and Use of Laboratory Animals 2011). The *Guide* has assumed this stance over time and with experience, and through the studying of animal behavior, it has been found that many species do not like to have their caging cleaned too frequently and it is actually stressful to the animals if you change bedding or caging too often. The proper equipment such as cage washers, tunnel washers, etc. to adequately clean and sanitize caging and accessories must be made available by the facility.

Enrichment

Enrichment programs for laboratory animals should be developed by each facility and approved by the IACUC. The amount and type of enrichment provided will depend upon the research being conducted or the testing with which the animals are involved. Ideally, for GLP studies, enrichment items should have a contaminant evaluation performed on them (certified) and a contaminant profile established, but practically this may be extremely cost prohibitive as well as severely limiting the types of items that can be used for enrichment. Therefore, at a minimum, items made of inert materials should be used, and for food enrichment, the items should be fit or acceptable for human consumption. Enrichment for various species can run the gamut of caging complexity and type to the manipulation of the variety of different food stuffs. Ideally items used as toys should be rotated regularly since animals will get bored with the same toys all the time, and this does not add to enrichment of the environment. Researchers must also be cognizant of the fact that if certain environmental changes are made, the model being studied may not work as expected since manipulation of the environment can affect the outcome of a study. It has also been found that some types of enrichment can be detrimental to the welfare of the animals causing injury or the development of a guarding type of behavior. When enrichment programs are being planned, research should be performed into the supply of the proper enrichment for the animals by using resources such as the scientific literature, the previous experience of peers, and/or observations recorded from actual in-house studies.

Veterinary Care

Veterinary care must be provided to all laboratory animals. This is a requirement of all agencies and programs that oversee laboratory animal care. The veterinary care program is the responsibility of the attending veterinarian (AV). The AV ideally should be board-certified in laboratory animal science and medicine, but veterinarians with suitable training or experience in laboratory animal science and medicine or those otherwise qualified in the care of the species are also considered adequate for the position. Keep in mind that a nonveterinarian cannot practice veterinary medicine. An adequate veterinary care program consists of the assessment of animal well-being and the effective management of animal procurement and transportation; preventive medicine; understanding of clinical disease, disability, or related health issues; protocol-associated disease, disability, or other sequelae; surgery and perioperative care; pain and distress; anesthesia and analgesia; and euthanasia (Committee for the Update of the Guide for the Care and Use of Laboratory Animals 2011). Trained personnel such as veterinary technicians, animal care technicians, research technicians, etc. can conduct many aspects of the program of veterinary care as long as they remain in timely contact with the veterinarian concerning any issues that may occur. The AV when reviewing protocols must assess the proper use of anesthetics and analgesics provided to the animals in the research proposal. The proper use constitutes selection of the appropriate anesthetic and/or analgesia for the type of research being conducted and species being used (Acred et al. 1994; Baumans et al. 1994). Improper selection can result in the less than adequate control of pain or the confounding or masking of study results. For example, if electroencephalograms (EEGs) are being studied to predict seizure activity, it would be inappropriate to use ketamine for any reason as this can reduce the seizure threshold in animals and actually cause seizure-like activity in animals that normally have a low seizure threshold. The use of ketamine in this situation would confound and or mask the study results. The frequency of dosing the animals must also be reasonable. If treatment is not frequent enough, breakthrough pain will occur, which does not provide adequate pain control, and too frequent dosing can lead to overdose and the development of adverse consequences such as severe respiratory depression or death as in the case of opioids. The AV should be knowledgeable with regard to the proper selection of analgesics and anesthetics in a wide variety of research situations, have a working knowledge of a potential drug and possible procedural interactions, and provide guidance to the investigators concerning these factors. The AV should also provide guidance to the investigators concerning the performance of the surgical procedures that are being conducted in research proposals. The assessment of proper pre-, intra-, and postsurgical techniques such as the use of proper aseptic technique, tissue handling, actual surgical methodology, appropriate post-op care, etc. is the responsibility of the AV. The assessment of the surgical procedure should include a review of the description of the procedure; direct oversight of the actual procedures; review of pre-op, surgical, and post-op records; assessment of animals postoperatively; and review of study of clinical observation records.

In addition to surgery and pain management in laboratory animals, the AV also provides guidance on animal procurement, appropriate transportation methods, husbandry, animal handling and restraint, medical treatment, euthanasia, dosing, and sample collection. Animals should be procured from reputable vendors that have been approved by the attending veterinarian. Animals obtained from approved vendors are least likely to have health problems or infectious disease issues. Following these simple procedures will in turn reduce the times for animal quarantine and avoid or minimize the possibility of an infectious agent from confounding the data. Animals from non-approved vendors should have extended quarantine time periods, and in some cases, special precautions should be used when handling these animals for the duration of the study in order to prevent the possible spread of any disease or disease agent (cases of subclinical disease) throughout the facility. In the case of animals that are going to remain in the facility for extensive lengths of time, scheduled health screens can be performed at multiple time points, and if infectious disease entities are found, the animals could be rederived. Acclimation times also need to be set to allow the animals to become accustomed to their new environment. Health surveillance programs as well as biosecurity protocols should be in place to ensure animal health as well as the collection of valid scientific data.

The AV should also be providing guidance on multiple aspects of study design and execution of technique. Dose volume limitations as well as blood volume collection limitations need to be established and are often set based on personal experience and the scientific literature (Morton et al. 2001; Diehl et al. 2001). Vehicle use should be monitored to ensure that the vehicles being used do not cause severe local irritation or systemic toxicity (Gad et al. 2006). Personnel handling of the animals and performing various techniques on them need to be properly trained. The AV is responsible for ensuring that personnel are receiving the appropriate training and that the methods are being performed properly. The AV is often involved in helping to develop new techniques and teaching others to perform these techniques. Animal restraint must be performed properly and be of minimal duration to get the job done. Animals should be acclimated to restraint devices prior to their regular use, and limits should be in place on the length of time that an animal can actually be physically restrained. The appropriateness of chemical restraint should also be considered for animals that pose a safety hazard to personnel and themselves, such as very large animals or nonhuman primates. Appropriate medical treatment should be prescribed by the AV as necessary. The condition of any animal requiring treatment needs to be assessed to determine if the condition is resolving, remaining the same, or getting worse. If the condition is not resolving, the treatment should be changed or the animal should be euthanized. Determination that a condition has resolved and treatment can be stopped should be made by the veterinarian or the veterinarian's designee. The AV is also responsible to ensure that the proper methods of euthanasia are being used and that personnel performing euthanasia are properly trained and proficient at the procedure.

Disaster Preparedness

All facilities should have a disaster preparedness plan in place. A disaster plan is required by USDA, OLAW, and AAALAC. Facilities can experience catastrophic events anytime whether from the forces of nature (i.e., hurricanes, tornados, severe winter storms, earthquakes, pandemics, etc.) or from human acts or error (i.e., vandalism, terrorist acts, prolonged power outages, fire). Plans must be in place on how to provide the animals with food, water, heating, cooling, and ventilation when a disaster strikes. While a copy of the plan should be on site, the original version should also be stored off-site. Provisions must also be made if the basic essentials for animals cannot be provided and/ or biosecurity has been breached. Responsible investigators should be involved in determining which animals should be relocated if relocation is an option. If animals can be relocated, what animals are going to be relocated and what priority, exactly how they are going to be transported, and to where they are to be transported are all questions that need to be addressed in the disaster plan. If animals cannot be relocated and cannot be provided for in an acceptable fashion during the disaster, they should be humanely euthanized. The possibility of the occurrence of animal injury also needs to be addressed, include the documentation of plans for treatment or euthanasia. The methods of euthanasia and personnel who will perform these methods need to be stated. Emergency contact information must be included in the document and readily and easily available to essential personnel. A chain of command needs to be established so employees know the proper steps to take in the event of a disaster. Personnel safety must be ensured. The disaster plan should be approved by the facilities administration or management. It is highly recommended that the disaster preparedness plan be rehearsed by essential personnel to ensure individuals have a working knowledge of their roles in the event of a disaster plan.

Domestic and International Terrorism

Animal rights (AR) groups are ubiquitous in countries all over the world, and how they get their message across covers the gamut of expression, from advertisements, media use, peaceful protests to vandalism, threats, and physical harm. Many of the animal rights groups outright identify themselves as such and include groups such as the People for the Ethical Treatment of Animals (PETA), the Animal Liberation Front (ALF), Stop Animal Exploitation Now (SAEN), National Anti-Vivisection Society (NAVS), Stop Huntingdon Animal Cruelty (SHAC), and the list goes on. Then there are those groups that do not outright identify themselves as animal rights groups in order to convince the public that they are either trying to improve animal welfare or human welfare. Examples of such covert groups are the Humane Society of the United States (HSUS) and the Physicians Committee for Responsible Medicine (PCRM). The goal of animal rights groups is to abolish the use of animals by humans and even the association of animals in a companion way with humans. The prohibition of the use of animals for research, testing, and in education is one of their primary goals. Different groups attempt to accomplish this in different way. HSUS tends to use the political arena and the media. This group is large enough and powerful enough, considering their budget is over $100 million dollars a year that it uses its influence to help introduce bills at the local, state, and federal levels. They use their money to help assure that government candidates that support their cause gain offices. Unfortunately HSUS tends to be misleading the public into thinking they are a humane society meaning they actually use the donations given to them to help animals by caring for them, feeding them, and finding homes for them. They do very little of this and contribute very little money to local humane society shelters. PETA is also attempting to expand their influence by methods other than sensationalism by buying shares in companies such as big pharmaceutical companies so that they can try to influence the shareholder votes concerning the use of animals in research and testing. PETA also uses local ordinances to file petty lawsuits against institutions that use animals for research and testing. They often use state sunshine laws in an attempt to get information on research projects from universities that use animals since universities are publicly funded. They then in turn use this information in sensationalistic and malicious ways to satisfy their own needs – *make money*. The interests that these organizations follow are concurrent with the money train. When the money on a given issue dries up, they are off to a new issue. The majority of the AR groups also like to use the media to further their cause. They often create outlandish campaigns to get the media and public's attention. They often take pictures and collect or make statements that are purposely taken out of context to convince the public of the horrible conditions and procedures to which laboratory animals are subjected. Government records such as USDA annual reports and inspection reports are available to the public and are the "golden fleece" for these organizations, since they use these reports and twist the information in them to "show" the public all of the "violations" that are occurring at research facilities and that should incense caring individuals. However they rarely if ever give the complete picture. The methods of protest described here are legal and not violent, but there are groups such as ALF and SHAC that have resorted to activities of harassment and violence to further their cause. ALF has openly and unapologetically made public claims to vandalizing institutions and harassing and physically attacking researchers. The members of SHAC relentlessly harassed Huntingdon Life Science (HLS) staff and other companies associated with Huntingdon that provided supplies or services in an attempt to shut the company down. In response to violent acts committed by these groups and others who claim their actions were in the best interests of animals, the United States passed the Animal Enterprise

Terrorism Act (AETA) (S.3880 2006) on November 27, 2006. This act allows the Department of Justice to apprehend, prosecute, and convict individuals committing acts of animal enterprise terror. Seven members of SHAC dubbed the SHAC 7 were the first individuals convicted of attempting to shut down an animal enterprise company, HLS, through harassment and threats. These individuals are currently serving various jail times. Other countries are currently passing laws to protect institutions that perform animal research, but there are governments that are buying into the animal rights movement as a result of public influence and infiltration of government officials by animal rights advocates. The research community needs to continue to educate the public with regard to the necessity of animal research as a benefit to both human and animal health. Organizations such as the National Association for Biomedical Research (NABR), Foundation for Biomedical Research (FBR) (Foundation for Biomedical Research 2012), and Americans for Medical Progress (AMP) (Americans for Medical Progres, 2012) are advocates for biomedical research. These organizations can be very helpful and can provide a copious supply of useful information with regard to animal rights activities and protection against such activities. They are making a concerted effort to educate the general public about the benefits of biomedical research through the use of various types of media such as educational pamphlets, television commercials, educational materials for schools, billboards, magazines, novels, etc. (Americans for Medical Progress, 2012).

References

Acred, P., Hennessey, T. D., MacArthur-Clark, J. A., Merrikin, D. J., Ryan, D. M., Smulders, H. C., Troke, P. F., Wilson, R. G., & Straughan, D. W. (1994). Guidelines for the welfare of animals in rodent protection tests: A report from the Rodent Protection Test Working Party. *Laboratory Animals, 28*(1), 13–18.

AAALAC: About AAALAC, "AAALAC International Mission Statement." (n.d.). *AAALAC*. Retrieved 20 Nov 2012 from http://www.aaalac.org/about/mission.cfm

AAALAC: About AAALAC, "What is AAALAC?" (n.d.). *AAALAC*. Retrieved 20 Nov 2012 from http://www.aaalac.org/about/index.cfm

AAALAC: Accreditation, "Benefits of AAALAC International Accreditation." (n.d.). *AAALAC*. Retrieved 20 Nov 2012 from http://www.aaalac.org/accreditation/benefits

American Association for Laboratory Animal Science: About AAALAS, "About AAALAS." (n.d.). *AALAS*. Retrieved 30 Nov 2012 from http://www.aalas.org/association/about.aspx

American Association for Laboratory Animal Science: Links (n.d.). *AALAS*. Retrieved 30 Nov 2012 from http://www.aalas.org/links.aspx

American Veterinary Medical Association. (2007). AVMA guidelines on Euthanasia. *Am. Vet. Med. Assoc.*

Americans for Medical Progress: "Because Research Needs Advocates" (n.d.). *AMP.* Retrieved 18 Dec 2012 from http://www.amprogress.org

Applied Research Ethics National Association, Office of Laboratory Animal Welfare. (2002). *Institutional animal care and use committee guidebook* (2nd ed.). Office of Laboratory Animal Welfare, National Institutes of Health.

Bennett, B. T. (2012). *Examining USDA's "age of enforcement".* Webinar: National Association for Biomedical Research. Bethesda, MD.

Baumans, V., Brain, P. F., Brugere, H., Clausing, P., Jeneskog, T., & Perretta, G. (1994). Pain and distress in laboratory rodents and lagomorphs: Report of the Federation of European Laboratory Animal Science Associations (FELASA) Working Group on Pain and Distress accepted by the FELASA Board of Management November 1992. *Laboratory Animals, 28*(2), 97–112.

Brewer, N. R.. (1999). Chapter 1 the architectonics of laboratory animal science. American Association for Laboratory Animal Science. Retrieved 30 Nov 2012 from http://www.aalas.org/association/history.aspx

Canadian Council on Animal Care. (1980). *Guide to the care and use of experimental animals volume 1.* Ottawa: Canadian Council on Animal Care.

Canadian Council on Animal Care. (1984). *Guide to the care and use of experimental animals volume 2.* Ottawa: Canadian Council on Animal Care.

Canadian Council on Animal Care. (1998). *Guidelines on: Choosing an appropriate endpoint in experiments using animals for research, teaching and testing.* Ottawa: Canadian Council on Animal Care.

Canadian Council on Animal Care. (2010). *CCAC guidelines on: Euthanasia of animals used in science.* Ottawa: Canadian Council on Animal Care.

Committee on Dogs, Institute of Laboratory Animal Resources, & Commission on Life Sciences. (1994). *Laboratory animal management: Dogs.* Bethesda, MD: National Academies Press.

Committee on Guidelines for the Use of Animals in Neuroscience and Behavioral Research, Institute for Laboratory Animal Research. National Research Council. Division on Earth and Life Studies, & National Academies Press. (2003). *Guidelines for the care and use of mammals in neuroscience and behavioral research.* Bethesda, MD: National Academies Press.

Committee on Long-Term Care of Chimpanzees. Institute for Laboratory Animal Research, Commission of Life Sciences, National Research Council. (1997). *Chimpanzees in research: Strategies for their ethical care, management, and use.* Bethesda, MD: National Academies Press.

Committee on Occupational Safety and Health in Research Animal Facilities, Institute of Laboratory Animal Resources, Commission on Life Sciences, National Research Council. (1997). *Occupational health and safety in the care and use of research animals.* Bethesda, MD: National Academies Press.

Committee on Pain and Distress in Laboratory Animals, Institute of Laboratory Animal Resources, & Commission on Life Sciences. (1992). *Recognition and alleviation of pain and distress in laboratory animals.* Bethesda, MD: National Academies Press.

Committee for the Update of the Guide for the Care and Use of Laboratory Animals, Institute for Laboratory Animal Research, Division of Earth and Life Studies, National Research

Council. (2011). *Guide for the care and use of laboratory animals* (8th ed.). Bethesda, MD: National Academies Press.

Committee on Well-Being of Nonhuman Primates, Institute for Laboratory Animal Research, Commission on Life Sciences, National Research Council. (1998). *The psychological well-being of nonhuman primates*. Bethesda, MD: National Academies Press.

Commission of the European Communities, Commission Staff Working Document. (2004). *Timetables for the phasing-out of animal testing in the framework of the 7th Amendment to the Cosmetics Directive (Council Directive 76/768/EEC)*. Retrieved 4 Dec 2012 from http://ec.europa.eu/consumers/sectors/cosmetics/animal-testin/index_en.htm.

Department of Defense, Directive No. 3216.01. (2012). Use of animals in DoD programs. Arlington, VA.

Department of Veterans Affairs, Veterans Health Administration, VHA Handbook 1200.7. (2011). *Use of animals in research*. Arlington, VA: Department of Veterans Affairs.

Diehl, K. H., Hull, R., Morton, D., Pfister, R., Rabemampianina, Y., Smith, D., Vidal, J. M., & van de Vorstenbosch, C. (2001). European Federation of Pharmaceutical Industries Association and European Centre for the validation of alternative methods. *Journal of Applied Toxicology, 21*(1), 15–23.

ETS 123: European Convention for the Protection of Vertebrae Animals used for Experimental and Other Scientific Purposes. (1986). Strasbourg 18.111.

Federal Register, Vol. 77, No. 250, rules and regulations. 2012, Dec 31. Department of Agriculture, Animal and Plant Health Inspection Service, 9 CFR Parts 2 and 3. *Handling of animals; contingency plans*.

Federation of Animal Science Societies (FASS). (2010). *Guide for the care and use of agricultural animals in research and teaching* (3rd ed.). Federation of Animal Science Societies. Bethesda, MD.

Foundation for Biomedical Research. (2012). Mission statement. Retrieved 18 Dec 2012 from http://www.fbresearch.org

Gad, S. C., Cassidy, C. D., Aubert, N., Spainhour, B., & Robbe, H. (2006). Nonclinical vehicle use in studies by multiple routes in multiple species. *International Journal of Toxicology, 25*, 499–521.

Gordon, H. S. (1999). Chapter 21 the history of the public health service policy on the humane care and use of laboratory animals. American Association for Laboratory Animal Science. Retrieved 30 Nov 2012 from http://www.aalas.org/association/history.aspx

H.R. 2256 (112): Pet Safety and Protection Act of 2011, 112th Congress, 1st Sess. (2011). *GPO*. http://www.gpo.gov

Middleton, C. C. (1999). Chapter 4 The History of the American College of Laboratory Animal Medicine. American Association for Laboratory Animal Science. Retrieved 30 Nov 2012 from http://www.aalas.org/association/history.aspx

Miller, J. G., Clark, J. D. (1999). Chapter 6 The History of the Association for Assessment and Accreditation of Laboratory Animal Care International. American Association for Laboratory Animal Science. Retrieved 30 Nov 2012 from http://www.aalas.org/association/history.aspx

Morton, D. B., Jennings, M., Buckwell, A., Ewbank, R., Godfrey, C., Holgate, B., Inglis, I., James, R., Page, C., Sharman, I., Verschoyle, L., Westall, L., & Wilson, A. B. (2001). *"Refining procedures for the administration of substances"*: A report of the BVAAWF/FRAME/RSPCA/UFAW Joint Working Group on Refinement. *Laboratory Animals, 35*, 1–41.

Mulder, J. B. (1999). Chapter 2 creation and development of AALAS programs. American Association for Laboratory Animal Science. Retrieved 30 Nov 2012 from http://www.aalas.org/association/history.aspx

National Association for Biomedical Research. Animal Law Section. (n.d.). *NABR*. Retrieved 4 Sep 2012 from http://www.nabranimallaw.org

National Institute of Mental Health. (2002). In A. R. Morrison, H. L. Evans, N. A. Ator, & R. K. Nakamura (Eds.), *Methods and welfare considerations in behavioral research with animals: Report of a National Institutes of Health Workshop.* NIH Publication No. 02–5083. Washington, DC: U.S. Government Printing Office.

National Research Council (2011). Guide for the Care and Use of Laboratory animals, National Academies of Science. Washington, DC.

Nosengo, N. (2012, 10 July). Italian scientists fight tightened rules on animal testing. *Nature.com.* Retrieved 7August 2012 from http://www.nature.com.

Office of Laboratory Animal Welfare, Office of Extramural Research, National Institutes of Health. (2002). *Public health service policy on humane care and use of animals.* Bethesda, MD: National Institutes of Health.

Office of Extramural Research (OER) Web Site. (n.d.). *PHS Policy on Humane Care and Use of Laboratory Animals, Frequently Asked Questions.* National Institutes of Health. Retrieved 11 Jul 2008 from http://grants.nih.gov/grants/olaw/faqs.htm

Organization for Economic Co-operation and Development. (2000). *Guidance document on the recognition, assessment, and use of clinical signs as humane endpoints for experimental animals used in safety evaluation.* Geneva: Organization for Economic Co-operation and Development.

Pennsylvania Veterinary Medical Association. Veterinary Laws & Regs. (n.d.). *pvma.* Retrieved 4 Sep 2012 from http://www.pavma.org

Rock, F. M., Jaslow, B. W., Peterson, A, Kaeppeli, M. K., Price, J. L. (2000). Preference of Single Housed Rats for Solid-Bottom or Wire-Bottom Stainless Steel Cage Floor. Poster Session (PS28) Contemporary Topics in Laboratory Animal Science, 39(4), July 2000. Bethesda, MD: American Association of Laboratory Animal Science.

Russell, W. S., & Burch, R. L. (1959). *The principles of humane experimental technique.* London: Methuen & Company.

S.810: Great Ape Protection and Cost Savings Act of 2011, 112th Cong., 1st Sess. (2011). *GPO.* http://www.gpo.gov

S.3880: Animal Enterprise Terrorism Act (2006; 109th Congress). (n.d.). *govtrack.us.* Retrieved 14 Dec 2012 from http://govtrack.us/congress/bills/109/s3880

Schofield, J. S. (2011). Animal-health pharmaceuticals: Research responsibilities and efforts in target animal safety and laboratory animal welfare. *Futures, 3*(7), 851–854.

Schwindaman, D. F. (1999). Chapter 20 the history of the Animal Welfare Act. American Association for Laboratory Animal Science. Retrieved 30 Nov 2012 from http://www.aalas.org/association/history.aspx

Silverman, J., Suckow, M. A., & Murthy, S. (Eds.). (2007). *The IACUC handbook.* CRC.

Society of Toxicology. Guiding principles in the use of animals in toxicology. (2008). *Society of toxicology.* Retrieved 28 Mar 12 from http://www.toxicology.org/ai/air/air6.asp

The European Parliament and the Council of the European Union. Directive 2010/63/EU of the European Parliament and of the Council of 22 Sep 2010 on the Protection of Animals Used for Scientific Purposes. Official Journal for the European Union. (2010). Brussels, Belgium.

United States Department of Agriculture. Animal and Plant Health Inspection Service. (2006). *The animal welfare act: An overview.* Washington, DC: US Department of Agriculture.

United States Department of Agriculture, Marketing and Regulatory Programs, Animal and Plant Health Inspection Service, Animal Care. (2011). *Animal care resource guide policies.* Washington, DC: US Department of Agriculture.

United States Department of Agriculture. Animal and Plant Health Inspection Service (2002), *Animal Welfare Act and Animal Welfare Regulations,* as found in Animal Welfare Act of May 13, 2002. As found in the United States Code. Title 7 – Agriculture, Chapter 54 – Transportation, Sale, and Handling of Certain Animals. Sections 2131–2159.

United States Department of Agriculture. Animal and Plant Health Inspection Service. Animal Care. (2012). *Animal care inspection guide.* Retrieved 8 Aug 2012 from http://www.aphis.usda.gov/animal_welfare/downloads/Consolidated_Inspection_Guide/AC%20Consolidated%20Inspection%20Guide%-%Complete.pdf.

United States Department of Health and Human Services, Public Health Service, Centers for Disease Control and Prevention, National Institutes of Health. (2009). *Biosafety in microbiological and biomedical laboratories* (5th ed.). HHS Publication No. (CDC) 21–112. Washington, DC.

United States Department of Health and Human Services, Public Health Service, National Institutes of Health. (1988). *Institutional Administrator's manual for laboratory animal care and use.* Office of Protection from Research Risks. Washington, DC.

United States Department of Health and Human Services. Office of Laboratory Animal Welfare. (n.d.) Position statements: OLAW responds to concerns regarding adoption of the care and use of laboratory animals: Eight Edition National Institutes of Health. Retrieved 1 Jun 2012 from http://grants.nih.gov/grants/olaw/positionstatement_guide.htm

Wolfle, T. L. (1999). Chapter 7 the history of the Institute of Laboratory Animal Resources 1953–1999. American Association for Laboratory Animal Science. Retrieved 30 Nov 2012 from http://www.aalas.org/association/history.aspx

The Inner Cro: Pathology – Necropsy and Gross Pathology

10

Charles B. Spainhour and Shayne C. Gad

Introduction and Basic Concepts

A well-managed necropsy operation provides a system that assures that all protocol-required tissues and gross lesions are observed, recorded, and properly fixed, for possible future histopathology evaluation. In regulated safety studies, a necropsy is performed to determine the possible cause of death and/or to detect induced or coincidental pathological alterations in tissues. Typically a complete necropsy includes examination of the external aspects of the body, all orifices; the cranial, thoracic, abdominal, and pelvic cavities and their contents; and the musculature, subcutis, and bone. However, gross observations only types of necropsies can also be performed depending upon the type of study, the objective of the study, or the limitations set by the protocol and the sponsor.

Pathology is defined as a field of medical science that studies the essential nature of disease, with particular attention being paid to the structural and functional changes in the tissues and organs of a living entity that occur as a

C. B. Spainhour
Spainhour Consulting Services, Scott Township, PA, USA

S. C. Gad
Gad Consulting, Cary, NC, USA

© Springer Nature Switzerland AG 2020
S. C. Gad et al., *Contract Research and Development Organizations-Their History, Selection, and Utilization*, https://doi.org/10.1007/978-3-030-43073-3_10

Table 10.1   Subdisciplines of pathology

Subspecialty of pathology	Area or focus of work
Cellular pathology	Changes that occur at the cellular level
Clinical pathology	Study of the use of laboratory methods and the data generated in the diagnosis of disease
Comparative pathology	Comparisons of the responses of organs or tissues to different diseases or insults and how these changes differ between various animal species
Experimental pathology	Examines the responses to artificially induced disease processes occurring in either tissues or organs
Functional pathology	Studies changes in organ or tissue function due to morbid changes occurring in either tissues or organs
Gross pathology	Evaluates large, macroscopic changes to organs that are visible to the naked eye or more readily observable with a dissecting microscope
Surgical of anatomic pathology	Evaluation of organs and tissues which are surgically accessible for diagnosis and treatment
Toxicologic pathology	An integration of the fields of toxicology and pathology requiring an understanding of all body systems and includes such disciplines as pathology (clinical, gross, anatomic), toxicology, biochemistry, physical chemistry, physiology, medicine, and more

result of disease or type of physical or chemical insult (Dorland 1994). Within the field of pathology, there are various subsets of the field (Table 10.1) (Haschek et al. 2002).

Medically, a necropsy is defined as the postmortem examination of a body, including the internal organs and other structures after thorough dissection to determine the cause of death and identify the existence of any pathological changes as well as the nature of those pathological changes (Dorland 1994). Sometimes, the necropsy is mistakenly referred to as an autopsy. By convention, the term necropsy is the examination of the bodies of animals, and the term autopsy is limited to the performance of the postmortem examination of humans.

The Necropsy Laboratory and Necropsy Tools

An area that is dedicated completely to necropsies is essential (Cooper 1994; Mayer 1995). The area should be well lit, permitting the accurate evaluation of the carcass and dissected parts. The most important aspect of lighting is that it be of such a type as to permit correct color presentation of, for example, internal organs. Tables, cabinets, and countertops preferably should be of high-quality stainless steel so that they are easy to clean and rust does not become a problem in the wet environment of the necropsy laboratory (Cooper 1994; Mayer 1995). Freezers for the storage of autoclaved and bagged carcasses need to be present in the necropsy room or in an adjacent room or contiguous area.

The tools to perform a necropsy will vary by species, the type of dissection that is required (e.g., eye only vs. whole body), and personal preferences (Feinstein and Waggie 2011). A typical necropsy work station will provide for the technician the items listed as follows:

- Sharp knife
- Scalpel blades
- Scalpel handle
- Dissecting/(sharp/blunt-nosed) scissors
- Small surgical scissors
- Forceps (large, small, serrated, and toothed)
- Bone-cutting scissors or pruning shears
- Syringes ($\leq$10 mL) with needles of various sizes
- Ligature or string or suture material
- Cutting boards
- Paper towels
- Plastic bags of various sizes
- Squeeze bottles of 10% neutral buffered formaldehyde
- Normal saline
- Cotton-tipped applicator sticks
- Leak-proof screw-top tissue containers
- Test tubes of various sizes for sample collection
- Container filled with fixative
- Tissue cards
- Plastic cassettes labeled to identify small individual or paired organs
- Weighing boats
- Multicompartment plastic tray
- Bucket for tissue and organ parts, cassettes, and animal identification

Balances will be needed within the necropsy room. An additional tool that needs to be available is an electrical drill, which can be used for some bone work. A hacksaw, a butcher's saw, and a Stryker precision oscillating tip saw are also necessary tools for bone work, especially the removal of the *calvaria*.

Finally, a high-quality stereoscopic microscope can be of great value in the examination of small organs, lesions, and small animals.

An appropriate level of personal protective gear should always be worn in the necropsy laboratory. Technicians should wear lab coats, protective eye wear, surgical gloves, and a surgical mask. Respirators are an option. Wristwatches, bracelets, rings, and other jewelry should not be worn by necropsy technicians while working. A passive dosimeter monitoring badge should be worn by all personnel in the necropsy laboratory for safety reasons.

Necropsy Setup

Careful thought and effort needs to go into the setup of a necropsy station to ensure a smooth flow of accurate and timely work. In preparation for the necropsy of small animal species, cover the work area with a piece of plastic covered by some sort of absorbent paper over it. This will absorb the blood and keep the work area neat and clean. For large animal species, the plastic and paper covering of the work area is not necessary as there is substantially more free blood, which should be allowed to drain through the perforated insert on the necropsy table.

Necropsy tissue containers need to display critical and select information to identify the study, the animal, and so on. Label information includes but is not limited to

1. The pathology specimen and fixative used
2. The pathology project number
3. The study number
4. The contractor number (if relevant and available)
5. The sex and species of the animal
6. Animal group number
7. Animal identification number
8. Date of sampling

Necropsy General Comments

For standard repeated-dose toxicity studies, the protocol describes the details of the study design. Near the end of the study protocol is a section generally labeled "Terminal Procedures and Anatomic Pathology" (or similar title). This section of the protocol contains critical information about the following study aspects: (1) termination, (2) gross necropsy, (3) organ weights, (4) tissue collection and preservation, (5) histology, and (6) histology evaluation.

Time delays in the proposed study schedule commonly occur, and for some strange reason, clients always feel that time can be made up at the pathology stage. An animal may or may not show changes in clinical signs, behavior, hematology, or clinical chemistry, but a complete pathological evaluation should not be accelerated or shortcuts taken because pathology and histopathology represent one of the most critical aspects for the evaluation of the *in vivo* response to the presence of a xenobiotic. The histopathological assessment needs to be of the highest quality and proper procedures followed with regard to the collection of pathology data.

Necropsy Personnel and Responsibilities

To successfully complete a necropsy, the following individuals are typically part of the necropsy team: study pathologist, study director, necropsy supervisor, senior pathology technician, pathology technical staff (animal transporters, blood collector/phlebotomist, dissector/prosector, weighing assistant), and quality assurance representative. Table 10.2 provides a complete listing of key individuals for the performance of necropsies and brief descriptions of their job responsibilities. The study sponsor may or may not be present. For any necropsy, the study director should be present and oversee the procedure. Depending upon the type of study involved, a study pathologist may be present. When a study is being terminated, the activity level in the necropsy laboratory can be intense, with technical staff and even the sponsor asking a lot of questions all at the same time of both the study director and the study pathologist.

In spite of this activity, the study director needs to be kept informed with regard to all observations and comments since the study director is ultimately the decision-maker for study conduct. However, the study director should listen to and consider the counsel of the study pathologist and other personnel involved in the nonclinical study. This relationship between the study director and the study pathologist is special. While it is unclear in this current regulatory climate just exactly how much written or verbal communication there should be between the study director and the study pathologist, in the author's experience, as long as everything is specifically documented so that an unambiguous trail can be

Table 10.2 Necropsy titles and functions

Title	Function/responsibilities
Pathologist or necropsy supervisor	(1) Analyzes information given by the sponsor to determine personnel and equipment requirements (2) Coordinates the necropsy setup, the selection of personnel, and the flow of work with the senior technician assigned to the necropsy (3) Records gross observations and conducts a tissue checkoff of all protocol-required tissues and is responsible to see that each cassette per animal has the proper tissue/organ, identification, and the animal's identification number on it (4) Capable of dissection of all species. NOTE: A sponsor may elect to have the study necropsy supervised by the study director, boarded pathologist, nonboarded pathologist or veterinarian after consideration of the length, anticipated findings, and complexity of the study. There is no GLP requirement in reference to this other than the fact that the individual must have the appropriate education, experience, and training to be in that position
Senior pathology technician	(1) Obtains the supplies and equipment to be used at the necropsy (2) Necropsy setup and assists in the selection of personnel (3) Assists the pathologist/necropsy supervisor in training personnel and in supervising personnel at the necropsy (4) May be designated as the overall necropsy supervisor to record gross observations at necropsy and conduct a tissue checkoff of all protocol-required tissues (5) Qualified in dissection of all species
Pathology technician	(1) Assists the senior pathology technician in necropsy setup and work flow (2) Capable of dissecting all species of animals
Prosector	(1) Dissection (2) Relate all gross observations to the pathologist and/or necropsy supervisor (3) Confirms each animal's identification number and writing that number on each tissue cassette for each animal
Phlebotomist	Collection of blood samples as required by the protocol
Weighing assistant	(1) Calibration of scales or confirmation that scales have been properly and acceptably calibrated (2) Confirms that tissues to be weighed have been properly trimmed of excess fat and connective tissue (3) Ensures that tissue weights are recorded properly and informs the pathologist or pathology associate of possible weight deviations from normal and have the deviations verified

followed from the initial observations to the recording of the data and the writing of the report, all should be well.

A few points need to be made with regard to the role and function of a study pathologist in nonclinical studies (US Food and Drug Administration [USFDA] 1988, 2000):

- The study pathologist should be allowed, and is encouraged, to provide input into the design of the study protocol, especially the sections involving necropsy, tissue collection, and histomorphological analysis.
- The study pathologist should be provided access to the test article information, pharmacology data, study protocol, amendments, deviations, in-life data, clinical pathology data, toxicokinetic data, and necropsy findings.
- The lines of communication between the study director and the study pathologist have to be open, clear, and unfettered at all times.
- If there is more than one pathologist, for example, light microscopic and electron microscopic pathologist, working on a study, clear lines of responsibility must be well-defined and clearly described.
- The study pathologist has the responsibility for the final interpretation of pathology data. However this does not mean that there cannot be spirited scientific discussion over interpretation involving the client, study pathologist, and study director.
- The study pathologist should be allowed to review all study tables and data in the report.
- The study pathologist will be responsible for writing the pathology report, but should assist the study director in preparing the final study report.
- The study pathologist should be cooperative in cases where a peer review of the pathology data is suggested or necessary for refinement of clarification of the pathology report (Morton et al. 2006, 2012; The Society of Toxicologic Pathologists 1991, 1997).

Necropsy teams can either be dedicated or comprised of suitably trained toxicology technicians, some of whom may have actually worked on the study being brought down. Dedicated necropsy teams can be very efficient in their activities, but add cost to an organization's operation.

The Prenecropsy Meeting

Prior to the initiation of any necropsy, a prenecropsy meeting with the members of the necropsy team should be held to ensure the best possible outcome for the activity. The following points should be discussed as required by the study protocol or at the sponsor's request:

1. The nature of any clinical or in-life findings
2. The list of protocol tissues required to be collected and potential target organs
3. The record of any clinical pathologic changes
4. The expected number of animals on which the necropsies to be performed
5. The animal species, sex, age, and strain
6. Group and animal numbering and identification scheme
7. What blood samples are required to be collected and details of collection (volume, route, etc.)
8. Any special requirements (e.g., organ weights, perfusions, bone marrow or blood smears, photography, electron microscopy sections)
9. Any precautions that need to be taken during the necropsy
10. Assignment and review of necropsy personnel and their responsibilities

A prenecropsy meeting is not usually necessary for studies which require only a gross necropsy, but this may depend on the overall purpose of the non-clinical study as well as the possible complexities that may exist in the necropsy.

Necropsy Data Collection

In preparation for the necropsy, the study protocol and a listing of animal numbers (by animal group and sex) from the study need to be obtained and a pathology project number assigned. Necropsy pathology data can be recorded on individual necropsy sheets or captured into an electronic database. The protocol-specific, species-specific, and sex-specific necropsy data sheet when generated (paper or electronic) will serve as the official necropsy record for each animal and would be referenced for future histopathology evaluation. The tissue/organ list is compiled when the form is prepared prior to the necropsy according to the protocol. Tissues need to be checked off as they are placed in fixative. If there is nothing to enter in a given space on the sheet, insert a dash or some other character to ensure that some entry is made so that there is no question as to whether or not something was overlooked. All lesions need to be recorded, and any missing tissue, for example, parathyroid and thymus, must be indicated. If a lesion is present in either organ of a paired set of organs, for example, kidney, this will need to be indicated along with whether it was present in the left or right organ. Overall, an entry is always required on the necropsy sheet, and all personnel involved in the necropsy should initial and date the form with electronic or penned signatures.

The Language of Pathology and Necropsy

All of the lesions that are observed during the course of the performance of a necropsy need to be documented in a precise and concise manner (Bucci 2002; King et al. 1989; Strafuss 1988). The written description must be able to generate in the mind of the reader a picture identical to that which was observed on the necropsy table. While this may seem simple, it is more often not a simple consideration. It is suggested to use descriptions that are familiar to help with the written observations, such as mahogany brown in color, cobblestone-appearance surface, lemon yellow color, glistening or shiny, sandpaper-like, or port wine red in color. The description of any lesion should incorporate not necessarily all of the following features, but those that are *appropriate*, such as the location, color, size/weight, shape, consistency, number (#) or percent (%) involved, time, severity, content, odor, or cause. The location of lesions should be described using well-defined anatomical reference points. Remember that sizes should be represented as best as possible in three dimensions. For hollow organs (e.g., gastrointestinal tract), the amount, appearance, and odor of the contents should be described. Be careful when ascribing a cause and always precede such documentation with the word "presumptive." It is important to be thorough, and it may be necessary to touch, squeeze, palpate, cut into (produce a cut surface), or put your nose near the carcass to gain a full appreciation of the sample and the moment. Use terminology correctly (see Tables 10.3 and 10.4 for a compendium of proper necropsy and pathology terminology).

Table 10.3 Terms for gross morphology and distribution of findings in necropsy

Gross morphology entries		Qualifiers for distribution	
		Distribution	Color
Accumulation	Laceration	Confluent	Black
Adhesion	Lesion	Diffuse	Blue
Alopecia	Mass	Multiple	Brown
Amputation	Nodule	Number	Clear
Calculus	Obstruction	Single	Cloudy
Crust	Parasite		Dark
Cyst	Perforation		Green
Deformity	Pigmentation		Gray or grey
Dilation	Prolapse		Mottled
Diverticulum	Rupture		Opaque
Emphysema	Scar		Pale
Enlarged	Small		Pink
Fluid	Thick		Purple
Focus	Thin		Red
Foreign body			Tan
Fracture			White
Hernia			Yellow
Intussusception			

Table 10.4 Necropsy terminology

Accumulation – A collection of material in a given area (e.g., dried blood, feces, etc.)

Adhesion – Abnormal fibrous union of an organ or part to another

Alopecia – Loss of hair, may be partial or total

Amputation – The removal of a limb or other appendage or outgrowth of the body

Anterior – Undesirable use in veterinary anatomy

Brittle – Liable to break or snap, friable

Calculus – A solid concretion composed chiefly of mineral substances and salts found in ducts, passages, hollow organs, and cysts

Caseous – Resembling cheese or curd; cheesy

Caudal – Pertaining to the tail

Clear – Absence of coloration; transparent

Cloudy – Obscured, not limpid or clear

Color – The following may be used; black, blue, brown, green, gray (or grey), pink, purple, red, tan, white, and yellow

Confluent – Becoming merged; not discrete

Coronal plane – A plane at right angles to a sagittal plane. Dividing the body into dorsal and ventral portions. Sometimes referred to as the frontal plane

(continued)

Table 10.4 (continued)

Cranial – Pertaining to the head

Crust – A bark-like hard covering, especially a dried exudate on the skin

Cyst – An enclosed space within a tissue or organ, lined by epithelium and usually filled with fluid or other material

Dark – Of a deep shade; black or almost black

Deformity – The state of being misshapen. Marked deviation from the normal in the size or shape of the body or part, congenital absence of a portion or all of a body part

Depressed – Sunk below the surface

Diffuse – Not definitely limited or localized, widely distributed

Dilation – The condition, as of an orifice or tubular structure, of being dilated or stretched beyond the normal dimensions

Distal – Situated away from the center of the body or from the point of origin

Diverticulum – A circumscribed pouch or sac of variable size occurring normally or created by herniation of the lining mucous membrane through a defect in the muscular coat of a tubular organ

Dorsal – Pertaining to the back or upper surface; nearer the back surface of the body

Emphysema – A pathological accumulation of air tissues or organs, applied especially to such a condition of the lungs. An anatomical alteration of the lungs characterized by abnormal enlargement of the air spaces distal to the terminal respiratory bronchiole often accompanied by destructive changes in the alveolar walls

Enlarged – Measurably larger than normal size

Fibrinous – Pertaining to or of the nature of fibrin. An elastic filamentous protein

Firm – Relatively solid, compact, or unyielding to touch

Flat – Smooth and regular with few or no hollows or depressions

Fluid – A fluid substance, such as any liquid secretion of the body

Focus – A small (usually <5 mm) circumscribed alteration of color or consistency; single site; foci (plural)

Foreign body – A substance occurring in any organ or tissue where it is not normally found

Fracture – A break in bone, cartilage, or solid organ usually caused by trauma

Friable – Easily crumbling or breaking into pieces (often used in reference to livers)

Gelatinous – Resembling gelatin or jelly

Granular – Composed of, like, or containing grains or granules

Gritty – Like, containing, or consisting of grit

Hard – Resisting indentation, incision, or compression; solid; unyielding

Hernia – Abnormal protrusion of an organ or a part through the containing walls of its cavity; beyond the normal confines

Intussusception – The prolapse of one part of the intestine into the lumen of an immediately joining part. The receiving of one part within another

Irregular – Lacking symmetry or uniformity

Laceration – A tear or wound made by tearing

(continued)

Table 10.4   (continued)

Lateral – On the side; farther from the median or midsagittal plane

Lesion – An alteration, structural or functional, due to disease. Any pathological or traumatic discontinuity of tissue or loss of function of a part. Very non-specific. Use more specific designations wherever possible

Linear – Of or pertaining to a line or lines

Lobulated – Made up of or divided into lobules

Mass – A circumscribed enlargement of an organ or tissue. May be irregular in shape. Usually applies to larger (>1 cm) lesions. See also Nodule.

Mottled – Marked with spots or blotches of different color or shades of color.

Medial – Relating to the middle or center

Multiple – More than one part, aspect, etc.

Nodule – A circumscribed enlargement or solid elevation of varying sizes. A nodule is relatively smaller than a mass (usually <1 cm).

Number – Use a whole number

Obstruction – The state of being occluded or stenosed, applied especially to hollow ducts and vessels; blockage or obstacle

Oily – Of, pertaining to, containing oil; greasy

Opaque – Impervious to light; not translucent or transparent; having no luster; dull

Oval – Having the shape of an egg

Pale – Of a very light shade of color; lacking in brightness or intensity of color

Papillary – Pertaining to or resembling a small nipple-shaped projection or elevation

Parasite – An organism that lives, during all or part of its existence, on or in another organism, its host at whose expense it obtains nourishment

Perforation – A hole made through a part of the wall of a cavity or tissue surface produced by a variety of means

Pigmentation – Coloration resulting from any normal or abnormal coloring matter of the body (i.e., bile, hematogenous (derived from blood) or ceroid pigment)

Plaque – Any patch or flat area

Polypoid – Resembling a polyp (a protruding growth especially from mucous membrane)

Posterior – Undesirable use in veterinary anatomy

Prolapse – The falling or sinking down of a part or organ, especially its appearance at a natural or artificial orifice

Proximal – Situated toward the center of the body or toward the point of origin

Punctate – Resembling or marked with points or dots

Raised – Elevated in low relief

Rostral – Pertaining to the nose. In a direction toward the nose (rostrad)

Round – Having a contour that is circular or approximately so

Rubbery – Having the consistency of a resinous elastic material

Rupture – A forcible tearing of a part or disruption of tissue; hernia

Sagittal plane – A plane at right angles to a coronal plane. The midsagittal (or median) plane divides the body into left and right halves. In contemporary usage, used for any plane parallel to the median, i.e., as a synonym for parasagittal

(continued)

Table 10.4 (continued)

Scaly – Scale-like; characterized by scales

Scar – A mark remaining after healing of a wound or other disease process. A permanent mark resulting from a wound or disease process in tissue, especially the skin

Single – Consisting of one only; individual

Size – Record dimensions in millimeters

Small – Measurably less than normal size

Soft – Less firm than normal

Spherical – Shaped like a sphere

Thick – Relatively greater than normal in depth or extent from one surface to the opposite

Thin – Having a relatively smaller distance than normal between opposite sides or surfaces. Not great in diameter or cross section

Transverse – Crosswise; lying across the long axis of the body or of a part

Ventral – Pertaining to the undersurface. Situated nearer the undersurface of the body

Viscous – Semi-fluid; sticky

Volume – Record volume of fluids in milliliters

Watery – Resembling water; thin or liquid

The Necropsy Procedure

Necropsy procedures are generally similar for all common laboratory animal species (rats, mice, guinea pigs, hamsters, rabbits, dogs, cats, ferrets, swine, and nonhuman primates), with some species-specific differences. Detailed procedures will not be presented here but can be found in veterinary pathology references (Ankel-Simmons 2000; AVMA 2007; Berringer et al. 1968; Elvang 2011; Everitt and Gross 2006; Feldman and Seely 1988; Getty 1975a, b; Gilbert 1968; Gray 1985; Hellebrekers and Hedenqvist 2011; King et al. 1989; Nickel et al. 1986; NRC 2011; Parkinson et al. 2011). These procedures can be modified based upon specific protocol or sponsor requirements; however, a few important points should be reiterated here.

First, before initiating necropsy, the animal's identification must be confirmed. If identification is missing or unreadable, it must be confirmed by other study personnel and a cage card or another method, and this alternative identification needs to be retained with the tissues. Generally, the necropsy should begin with a complete examination of the external body and including orifices, although this is often overlooked. The pelage can be wetted with normal saline to keep fur from becoming airborne and contaminating internal organs when incisions are made. Incisions are made to expose the subcutis, chest, neck, abdomen, retroperitoneum, pelvis, musculature, bone, brain, spinal column, and eyes in that order. For males, the testes should always be expressed from the scrotum into the abdominal cavity. Some species-specific differences in necropsy procedures and organ/tissue collection are outlined as follows:

For dogs and swine:

- Remove mandibular salivary glands and a pair of cervical lymph nodes.
- Remove thyroids and parathyroids; trim away any extraneous tissue and place in a cassette.
- Strip the jejunum from the mesentery, carefully open it, and examine the mucosal surface. Remove and save a 10- to 20-cm piece.
- Remove the ileum, cecum, colon, and mesenteric lymph nodes. Open these tubular organs, and rinse away the contents with normal saline, and examine the mucosal surfaces.
- Remove lacrimal glands and/or the third eyelid.
- Remove eyes with approximately 0.5 cm of optic nerve attached.

For nonhuman primates:

- Leave thyroids and parathyroids attached to the trachea.
- Dissect away the trachea and bronchial lymph nodes from the thoracic "pluck" if they are to be weighed and place in a cassette.
- Remove lacrimal glands and/or the third eyelid.
- Remove eyes with approximately 0.5 cm of optic nerve attached.

For rabbits:

- Remove submaxillary salivary glands and a pair of cervical lymph nodes.
- Leave thyroids and parathyroids attached to the trachea.
- Remove the mesenteric lymph nodes with a segment of the descending colon (forms a "horseshoe" circle around the lymph nodes), and remove an 8-cm-long piece of appendix with jejunum attached.
- The pelvic cavity *must* be opened completely to examine the male accessory reproductive organs and to obtain sections of the prostate and the seminal vesicles.
- Remove both eyes with approximately 0.5 cm of optic nerve attached and the lacrimal/Harderian glands for each eye.
- The pituitary gland is covered by a thin plate of bone, which should be very carefully dissected away in order to expose the gland for removal. Cut the

bone on each side and along the posterior border, and then carefully lift the flap superiorly.

For rats:

- Skeletal (thigh) muscle should be removed from the posterior aspect of the right leg.
- The sciatic nerve should be removed from the right leg and placed in a cassette or can be left attached to the skeletal (thigh) muscle.
- The skin and muscle of the right leg should be removed and the tibia transected at a point near the tibiotarsal joint (knee including articular surfaces).

For mice:

- The skeletal (thigh) muscle should remain intact with the femur.
- The sciatic nerve should be left attached to the leg skeletal muscle.

  When the right leg is removed, only the skin should be dissected free from the leg. The leg muscles and sciatic nerve remain attached and the tibia, which is transected near the tibiotarsal joint (knee with articular surfaces is saved for evaluation).

Tissue Collection in Necropsy

There is a "best practices" section available on the website of the Society of Toxicologic Pathology (http://www.toxpath.org) and published enumerating the tissues that should be collected from Good Laboratory Practice (GLP)-quality repeated-dose toxicity studies that are supportive of the registration (Food and Drug Administration [FDA]) of new pharmaceutical products (Bregman et al. 2003). This tissue list can be used for all types of repeated-dose toxicity studies, regardless of duration, route of administration, species or strain of animal, or the type of test article. However, the route of administration may suggest that additional tissues be collected, such as nasal cavity, nasal turbinates, pharynx, larynx, and tracheobronchial lymph nodes for inhalation studies. Tissues that are known targets of the test article must be added to the list. Finally, the presence or absence of some organs or tissues might be unique to a given species and should be added to or deleted from the list as necessary. Some specific examples are:

- Minipigs: spiral, transverse, and descending colon; vesicular gland instead of seminal vesicles; bulbourethral gland (urogenital); no parathyroids
- Rats: no gallbladder
- Rabbits: appendix, sacculus rotundus
- Dog: no seminal vesicles
- Nonhuman primate: diaphragm, axillary lymph nodes, tracheobronchial lymph nodes, tonsils, lip

For all species, the stomach can be listed by its component parts (cardia, fundus, and pylorus).

Not all tissues or organs are represented in the abovementioned list, because agencies expect only a representative sampling to maximize detection, resources, and safety (Bregman et al. 2003). There are additional tissues that are recommended for collection and evaluation by other regulatory agencies, and these include the optic nerve, oviduct, ureter, nasal cavity, Zymbal's gland, clitoral/preputial gland, diaphragm, extraorbital lacrimal gland, rectum, three different salivary glands, larynx, pharynx, coagulating gland, and tongue. The basis for lack of inclusion of these tissues into the basic core list is:

- Historical data support the expression of toxicity, or neoplasia rarely occurs in these additional tissues.
- Tissues currently on the list already provide adequate screening for specific organ systems (e.g., single salivary gland vs. three salivary glands).
- While routine examination may not be required for some tissues, gross examination may suggest the addition of other tissues to the list.
- Some animal tissues such as Zymbal's gland and clitoral/preputial glands do not have human counterparts, and therefore findings in these tissues or organs do not translate to human safety.

Weighing and Necropsy

An important part of the necropsy and pathology evaluation is the collection of organ weights (Sellers et al. 2007). Organ weights are a commonly used parameter in toxicology evaluations. Ideally, a complete understanding of a test article metabolism, pharmacokinetics, and mechanism of action coupled with an understanding of the biochemistry, molecular biology, and physiology of the animal model will aid in predicting and understanding potential organ weight changes. If organs are not to be weighed, they should be placed in fixative immediately. If organs are to be weighed, they should be kept moist by misting with normal saline until they are weighed. Organs that exist in pairs (e.g., adrenals and kidneys) should be weighed together and not individually for studies being submitted to the FDA or European Union (EU). It is never appropriate to compare the weights of fixed versus fresh organ weights of the same tissues.

When tissues are required by the protocol to be weighed prior to fixation at necropsy, the following procedure should be used: (1) remove the organ to be weighed from the animal; (2) trim away excess fat and connective tissue from the organ or tissue; (3) place the material to be weighed in a weighing boat (tared and calibrated balance) which has been identified with the animal number or in separate compartment in the individual animal tissue collection tray, keeping the tissue moist (not immersed) with saline; (4) record the weight on a paper or electronic necropsy sheet or other authorized form; and (5) return the tissue or organ to the collection tray.

Some organs such as the liver may actually demonstrate changes in weight in studies of less than 7 days' duration, so the weighing of organs may be a very sensitive indicator of toxicologic activity. Changes in brain weights are not usually associated with the development of neurotoxicity; however, the value of brain weights can be used for the calculation of organ-to-brain weight ratios. If terminal body weights of animals are highly variable as a result of test article effects, the use of organ-to-brain weight ratios can significantly reduce numeric scatter. Indeed, organ-to-brain weight ratios should be routinely determined for all repeated-dose toxicity studies. Changes in heart weights may well be predictive of the development of myocardial hypertrophy that could be extremely difficult if not impossible to pick up with macroscopic or even microscopic examination (Bregman et al. 2003; Sellers et al. 2007). Similarly for the liver, increases in weight may be reflective of hepatocellular hypertrophy secondary to peroxisome proliferation or enzyme induction (Bregman et al. 2003; Sellers et al. 2007). Changes in kidney weight may indicate renal toxicity or tubular hypertrophy. Finally, changes in the weight of the adrenal glands may indicate test article toxicity, stress, hyperplasia, hypertrophy, or a general endocrinopathy (Bregman et al. 2003; Sellers et al. 2007).

Thyroid and pituitary gland weights should be collected for all species except mice; due to their sizes, weighing the thyroid and pituitary glands in mice may lead to artifacts that could confound microscopic data interpretation. When dealing with rodents, the fixation of thyroid and pituitary glands before weighing may lead to the generation of more accurate weights.

Inflammation or changes in the production of sperm may be reflected in weight changes for the epididymides, and testicular weight changes may indicate the presence of edema or changes in the seminiferous tubules. Prostate weights can be affected by test articles demonstrating androgenic, antiandrogenic, or estrogenic activity. In repeated-dose toxicity studies involving rats, the testes, epididymides, and prostate should always be weighed. Testes should always be weighed in mice, but the prostate and epididymides may be weighed on an individual basis only. In general, the weights of seminal vesicles will add little value gained from the weights of the prostate gland alone. For nonrodents, testes should always be weighed, but the epididymides and prostate should only be weighed on an individual basis. It is important to recognize that the weights of the prostate, epididymides, and other male accessory organs are only of significant value when the organs are collected from sexually mature animals.

For GLP repeated-dose toxicity studies in rodents of durations greater than 7 days, splenic and thymic weights should always be captured. For nonrodents, postpubertal dogs, and nonhuman primates, thymic weights can provide valuable information, but the normal involution of the thymus can complicate the interpretation of thymic weight data, especially when studies are of greater than 3 months' duration. Splenic weights in nonrodents can be influenced by the quality of exsanguinations and the method of euthanasia. Lymphoid organ weights can exhibit a high degree of variability for a variety of reasons, and so the weights of spleens and thymuses need to be viewed concurrently with their histomorphologic evaluation. Lymph nodes are difficult to dissect from all fat and can also vary markedly in size, making the collection of weights from these structures a task of questionable value.

There are some organs that are not routinely weighed but can be weighed depending upon the known or expected toxicity of the test article. Histopathology is typically sufficient to detect toxicity in salivary glands, but if a test article has specific effects on secretory glands, then weighing those may be useful. For rodents, isolating the pancreas is extremely difficult; thus, weighing the pancreas may not be appropriate, whereas the pancreas is readily isolated from nonrodents, so weighing the pancreas from nonrodents could be useful. Dissection and trimming of the gastrointestinal tract can be problematic and tend to be inconsistent (e.g., gut not emptied and cleaned) causing weight collection data to be highly variable. The uterus and ovaries can be weighed if necessary but are not organs that are routinely scheduled for weighing due to normal reproductive cycling and age (Bregman et al. 2003; Sellers et al. 2007). Lung weights can provide critically important information in inhalation studies. However, if the route of administration is by some pathway other than inhalation, then the collection of lung weights may not be necessary if there is no suspicion of pulmonary toxicity (e.g., paraquat), and adequate evaluation may be gained from just the histomorphological analysis.

Organ weights should not be collected from animals that are euthanized or suffer untimely deaths because there are no matched controls and there might be significant differences (e.g., nutritional state and congestion) that will undoubtedly confound the data interpretation. Finally, the study pathologist should review all of the organ weight data and provide an interpretation of those data. The study pathologist is generally the most qualified person to evaluate organ weight changes and correlate those data with the clinical chemistry, hematology, gross pathology, and histomorphology.

Missing Tissues

Tissues or organs can be missing because of agenesis, maceration, or destruction in the dissection process, or the tissue or organ is lost because of the activity that occurs during the performance of the necropsy. In cases of agenesis and destruction of the tissue or organ, it is critical to thoroughly document the situation. However, when a tissue or organ is missing, every effort must be made to try and find the missing tissue or organ. Sometimes tissues or organs get placed in the wrong compartment of an animal tissue or organ tray. If the tissue or organ is found, place it in its appropriate place and document the occurrence. If the tissue or organ is not found, document that it was lost during necropsy. If tissues or organs are frequently misplaced or become lost during the necropsy, the necropsy process might be flawed, or participants are working too quickly, or the necropsy personnel are not paying attention to the details of their task and need to be counseled. Retraining of personnel may well be in order, or a reevaluation of the flow of work during necropsy can be useful in resolving the problem.

Unscheduled Deaths

It cannot be emphasized enough that once animals are terminated, necropsy should immediately follow in order to avoid the effects of autolysis. If this is not possible, then refrigeration of the carcass is the next best option. Never should a carcass be frozen because freezing and the ultimate thawing will produce significant tissue damage and complicate the histopathology assessment.

Various scenarios may occur leading to the unscheduled deaths of animals during a study and are illustrated as follows

Scenario A

If an animal is found dead, it should be subjected to necropsy as soon as possible using typical normal necropsy techniques. However, due to the presence of autolysis and cell death, the value of any biological samples collected will be questionable. These fluids can be collected if desired and saved or even analyzed but need to be appropriately marked and annotated in the study record that the samples came from a dead animal. To avoid or lessen the frequency of these types of situations, the study director needs to understand the pharmacology and toxicology of the test article and educate the technical staff for the potential of unscheduled death and possibly change the schedule (i.e., frequency and timing) for performing observations of the animals with special emphasis on the development of any premonitory signs suggesting death. Additionally, a pathologist can assist in discerning the differences in changes in tissue as a result of agonal change, autolysis, or trauma.

Scenario B

At times, an animal must be terminated in extremis as a result of a handling-induced injury (i.e., gavage error, significant skeletal injury [broken bone], and getting crushed between a cage and the cage rack). It is important to have a plan for unscheduled deaths so that the necropsy can be performed as close as possible to the time of death minimizing the contribution of tissue autolysis. The animal will need to be euthanized, and with proper planning, the necropsy can be performed shortly after then animal has been euthanized using normal necropsy procedures. Also, any required biological fluids, for example, blood, may be collected. It is important to appreciate that the biochemistry and physiology of the animal is not normal. There are two schools of thought with regard to the handling of these types of animals. One position is that no samples of any biological fluids should be collected because of the altered biochemistry and physiology. The alternative view is that the animal is still alive, and every effort should be made to collect as much information as possible and, accordingly, any biological fluid required by the protocol. While insights may be gained from these samples with regard to a mechanism of death, most likely the data generated from these samples will be aberrant. Regardless of one's position, if the data from such an animal is used, there needs to be NO ambiguity in the study record with regard to documentation of the nature of the sample and the state of the animal and that any biological fluid samples collected are not normal samples. Normal necropsy procedures should be followed for harvesting tissues; however, one big difference with scheduled versus unscheduled deaths is that the study pathologist or a pathologist may not be present for the necropsy.

Scheduled Deaths

At times, highly detailed procedures regarding the execution of a necropsy will be delineated in the study protocol. However, when procedures are not specified by the study protocol, animals should be terminated in numerical order, across the consecutive study groups to minimize the confounding effects of potential group-to-group variation and intradiurnal physiologic and biochemical changes within animals (Doerning and Cruze 1997). In cases of a very large study where terminations are scheduled across a period of several days, after day 1, animals should continue to be terminated in numerical order, across the consecutive study groups, to minimize the confounding effects, keeping as many other parameters alike as much as possible (e.g., start times). Also, the order of removal of tissues should follow a standard necropsy procedure such as described here, but techniques may vary slightly depending on the study design, the protocol, or if extensive lesions in one or more organ systems require a specialized and detailed dissection and/or description. Terminal body weights should be collected at an appropriate time from all animals at the end of a study. These weights are very central to the determination of accurate and meaningful organ-to-body weight ratios. To minimize variation, these weights should be collected at the time of necropsy. Special considerations for the performance of necropsy may include the following:

1. Target organs may be removed first (e.g., in an inhalation study, the lungs should be removed first).
2. Tissues are to be removed with forceps by grasping the surrounding, attached, or contiguous membrane to prevent handling artifacts.
3. Tissues may need to be incised in such a fashion as to provide the maximum exposure to the fixative (e.g., liver lobes may be incised to ensure proper fixation; the brain may be fixed *in toto*).
4. A fixative other than the standard fixative which is 10% neutral buffered formalin (NBF) may be used.

Tissue Fixation and Necropsy

Fixation is performed to kill the tissue, prevent the development of *postmortem* decay (autolysis), and preserve the biological material in a state that is as close to its natural state as is possible (Carson 1997; Culling et al. 1985; Kiernan 2000; Preece 1972). A fixative denatures or destroys biological molecules especially proteolytic enzymes, thereby preventing degradation, as well as protects a sample from the decay and damage from microorganisms. Since fixatives alter cells and tissues on a molecular level, their mechanical strength, rigidity, and stability preserve morphology as the tissue sample is processed. Fixation is the first step of a multistep process preparing biological materials for microscopic evaluation. There are multiple types of fixation, such as heat fixation, perfusion, and immersion. Immersion is the most commonly used method of fixation, and in this procedure, a tissue is immersed in a fixative of volume that is 15–20 times greater than the volume of the tissue to be fixed. To become fixed, the fixative must diffuse through the tissue. Therefore, tissue size, density, surface area, thickness, and the type of fixative must be considered. The larger the sample, the longer it takes for the fixative to reach the deeper parts of the tissue and the longer it takes for a material to become fixed, so the higher the level of autolysis that will be found in the sample. A concise summary of common fixatives is presented in Table 10.5.

There are multiple factors that can affect fixation, and these include pH (kept within the physiological range of pH 4–9 with ultrastructure preservation kept at pH 7.2–7.4), osmolarity (hypertonic solutions cause cell shrinkage and hypotonic solutions cause cell swelling), specimen size (1–4 mm), volume of

Table 10.5 Fixatives

Fixative	Features/example
Formaldehyde	(1) Most commonly used
	(2) Formalin (10% neutral buffered formalin)
	(3) Acts as cross-linker, creates covalent bonds between proteins providing rigidity
	(4) Fixative of choice for proteins
	(5) Karnovsky's (paraformaldehyde + NaOH + cacodylate + glutaraldehyde)
Alcohols	90% isopropyl alcohol
	Fixative of choice for nucleic acids
	Davidson's (ethanol + acetic acid + formaldehyde)
	Davidson's favored for fixation of ophthalmic tissues
Oxidizing agents	Potassium dichromate
Mercurials	Zenker's I solution
Picrates	Picrate salts
	Bouin's solution
	The fixative of choice for biogenic amines is Bouin's
HOPE	Hepes-glutamic acid buffer-mediated organic solvent protection effect
	Fixative of choice for nucleic acids
Frozen section	Fixative of choice for enzymes
	Fixative of choice for mucopolysaccharides
Glutaraldehyde/osmium tetroxide	Fixative of choice for lipids

fixative (15–20 times the tissue volume), and duration of immersion or fixation (1 h/mm of tissue) (Carson 1997; Kiernan 2000).

In some studies, a more detailed dissection of the eye will be requested (Maggs et al. 2008; Slatter 2001). Regardless of species, the removal of the eyes commences with the removal of the palpebral and bulbar conjunctiva. When this tissue is elevated with forceps and dissected free of the globe, the eye is carefully removed with a pair of forceps, being careful to transect the optic nerve at a point as distal as possible from the eye. After the eye with the optic nerve attached is removed, remove the aqueous humor. This is accomplished by inserting a 1-mL syringe with 25–27G 1-in. needle into the anterior chamber of the eye. Next, remove the cornea. This is done by making a deep incision that follows the demarcation between the sclera (white part of the eye) and the cornea (clear part of the eye). Trim and gently remove the cornea. Next, trim the iris and ciliary body from the eye and remove the lens. Collect the vitreous humor using a 1-mL syringe or a small spatula. Peel or scrape the choroidal-retinal tissue from the posterior interior surface of the globe (*Note*: In the rat, the retina often comes out with the vitreous humor). One can tell the difference between the two tissues by the fact that the vitreous humor is clear and colorless and the retinal tissue is pink. Trim the optic nerve from the rear of the exterior of the eyeball. If the pigmented portion of the retina is also required, the posterior portion of the globe will be submitted intact with or without the neuroretina since the pigmented layer of the retina is generally tightly adhered to the sclera.

Blood and Bone Marrow Smears

If a protocol requires blood or bone marrow smears to be made and does not specify from which location, the following procedure can be used. To prepare a blood smear from a rodent, anesthetize or asphyxiate the animal by carbon dioxide asphyxiation, and place the animal in dorsal recumbency. Collect blood using a syringe and needle (3-mL syringe and 22G 1-in. needle) via percutaneous cardiocentesis. Alternatively, open the chest, expose the heart, and collect blood via direct cardiocentesis. For other species, blood can be collected via access to any suitable peripheral vein. For details on blood smear preparation, references are readily available (Bessis 1976).

Special Considerations

It would be a rare event for a necropsy to be performed under sterile conditions. This type of procedure would most likely be invoked only in cases where there is a severe complicating fungal infestation, bacterial or viral infection, a highly infectious or toxic test article (e.g., live virus), or in cases where samples are to be collected for polymerase chain reaction (PCR) analysis. There are many resources available addressing aseptic technique (for details, see Slatter 1993).

When working with gene therapy products, where PCR analysis will be required as part of the study protocol, a necropsy will need to be performed in such a fashion as to preclude the intertissue contamination with foreign nucleic acids, proteases, nucleases, and so on from other tissues (Compton and Riley 2001; Feinstein and Waggie 2011). While many aspects of the necropsy will remain unchanged from a standard necropsy, molecular techniques such as PCR analysis are of very high sensitivity, and steps must be taken to eliminate the potential for cross-contamination between specimens collected for such analysis. Strict control of the environment is necessary to prevent potential contamination. One way to address this is for necropsy technicians to collect their samples from animals, tissues, or organs for PCR analysis in laminar flow hoods. As a general rule for the collection of samples for PCR analysis, no instrument should touch any more than a single point of a single tissue or organ at any time. Gloves and table coverings need to be changed frequently, at a minimum between tissues or organs and even between procedures. Instruments need to be continually replaced and replenished with fresh, clean instruments, which have been sterilized by heat or submerged in a 10% solution of bleach or some other suitable disinfectant for a period of contact time of 5 min and rinsed (phosphate-buffered saline solution) and dried before using again. Specific procedures such as priority of order of organ or tissue collection will, in most cases, be dictated by the individual client or preferences for collection stated by the laboratory performing the actual PCR analysis. Any specimens collected should be immediately placed in sterile tubes or containers and frozen rapidly at −80 °C.

Whole-Animal or Whole-Organ Perfusion

Another specialty technique that may be used occasionally in necropsy is whole-animal or isolated-organ vascular perfusion fixation (McMenamine 2000; Rostgaard et al. 1993; Scouten et al. 2006; Simmons et al. 1996; Stickrod and Stansifer 1981; Stretch et al. 1999; Spector and Goldman 2005). While this performed usually in rats or mice, it can be performed in most any species. The advantages of this procedure are the following: (1) fixation begins immediately after the arrest of systemic circulation, minimizing the alteration of cell structure resulting from *postmortem* effects; (2) vascular perfusion under *in situ* conditions results in a uniform and rapid dissemination of fixative into all parts of the tissue via the vascular bed, resulting in an increased depth and rate of actual fixation; (3) the manipulation of tissues after circulatory arrest and prior to fixation is minimized thereby resulting in fewer artifacts; (4) many organs and tissues can be fixed concurrently; and (5) for immunocytochemical procedures utilizing relatively mild fixation conditions, fewer changes from autolysis result; greater immunocytochemical activity is retained, and the redistribution or translocation of cellular components is minimized. There are a variety of possible routes for vascular perfusion and include the portal vein, aorta via the left ventricle, descending aorta, and vena cava.

Virtually any organ-specific perfusion procedure can be readily modified to effect fixation (Mehendale 2008). Typically, the perfusion procedure is composed of two parts: the preperfusion portion and the actual perfusion portion. For preperfusion, the animal is weighed and injected with a suitable anesthetic. An inhalational anesthetic such as Metofane can also be used. Before beginning the perfusion procedure, animals should be checked for a suitable plane of anesthesia by a person that is qualified to perform such an assessment. There should be no deep pain reflex present in the animal. During the perfusion procedure, every attempt should be made to keep the animal warm (body temperature), as in this anesthetized state, the animal will be prone to hypothermia. Typically, the animal will painlessly expire during the perfusion process, but if the animal survives or lingers, euthanasia should be administered promptly.

Prior to the initiating perfusion, a flow rate must be set. Flow rates vary according to species: rat, 50 mL/min; mouse, 5 mL/min; dog (adult beagle), 400 mL/min; dog (adult hound), 500 mL/min; nonhuman primate, 350 mL/min; rabbit, 250 mL/min; sheep, 600 mL/min; and pig, 600 + mL/min, depending upon size. The times for perfusion also vary. Flushing should take place for 2–4 min, 2 min for rodents and 4 min for nonrodents. Fixative should be allowed to perfuse for 8–10 min, generally 8 min for rodents and 10 min for nonrodents.

One needs to assess the quality of the perfusion when fluid administration is complete. A high-quality perfusion has occurred when the intended tissues all appear to be fixed and firm, most of the circulatory system is devoid or emptied of blood, and the brain is paler than that of a nonperfused animal. An acceptable but not the ideal level of perfusion has occurred when there is some evidence of perfusion fixation as demonstrated or judged by the tissues being only slightly less malleable than those of a nonperfused animal, the brain not being firm, and the brain not having pallor. Finally, an unacceptable level of perfusion fixation has occurred when there is no evidence of perfusion fixation in any tissues, tissues are soft, the brain is soft, the brain is pink, and all tissues resemble those of a nonperfused animal.

Photography

One final special topic in necropsy and gross pathology is photography (Edwards 1988; McGavin 1988; Saikia et al. 2008; Stack et al. 2001; Weinberg 1997). The photographing of tissue and organ specimens can be highly useful for purposes of illustration and explanation as well as measurements. Photographs coupled with modern communication technology permit a distant observer to easily visualize images of gross lesions and even histological sections, enhancing the quality of any pathology-based discussions. However, despite the utility of using cameras in the necropsy, their use is fraught with various challenges. To take pictures, the cameras need to be of good quality and hence not of insignificant expense. One needs to be careful of using such equipment in a wet environment so as not to damage it with moisture. Finally, most, if not all, contract research organizations and pharmaceutical companies forbid or stringently regulate (SOPs) the presence and use of cameras (including cell phones) on site. Due to the sensitivity and the nature of the work performed in a necropsy laboratory, any camera used should be the property of the hosting organization (not the client or visitor), stored in a secure location, and, when used, should be in the indisputable possession and control of a suitable individual employed by the host organization. These simple guidelines can prevent downstream embarrassing events and troublesome animal rights activities.

Use of Image Data in Necropsy/Pathology

The Society of Toxicologic Pathology has published a very useful reference on the use of image data in pathology (Tuomari et al. 2007). In general, images that are used for the generation of data are considered to be raw data. Alternatively, images that are not used to generate actual data are not considered to be raw data. For example, an image that is generated for use in illustrative purposes is not considered to be raw data. On the other hand, images that are generated for the purposes of diagnosis or morphometric analysis are considered raw data. Under current technology, any image that is used for the purpose of generation of data becomes raw data at the moment in time of the generation of the actual data. Each image, as it becomes raw data, must be suitably documented, indicating the person that generated it and time that the image was generated for data. Each photograph should always include a reference marker indicating scale or size. Those images that become raw data must be archived, and the relevant SOP must be in place for the collection and use of images and the generation of data from such. Any equipment used must be appropriately qualified, tested, and validated. Relevant training records and procedures for those performing the procedures must be in place. Any GLP exceptions must be stated as deviations in the compliance statement portion of the study protocol. Images that are not used to generate raw data do not have to be archived, unless they are somehow referenced or used in the study report. One final point is that since illustrative images are not used for purposes of diagnosis, interpretation, or measurement, they cannot be used to override the study pathologist's written and recorded observations obtained from the first-hand examination of the tissues at the time of necropsy.

Clinical Pathology

The opinions expressed in this chapter are the personal opinions of a previously practicing veterinarian, who set up a clinical pathology laboratory in his veterinary clinic to assess the health status of veterinary patients along with those of fellow safety consultants with collective experience in excess of 125 years. These opinions also happen to be in complete compliance with the expectations of regulatory agencies (Aiello and Moses 2016; Gad 2017a, b, c, d; Goldenthal 1968; Hastings 2007; ICH 1997, 2008a, b; Mathieu 2000, 2005 and Rang 2006). Clinical pathology is a medical specialty concerned with the diagnosis of disease or interpretation of toxicological effects based upon the analysis of bodily fluids such as blood or urine. Typical clinical pathology measurements are listed in Table 10.6. A basic clinical pathology laboratory needs at the minimum two full-time technicians. The technicians should be either a medical technologist or medical laboratory scientist. They should have a bachelor's degree in either biology or chemistry. They can also have a bachelor's of medical laboratory science. They should be certified by the American Society of Clinical Pathology and have completed a clinical rotation in clinical chemistry, hematology, coagulation analysis, urinalysis, serology, blood banking procedures, bacteriology, parasitology, and mycology.

Table 10.6 Clinical pathology measures

Clinical chemistry	Hematology	Urinalysis
Albumin	Erythrocyte count (RBC)	Chloride
Alkaline phosphatase (ALP)	Hemoglobin (HGB)	Bilirubin
Blood urea nitrogen (BUN)	Hematocrit (HCT)	Glucose
Calcium	Mean corpuscular hemoglobin (MCH)	Occult blood
Chloride	Mean corpuscular volume (MCV)	pH
Creatine	Platelet count	Phosphorus
Creatine phosphokinase (CPK)	Prothrombin time	Potassium
Direct bilirubin	Reticulocyte count	Protein
Gamma glumly transferees (GGT)	White cell count (WBC)	Sodium
Globulin	White cell differential count	Specific gravity
Glucose		Volume
Lactic dehydrogenase (LDH)		
Phosphorus		
Potassium		
Serum glutamic oxaloacetic transaminase (SGOT)		
Serum glutamic pyruvic transaminase (SGPT)		
Sodium		
Total bilirubin		
Total cholesterol		
Total protein		
Triglycerides		

The basic laboratory should have the following equipment:

- Hematology analyzer
- Clinical chemistry analyzer
- Coagulation analyzer
- Urine analyzer
- Centrifuge
- Slide stainer
- Computers and printers
- Tube labeler

The clinical chemistry analyzer should be capable of running electrolytes, proteins, lipids, lipoproteins, enzymes, and various biomarkers. It should also be capable of doing quantitative urine chemistry testing of sodium, potassium, chloride, urea nitrogen, calcium, creatinine, and total protein. Although qualitative testing of urine is acceptable, semiquantitative and quantitative testing is preferable to agencies despite the fact that there are no guidelines mandating such. Probable conditions that can affect hematological changes are listed in Table 10.7, and changes in biochemical parameters and their association with specific target organs are listed in Table 10.8.

The electrolytes are vital in maintaining fluid- and acid-based balance. The following are typically used to monitor kidney function:

- Sodium
- Potassium
- Chloride

The following is generally used to monitor bone, heart, nerves, and kidney status:

- Calcium

The following are used to monitor kidney, liver, and gastrointestinal function:

- Inorganic phosphorus
- Magnesium

Proteins serve as enzymes, antibodies, coagulation factors, hormones, or molecular transport. Total protein monitors liver, kidney, and bone marrow disorders. Albumin helps transport large molecules and screens for liver disease and dehydration.

Lipids are a group of molecules with poor water solubility that have various functions such as providing cellular metabolic energy, making up components of cellular membranes, hormones, and vitamin D. Cholesterol is a component of cell membranes, and the test helps monitor plaque buildup in arteries. The triglyceride test serves to indicate cardiovascular status. Low-density lipoprotein transports cholesterol from the liver to other tissues. It is associated with

Table 10.7 Some probable conditions affecting hematological changes

Parameter	Elevation	Depression	Parameter	Elevation	Depression
Red blood cells	1. Vascular shock 2. Excessive diuresis 3. Chronic hypoxia 4. Hyperadrenocorticism	1. Anemias (a) Blood loss (b) Hemolysis (c) Low RBC production	Platelets		1. Bone marrow depression 2. Immune disorder
Hematocrit	1. Increased RBC 2. Stress 3. Shock (a) Trauma (b) Surgery 4. Polycythemia	1. Anemias 2. Pregnancy 3. Excessive hydration	Neutrophils	1. Acute bacterial infections 2. Tissue necrosis 3. Strenuous exercise 4. Convulsions 5. Tachycardia 6. Acute hemorrhage	
Hemoglobin	1. Polycythemia (increase in production of RBC)	1. Anemias 2. Lead poisonings	Lymphocytes	1. Leukemia 2. Malnutrition 3. Viral infections	
Mean cell volume	1. Anemias 2. B-12 deficiency	1. Iron deficiency	Monocytes	1. Protozoal infections	
Mean corpuscular hemoglobin	1. Reticulocytosis	1. Iron deficiency	Eosinophils	1. Allergy 2. Irradiation 3. Pernicious anemia 4. Parasitism	
White blood cells	1. Bacterial infections 2. Bone marrow stimulation	1. Bone marrow depression 2. Cancer chemotherapy 3. Chemical intoxication 4. Splenic disorders	Basophils	1. Lead poisoning	

RBC red *blood* cell

Table 10.8 Association of changes in biochemical parameters with actions at particular target organs

Parameter	Blood	Heart	Lung	Kidney	Liver	Bone	Intestine	Pancreas	Notes
Albumin				↓	↓				Produced by the liver. Very significant reductions indicate extensive liver damage
ALP					↑	↑	↑		Elevations usually associated with cholestasis. Bone alkaline phosphatase tends to be higher in young animals
Bilirubin (total)	↑				↑				Usually elevated due to cholestasis, either due to obstruction or hepatopathy
BUN				↓	↑				Estimates blood filtering capacity of the kidneys. Doesn't become significantly elevated until the kidney function is reduced 60–75%
Calcium				↓					Can be life threatening and result in acute death
Cholinesterase				↓	↓				Found in the plasma, brain, and RBC

								Comments
CPK	↑							Most often elevated due to skeletal muscle damage but can also be produced by cardiac muscle damage. Can be more sensitive than histopathology
Creatinine			↑					Also estimates blood filtering capacity of kidney as BUN does
Glucose							↑	Alterations other than those associated with stress are uncommon and reflect an effect on the pancreatic islets or anorexia
GGT				↑				Elevated in cholestasis. This is a microsomal enzyme, and levels often increase in response to microsomal enzyme induction
HBDH	↑	↑		↑				
LDH	↑	↑	↑	↑				Increase usually due to skeletal muscle, cardiac muscle, or liver damage. Not very specific

(continued)

Table 10.8 (continued)

Parameter	Blood	Heart	Lung	Kidney	Liver	Bone	Intestine	Pancreas	Notes
Protein (total)				↓	↓				Absolute alterations are usually associated with decreased production (liver) or increased loss (kidney). Can see increase in case of muscle "wasting" (catabolism)
SGOT		↑		↑	↑			↑	Present in the skeletal muscle and heart and most commonly associated with damage to these
SGPT					↑				Elevations usually associated with hepatic damage or disease
SDH					↑↓				Liver enzyme which can be quite sensitive but is fairly unstable. Samples should be processed as soon as possible

↑ increase in chemistry values; ↓ decrease in chemistry values

ALP alkaline phosphatase, *BUN* blood urea nitrogen, *CPK* creatinine phosphokinase, *GGT* gamma-glutamyl transferase, *HBDH* hydroxy-butyric dehydrogenase, *LDH* lactic dehydrogenase, *RBC* red blood cells, *SDH* sorbitol dehydrogenase, *SGOT* serum glutamic oxaloacetic transaminase (also called AST: [aspartate aminotransferase]), *SGPT* serum glutamic pyruvic transaminase (also called ALT [alanine aminotransferase]) coronary artery disease. High-density lipoprotein transports cholesterol from peripheral tissues to the liver. It is used to assess coronary artery disease.

Biomarkers such as glucose, total bilirubin, creatinine, and blood urea nitrogen are measurable parameters that can indicate a normal biological state, pathogenic state, or pharmacologic process. Glucose monitors carbohydrate metabolism. Total bilirubin monitors liver function. Creatinine and BUN monitor kidney function.

Coagulation also known as clotting is the process by which blood changes from a liquid to a gel, forming a clot. It potentially results in hemostasis which is the cessation of blood loss. The coagulation analyzer should be capable of doing at least the following tests.

– Prothrombin time (PT) – measures intrinsic and extrinsic pathways of coagulation cascade
– Activated partial thromboplastin time (APTT) – measures intrinsic pathway
– Fibrinogen (FIB) – functions primarily to occlude blood vessels and thereby stop excessive bleeding
– Thrombin time (TT) – elapsed time for clot formation

Urinalysis is the analysis of urine in order to evaluate renal function and dysfunction. Urinalysis can be qualitative, semiquantitative, or quantitative. Ideally, the urine analyzer should be able to perform qualitative urine chemistry analysis via use of a dipstick to measure amounts of leukocytes, nitrates, pH, blood, glucose, ketones, urobilinogen, bilirubin, specific gravity, color, and clarity. The urine analyzer should also be able to perform semiquantitative automated microscopic analysis for formed elements such as cells, crystals, sperm, and casts. As stated previously, the clinical chemistry analyzer should also be capable of doing quantitative urine chemistry testing of sodium, potassium, chloride, urea nitrogen, calcium, creatinine, and total protein.

All testing and data collection should be done in compliance with regulatory guidelines of the FDA and Good Laboratory Practice (GLP). Regular internal inspections should be performed by the quality assurance department. All maintenance, calibrations, and data evaluation are done by the technicians as per standard operating procedures (SOP) (Gad 2017a, b, c, d; Goldenthal 1968; Hastings 2007; ICH 1997, 2008a, b; Mathieu 2000, 2005 and Rang 2006). Finally, it is very desirable for the clinical pathology laboratory to participate in some sort of extramural proficiency and linearity testing program (e.g., Veterinary Laboratory Association™ Quality Assurance Program).

References

Aiello, S. E., & Moses, M. A. (Eds.). (2016). Clinical pathology and procedures. In *The Merck veterinary manual* (11th ed., pp. 1584–1729). Kenilworth: Merck and Co, Inc.

Ankel-Simmons, F. (2000). *Primate anatomy an introduction* (2nd ed.). San Diego: Academic Press.

AVMA (American Veterinary Medical Association). (2007). *AVMA guidelines on euthanasia*. Schaumburg: AVMA.

Berringer, O. M., Browning, F. M., & Schroeder, C. R. (1968). *An atlas and dissection manual of rhesus monkey anatomy*. Tallahassee: Anatomy Laboratory Aids.

Bessis, M. (1976). *Blood smears reinterpreted* (Vol. 10, pp. 217–236). Translated by George Brecher (1977). Springer: New York.

Bregman, C. L., Adler, R. R., Morton, D. G., Regan, K. S., & Yano, B. L. (2003). Recommended tissue list for histopathologic examination in repeat-dose toxicity and carcinogenicity studies: A proposal of the Society of Toxicologic Pathology (STP). *Toxicologic Pathology, 31*, 252–253.

Bucci, T. J. (2002). Basic techniques. In W. M. Haschek, C. G. Rousseaux, & M. A. Wallig (Eds.), *Handbook of toxicologic pathology* (Vol. I, 2nd ed., pp. 171–186). Orlando: Elsevier Press.

Carson, F. L. (1997). *Histotechnology: A self-instructional text* (2nd ed.). Chicago: American Society of Clinical Pathologists.

Compton, S. R., & Riley, L. K. (2001). Detection of infectious agents in laboratory rodents: Traditional and molecular techniques. *Comparative Medicine, 51*, 113–133.

Cooper, E. C. (1994). Animal facilities. In E. C. Cooper (Ed.), *Laboratory design handbook* (pp. 99–110). Boca Raton: CRC Press.

Culling, C. F. A., Allison, R. T., & Barr, W. T. (1985). *Cellular pathology technique* (4th ed.). London: Butterworths.

Doerning, B. J., & Cruze, C. (1997). The effects of routine animal husbandry and experimental procedures upon physiological parameters of rats. In *Abstracts of Scientific Papers, Platform and Poster Presentations, 1997 AALAS National Meeting*. Anaheim.

Dorland, W. A. N. (Ed.). (1994). *Dorland's illustrated medical dictionary* (28th ed., p. 1103). Philadelphia: W.B. Saunders Company, 1244.

Edwards, W. D. (1988). Photography of medical specimens: Experiences from teaching cardiovascular pathology. *Mayo Clinic Proceedings, 63*, 42–52.

Elvang, H. (2011). *Necropsy. A handbook and atlas* (1st ed.). Copenhagen: Samfundslitteratur.

Everitt, J. I., & Gross, E. A. (2006). Euthanasia and necropsy (Chapter 20). In M. A. Suckow, S. H. Weisbroth, & C. L. Franklin (Eds.), *The laboratory rat* (2nd ed., pp. 665–678). Burlington: Elsevier Academic Press.

Feinstein, R. E., & Waggie, K. S. (2011). Post mortem procedures (Chapter 21). In J. Hau & S. J. Schapiro (Eds.), *Handbook of laboratory animal science, Volume I: Essential principles and practices* (3rd ed., pp. 613–634). Boca Raton: CRO Press.

Feldman, D. B., & Seely, J. C. (1988). *Necropsy guide : Rodents and the rabbit* (1st ed.). Boca Raton, FL: CRC Press.

Gad, S. C. (2017a). The drug development process and the global pharmaceutical market-place. In *Drug safety evaluation* (3rd ed., pp. 1–12). Hoboken: Wiley.

Gad, S. C. (2017b). Regulation of human pharmaceutical safety: Routes to human use and market. In *Drug safety evaluation* (3rd ed., pp. 13–58). Hoboken: Wiley.

Gad, S. C. (2017c). Nonclinical manifestations, mechanisms, and end points of drug toxicity. In *Drug safety evaluation* (3rd ed., pp. 115–128). Hoboken: Wiley.

Gad, S. C. (2017d). Repeat-dose toxicity studies. In *Drug safety evaluation* (3rd ed., pp. 159–168). Hoboken: Wiley.

Getty, R. (1975a). *Sisson and Grossman's the anatomy of the domestic animals* (Vol. I, 5th ed.). Philadelphia: W. B. Saunders.

Getty, R. (1975b). *Sisson and Grossman's the anatomy of the domestic animals* (Vol. II, 5th ed.). Philadelphia: W. B. Saunders.

Gilbert, S. G. (1968). *Pictorial anatomy of the cat* (Rev. ed.). Seattle: University of Washington Press.

Goldenthal, E. (1968). Current view on safety evaluation of drugs. *FDA Papers*, pp. 13–18.

Gray, H. (1985). *Anatomy of the human body*. C. D. Clemente (Ed.), (Thirtieth American ed., 1–18, 1–1608). Philadelphia: Lea & Febiger.

Haschek, W. M., Rousseaux, C. G., & Wallig, M. A. (2002). Toxicologic pathology: An introduction. In W. M. Haschek, C. G. Rousseaux, & M. A. Wallig (Eds.), *Handbook of toxicologic pathology* (Vol. I, 2nd ed., pp. 3–14). Orlando: Elsevier Press.

Hastings, K. L. (2007). Nonclinical safety evaluation of biotechnology-derived pharmaceuticals. *FDA*. www.fda.gov

Hellebrekers, L. J., & Hedenqvist, P. (2011). Laboratory animal analgesia, anesthesia, and euthanasia (Chapter 17). In J. Hau & S. J. Schapiro (Eds.), *Handbook of laboratory animal science, Volume I: Essential principles and practices* (3rd ed., pp. 485–534). Boca Raton: CRO Press.

ICH. (1997). S6 Preclinical safety evaluation of biotechnology-derived pharmaceuticals.

ICH. (2008a). M3 (R2) Nonclinical safety studies for the conduct of human clinical trials for pharmaceuticals.

ICH. (2008b). M3 (R2) Nonclinical safety studies for the conduct of human clinical trials and marketing authorization for pharmaceuticals.

Kiernan, J. A. (2000). Formaldehyde, formalin, paraformaldehyde and glutaraldehyde: What they are and what they do. *Microcoscopy Today, 00-1*, pp. 8–12. Miami: Today Enterprises.

King, J. M., Dodd, D. C., Roth, L., & Newson, M. E. (1989). *The necropsy book*. Gurnee: Charles Louis Davis, DVM Foundation.

Maggs, D. J., Miller, P. E., & Ofri, R. (2008). *Slatter's fundamentals of veterinary ophthalmology* (4th ed.). St. Louis: Saunders Elsevier.

Mathieu, M. (2000). *New drug development: A regulatory overview* (5th ed.). Waltham: Parexal.

Mathieu, M. (2005). *New drug development: A regulatory overview* (7th ed.). Waltham: Parexal.

Mayer, L. (1995). Animal facility criteria. In L. Mayer (Ed.), *Design and planning of research and clinical laboratory facilities* (pp. 161–186). New York: Wiley.

McGavin, M. D. (1988). *Specimen dissection and photography: For the pathologist, anatomist and biologist*. Springfield: Charles C. Thomas, Ltd.

McMenamine, P. G. (2000). Optimal methods for preparation and immunostaining of iris, ciliary body and choroidal wholemounts. *Investigative Ophthalmology & Visual Science, 41*(10), 3043–3048.

Mehendale, H. M. (2008). Application of isolated organ perfusion techniques in toxicology. In A. W. Hayes (Ed.), *Principles and methods of toxicology* (5th ed., pp. 1865–1922). Boca Raton: CRC Press.

Morton, D., Kemp, R. K., Francke-Carroll, S., Jensen, K., McCartney, J., Monticello, T. M., Perry, R., Pulido, O., Roome, N., Schafer, K., Sellers, R., & Snyder, P. W. (2006). Society of Toxicologic Pathology Position Paper: Best practices for reporting pathology interpretations within GLP toxicology studies. *Toxicologic Pathology, 34*, 806–809.

Morton, D., Sellers, R., Barale-Thomas, E., Bolon, B., George, C., Hardisty, J. F., Irizarry, A., McKay, J. S., Odin, M., & Teranishi, M. (2012). Society of Toxicologic Pathology. http://www.toxpath.org: Best practices.

Nickel, R., Schummer, A., Seiferle, E., Frewein, J., Wilkens, H., & Wille, K-H. (1986). *The anatomy of the domestic animals. Volume I: The Locomotor system of the domestic mammals*. (Translated by Walter G. Siller and William M. Stokoe) (Founded by Richard Nickel, August Schummer, and Eugen Seiferle). Berlin: Verlag Paul Parey/New York: Springer.

NRC (National Research Council). (2011). Chapter 3, 56–70. Veterinary care. In *Guide for the care and use of laboratory animals* (8th ed.). Washington, DC: The National Academies Press.

Other Readings

Parkinson, C. M., O'Brien, A., Albers, T. M., Simon, M. A., Clifford, C. B., & Pritchett-Corning, K. R. (2011). Diagnostic necropsy and selected tissue and sample collection in rats and mice. *Journal of Visualized Experiments (JoVE)*, (54), e2966. https://doi.org/10.3791/2966, Boston, MA.

Popesko, P., Rajtova, V., & Horak, J. (1992a). *A colour atlas of the anatomy of small laboratory animals. Volume one (rabbit and guinea pig)*. London: Wolfe Publishing, Ltd.

Popesko, P., Rajtova, V., & Horak, J. (1992b). *A colour atlas of the anatomy of small laboratory animals. Volume two (rat, mouse and golden hamster)*. London: Wolfe Publishing, Ltd.

Preece, A. (1972). *A manual for histologic technicians* (3rd ed.). La Jolla: Little Brown.

Rang, H. P. (2006). *Drug discovery and development*. Edinburgh: Churchill Livingstone.

Rostgaard, J., Qvortrup, K., & Poulsen, S. (1993). Improvements in the technique of vascular perfusion-fixation employing a fluorocarbon-containing perfusate and a peristaltic pump controlled by pressure feedback. *Journal of Microscopy, 172*, 137–151.

Saikia, B., Gupta, K., & Saikia, U. M. (2008). The modern histopathologist: In the changing face of time. *Diagnostic Pathology, 25*, 3–10.

Schummer, A. (1977). *The anatomy of the domestic animals. Volume IV: Anatomy of the domestic birds*. (Translated by Walter G. Siller and Peter A. L. Wright) (Founded by Richard Nickel, August Schummer, and Eugen Seiferle). Berlin: Verlag Paul Parey/New York: Springer.

Schummer, A., Nickel, R., & Sack, W. O. (1979). *The anatomy of the domestic animals. Volume II: The viscera of the domestic mammals.* (Translated by Walter G. Siller and William M. Stokoe) (Founded by Richard Nickel, August Schummer, and Eugen Seiferle). Berlin: Verlag Paul Parey/New York: Springer.

Schummer, A., Wilkens, H., Vollmerhaus, B., & Habermehl, K-H. (1981). *The anatomy of the domestic animals. Volume III: The circulatory system, the kin, and the cutaneous organs of the domestic mammals.* (Translated by Walter G. Siller and Peter A. L. Wight) (Founded by Richard Nickel, and August Schummer). Berlin: Verlag Paul Parey/New York: Springer.

Scouten, C. W., O'Connor, R., & Cunningham, M. (2006). Perfusion fixation of research animals. *Microscopy Today, 14,* 26–33.

Sellers, R. S., Morton, D., Michael, B., Roome, N., Johnson, J. K., Yano, B. L., Perry, R., & Schafer, K. (2007). Society of Toxicologic Pathology position paper: Organ weight recommendations for toxicology studies. *Toxicologic Pathology, 35,* 751–755.

Simmons, M. M., Blamire, I. W., & Austin, A. R. (1996). Simple method for the fixation of adult bovine brain. *Research in Veterinary Science, 60*(3), 247–250.

Slatter, D. (1993). *Textbook of small animal surgery* (Vol. I, 3rd ed.). Philadelphia: W. B. Saunders.

Slatter, D. (2001). *Fundamentals of veterinary ophthalmology* (3rd ed.). Philadelphia: W. B. Saunders.

Spector, D. L., & Goldman, R. D. (2005). *Basic methods in microscopy: Protocols and concepts from cells: A laboratory manual.* Cold Spring Harbor: Cold Spring Harbor Laboratory Press.

Stack, L. B., Storrow, A. B., Morris, M. A., & Patton, D. R. (2001). *Handbook of medical photography.* Philadelphia: Hanley & Belfus.

Stickrod, G., & Stansifer, M. (1981). Perfusion of small animals using a mini-peristaltic pump. *Physiology & Behavior, 27*(6), 1127–1128.

Strafuss, A. C. (1988). *Necropsy procedures and basic diagnostic methods for practicing veterinarians.* Springfield: Charles C. Thomas.

Stretch, G. L., Nation, R. L., Evans, A. M., & Milne, R. W. (1999). Organ perfusion techniques in drug development. *Drug Development Research, 46,* Wiley, New York, 3–4.

The Society of Toxicologic Pathologists. (1997). Position paper of the Society of Toxicologic Pathologists: Documentation of pathology peer review. *Toxicologic Pathology, 25*(6), 655.

The Society of Toxicologic Pathologists. (1991). Peer review in toxicologic pathology: Some recommendations. *Toxicologic Pathology, 19*(3), 290–292.

Tuomari, D. L., Kemp, R. K., Sellers, R., Yarrington, J. T., Geoly, F. J., Fouillet, X. L., Dybdal, N., Perry, R., & Long, P. (2007). Society of Toxicologic Pathology position paper on pathology image data: Compliance with 21 CFR Parts 58 and 11. *Toxicologic Pathology, 35,* 450–455.

U.S. Food and Drug Administration (FDA). (1988). Good laboratory practices. CFR 21 Part 58, April 1988.

U. S. Food and Drug Administration (FDA). (2000). Redbook 2000: Guidance for industry and other stakeholders toxicological principles for the safety assessment of food ingredients Redbook 2000. Chapter IV.B.3. Pathology considerations in toxicity studies, July 2000.

Weinberg, D. S. (1997). Digital imaging as a teaching tool for pathologists. *Clinics in Laboratory Medicine, 17,* 229–239.

Electronic Reporting Requirements (SEND and eCTD)

11

Robin C. Guy

Introduction

The Federal Food, Drug, and Cosmetic Act was legislated in 1938. This Act provided much-needed standards for quality for foods, pharmaceuticals, and cosmetics. The Food, Drug, and Cosmetics Act was amended in 1962. Part of the amendment contains grounds for refusing an application if the applicant does not provide proof that a product is both efficacious and safe before receiving FDA approval (Public Law 1962). This amendment forged the way for regulatory submissions, including Investigative New Drugs (NDA), New Drug Applications (NDA), and Center for Biologics Evaluation and Research (BLA). These regulatory submissions were historically paper-based and were generally voluminous (sometimes as much as 30–60 volumes of summaries, data, and reports), difficult to organize and maintain, and certainly challenging to store and then mail the three required copies to the FDA!

Section 745A(a) of the Federal Food, Drug, and Cosmetic Act (FD&C Act), added by Section 1136 of the Food and Drug Administration Safety and Innovation Act (FDASIA), became effective on October 1, 2012. The FDASIA includes the fifth reauthorization of the Prescription Drug User Fee Act

R. C. Guy
Robin Guy Consulting LLC, Toxicology, Safety Assessment & GLP Consulting,
Lake Forest, IL, USA
e-mail: robinguy@robinguy.com

© Springer Nature Switzerland AG 2020
S. C. Gad et al., *Contract Research and Development Organizations-Their History, Selection, and Utilization*, https://doi.org/10.1007/978-3-030-43073-3_11

(PDUFA V) that provides FDA with resources, including electronic data, necessary to produce a more efficient review of applications for human drug and biologic products, including New Drug Applications (NDAs), Abbreviated New Drug Applications (ANDAs), Biologics License Applications (BLAs), and Investigational New Drug Applications (INDs) to the Center for Drug Evaluation and Research (CDER) or the Center for Biologics Evaluation and Research (CBER).

The FDA determined that multiple guidance documents were needed to describe and implement all of the submissions and details needed to cover electronic formatting. These documents will be discussed throughout the chapter.

On December 17, 2014, the binding guidance "Providing Regulatory Submissions in Electronic Format — Submissions Under Section 745A(a) of the Federal Food, Drug, and Cosmetic Act" was published. This guidance describes how FDA interprets and plans to implement the requirements of Section 745A(a), by implementing additional statutory electronic submission requirements, describing the submission types that must be submitted electronically, exemptions from and criteria for waivers of the electronic submission requirements, and the timetable and process for implementing the requirements. As a result, all commercial INDs (as of December 17, 2017) and all NDAs and BLAs (as of December 17, 2016) must be in eCTD format.

The standardized format used for eCTDs in the United Sates is in the same format that is required for other countries, primarily countries that are Organisation for Economic Co-operation and Development (OECD) members. The eCTD is arranged in five modules (although Module 1 is not technically part of the eCTD), with each containing an explicit type of material:

- Module 1: region-specific administrative information
- Module 2: CMC (chemistry, manufacturing, controls), nonclinical and clinical overviews and summaries
- Module 3: detailed manufacturing information
- Module 4: nonclinical study reports
- Module 5: clinical study reports

Additional guidances were published while individual guidances (e.g., "Providing Regulatory Submissions in Electronic Format – Standardized Study Data," and "Providing Regulatory Submissions in Electronic Format –

Human Pharmaceutical Product Applications and Related Submissions Using the eCTD Specifications") will be developed to specify the formats for specific submissions and corresponding timetables for implementation. As will be discussed later in this chapter, the FDA issued "Providing Regulatory Submissions in Electronic Format – Standardized Study Data: Guidance for Industry" in December 2014. According to the Food, Drug, and Cosmetic Act Section 745A(a), applications must utilize specific standards as defined in the FDA Data Standards Catalog starting 24 months after the final guidance is announced for NDAs and BLAs and 36 months after the final guidance is announced for INDs.

There is also a requirement to supply the FDA with electronic data from certain nonclinical studies. For submission of study data, all commercial INDs (as of December 17, 2017) and all NDAs and BLAs (as of December 17, 2016) must include Standard for Exchange of Nonclinical Data (SEND) electronic format for specified studies. Submissions may not be filed or received if they do not adhere to the eCTD Guidance.

This chapter will not cover detailed scientific content, as each submission will differ and is not possible to be included in a single chapter. Refer to the M4 series of guidances for more information.

Where to Start

The "good old days" of paper submissions are gone, as we move into more technically advanced systems for submissions. Fortunately, the FDA has instructions on multiple areas of their website (www.fda.gov). It is highly suggested that the sponsor review the website for appropriate documents and guidances, including the proper headings and hierarchy/granularity for regulatory submission.

It is suggested to start obtaining FDA Electronic Submissions Gateway (Gateway) access as soon as practical. The Gateway is the software system that the FDA uses to accept the submissions. Currently, all submissions 10 gigabytes or smaller must be submitted via the Gateway. It is also suggested that the Gateway system be tested in your own business environment by sending a sample submission prior to your actual submission. It is better to check for errors and learn the system prior to your company's deadline for submission, so that any issues may be resolved in advance.

Preparing the Nonclinical Section of the eCTD

Format and Content

Module 2 of the eCTD is where the nonclinical summaries reside. The summaries in Module 2 may be expansive and can be time-consuming. Sponsors must follow the formatting as described in the 2017 FDA final guidance document: M4 Organization of the Common Technical Document for the Registration of Pharmaceuticals for Human Use (FDA 2017). See Fig. 11.1 for this formatting.

Each document in the eCTD should be numbered starting at page one, with the exception that each published literature references would have its own numbered pages. In addition, all pages of a document should include a unique header or footer that briefly identifies its subject matter.

For subheadings in each document, numbering can theoretically become extremely long. The M4 Guidance suggests that in order to avoid level subheading numbering longer than four digits (e.g., 2.6.6.3.2.1) within a document, which is acceptable but cumbersome, the applicant may use a shortened numbering string. In this case, the document number and the name (e.g., 2.6.6 Toxicology Written Summary) should appear in page headers or footers, and then section numbering within the document can be used, for example, 1, 1.1, 2, 3, 3.1, 3.2, etc. (FDA 2017).

The sponsor is directed to ICH M4 Safety (M4S) – The Common Technical Document for the Registration of Pharmaceuticals for Human Use: Safety – M4S(R2) (EMA 2003a), which details the nonclinical overview and nonclinical summaries of Module 2 and the organization of Module 4. It states that section headings should be maintained in the eCTD document; however, if a study has not been performed in a certain category, a brief explanation should be provided as to why these studies were not conducted (EMA 2003b). In addition, the sponsor needs to review ICH M4 Quality (M4Q), Module 2 Quality Overall Summary, and also Module 3 Format of the Quality Section of the

Organization of the Common Technical Document for the
Registration of Pharmaceuticals for Human Use

Module 1: Administrative Information and Prescribing Information

1.1 Table of Contents of the Submission Including Module 1

1.2 Documents Specific to Each Region (for example, application forms, prescribing information)

Module 2: Common Technical Document Summaries

2.1 Table of Contents of Modules 2-5

2.2 CTD Introduction

2.3 Quality Overall Summary

2.4 Nonclinical Overview

2.5 Clinical Overview

2.6 Nonclinical Written and Tabulated Summaries

Pharmacology

Pharmacokinetics

Toxicology

2.7 Clinical Summary

Biopharmaceutic Studies and Associated Analytical Methods

Clinical Pharmacology Studies

Clinical Efficacy

Clinical Safety

Literature References

Synopses of Individual Studies

Module 3: Quality

3.1 Table of Contents of Module 3

3.2 Body of Data

3.3 Literature References

Module 4: Nonclinical Study Reports

4.1 Table of Contents of Module 4

4.2 Study Reports

4.3 Literature References

Module 5: Clinical Study Reports

5.1 Table of Contents of Module 5

5.2 Tabular Listing of All Clinical Studies

5.3 Clinical Study Reports

5.4 Literature References

Fig. 11.1 Common Technical Document Organization from the M4 guidance (FDA 2017)

eCTD. Nonclinical sections of the eCTD are mainly found in Modules 2.4 and 2.6 and Module 4.

Module 2.4 is the Nonclinical Overview. The Nonclinical Overview provides an integrated analysis of the overall information in the eCTD. In general, the Nonclinical Overview should not exceed about 30 pages. It should contain appropriate references and links to the tabulated summaries, in the following format: (Table X.X, Study/Report Number). The Nonclinical Overview should be presented in the following order:

- Overview of the nonclinical testing strategy
- Pharmacology
- Pharmacokinetics
- Toxicology
- Integrated overview and conclusions
- List of literature references

Module 6.6 is where the written and tabulated summaries are inserted in the document. Generally, the sponsor will prepare these sections, but often, the CRO will prepare the tabulated summaries and present them in an appendix to the report. This would need to be discussed in the contract between the CRO and the sponsor, or it may be added to the items listed in the protocol that will be prepared for the study report.

Order of Presentation Within a Section (EMA 2003b)

3.2.1 In vitro studies before in vivo studies
3.2.2 Ordered by species, by route, and then by duration (shortest duration first)
3.2.3 Order of species is as follows:

- Mouse
- Rat
- Hamster

- Other rodent
- Rabbit
- Dog
- Nonhuman primate
- Other nonrodent mammal
- Non-mammals

3.2.4 Routes of administration should be ordered as follows:

- The intended route for human use
- Oral
- Intravenous
- Intramuscular
- Intraperitoneal
- Subcutaneous
- Inhalation
- Topical
- Other

Module 4 Study Reports and Data

Module 4 is where the study reports are located. The study director will be the one to sign the final report for studies conducted at their facility. The study director's facility, the contract research organization (CRO), will then circulate the final report to the sponsor. If the study was conducted, in-house, then, of course, the study director would issue their final report. The SEND data, as appropriate, must be included in Module 4 with the corresponding report. SEND data are the individual data that are collected throughout the study. They are a combination of actual numeric data, more complicated data like clinical observations or pathology findings, and metadata. SEND will be detailed later in this chapter. The following is the order of the eCTD Module number and corresponding Section for Module 4 reports (EMA 2003b):

4.1 *Table of Contents of Module 4*
4.2 *Study Reports:*

4.2.1 *Pharmacology*

    4.2.1.1 *Primary Pharmacodynamics*
    4.2.1.2 *Secondary Pharmacodynamics*
    4.2.1.3 *Safety Pharmacology*
    4.2.1.4 *Pharmacodynamic Drug Interactions*

4.2.2 *Pharmacokinetics*

    4.2.2.1 *Analytical Methods and Validation Reports (if separate reports are available)*
    4.2.2.2 *Absorption*
    4.2.2.3 *Distribution*
    4.2.2.4 *Metabolism*
    4.2.2.5 *Excretion*
    4.2.2.6 *Pharmacokinetic Drug Interactions (nonclinical)*
    4.2.2.7 *Other Pharmacokinetic Studies*

4.2.3 *Toxicology*

    4.2.3.1 *Single-Dose Toxicity (in order by species, by route)*
    4.2.3.2 *Repeat-Dose Toxicity (in order by species, by route, by duration; including supportive toxicokinetics evaluations)*
    4.2.3.3 *Genotoxicity*

        4.2.3.3.1 *In vitro*
        4.2.3.3.2 *In vivo (including supportive toxicokinetics evaluations)*

    4.2.3.4 *Carcinogenicity (including supportive toxicokinetics evaluations)*

        4.2.3.4.1 *Long-term studies (in order by species; including range-finding studies that cannot appropriately be included under repeat-dose toxicity or pharmacokinetics)*

4.2.3.4.2 *Short- or medium-term studies (including range-finding studies that cannot appropriately be included under repeat-dose toxicity or pharmacokinetics)*

4.2.3.4.3 *Other studies*

4.2.3.5 *Reproductive and Developmental Toxicity (including range-finding studies and supportive toxicokinetics evaluations) (If modified study designs are used, the following sub-headings should be modified accordingly.)*

4.2.3.5.1 *Fertility and early embryonic development*

4.2.3.5.2 *Embryo-fetal development*

4.2.3.5.3 *Prenatal and postnatal development, including maternal function*

4.2.3.5.4 *Studies in which the offspring (juvenile animals) are dosed and/or further evaluated.*

4.2.3.6 *Local Tolerance*

4.2.3.7 *Other Toxicity Studies (if available)*

4.2.3.7.1 *Antigenicity*

4.2.3.7.2 *Immunotoxicity*

4.2.3.7.3 *Mechanistic studies (if not included elsewhere)*

4.2.3.7.4 *Dependence*

4.2.3.7.5 *Metabolites*

4.2.3.7.6 *Impurities*

4.2.3.7.7 *Other*

4.3 *Literature References*

Hints

To assist the FDA reviewers in reviewing your application, the following may help accelerate their review:

- Use bookmarks and link to references, tables, and figures, and link these to the Table of Contents.

- The Table of Contents should be easily understood (e.g., don't just reference a table number or appendix number, use the title in the table of contents).
- Use blue text for links so that they stand out.
- Any scanned item should be searchable.

Submission of the eCTD

This section is devoted to the eCTD submission, in general, through the Gateway. Submission of the study data in SEND files is discussed in section "Submission of SEND Data in Module 4 of the eCTD".

Electronic Submissions Gateway

The Food and Drug Administration (FDA) Electronic Submissions Gateway (Gateway; also called "ESG" by the FDA) is the system that the agency uses for accepting electronic regulatory submissions. The FDA Gateway does not open or review submissions. It is the pathway that transmits the secure submission of regulatory information so that it reaches the proper FDA Center or Office for review.

Validation and Issues with Validation

The submission is checked, or validated, once received. For example, CDER retrieves the submission from Gateway and checks the following:

- The presence of a us_regional.xml file
- Valid application number
- Non-duplicate sequence number for the application
- Submission is not a single file
- Application type/number in the form (e.g., 356 h, 1571) matches application/type in the us_regional.xml

If initial validation is successful, the eCTD validation tool is used to check for any high errors in the eCTD submission. Additional information may be found in the "Specifications for eCTD Validation Criteria" at https://www.fda.gov/media/87056/download.

If the submission is not up to the current regulations, it may not be accepted. Some issues with validation are indicated below. These should be checked for correctness prior to submission to avoid delays.

- Duplicate submissions caused by submission of the same sequence more than once.
- Submission to the incorrect FDA Center. Ensure that the either CDER or CBER is selected correctly when using the Gateway.
- Submitting zip or exe files, for example, which are not considered valid file types.
- Did not use the standard eCTD format.

Acknowledgment

Acknowledgment from the Gateway occurs when validation and processing of the submission is successfully completed and has been sent to the appropriate Review Division.

The FDA website contains a complete listing of all documents and supportive files needed to submit electronically. This may be found on the eCTD web page at https://www.fda.gov/Drugs/DevelopmentApprovalProcess/FormsSubmissionRequirements/ElectronicSubmissions/ucm153574.htm.

Submission of SEND Data in Module 4 of the eCTD

SEND is an acronym for Standard for Exchange of Nonclinical Data. Study data and supporting information (metadata) will have electronic files appropriately placed in the eCTD in a predetermined location in Module 4. This is a mandatory part of each eCTD application.

SEND Background

SEND is a data exchange standard developed and maintained by CDISC (Clinical Data Interchange Standards Consortium), a nonprofit organization that develops data standards to streamline clinical research and enable connections to healthcare. It assists the FDA reviewer as it standardizes data and, since the data is all electronic, also assists with streamlining the review process.

SEND organizes a nonclinical study, including the study protocol, dosing information, and collected test results and observations, and metadata into a series of machine-readable files, called datasets. Each dataset has a specific purpose, naming convention and organization, with certain datasets that contain similar information having a similar organization. A detailed description of each dataset's organization and examples of how common study data is represented and is published in a SENDIG (SEND Implementation Guide). As the standard changes, there is a public review, then new versions of the SENDIG are published on the CDISC website. Currently, SENDIG version 3.0 and 3.1 are available.

SEND Regulatory

When the guidance "Providing Regulatory Submissions in Electronic Format — Submissions Under Section 745A(a) of the Federal Food, Drug, and Cosmetic Act" was published in December, 2014, an offshoot of the guidance "Providing Regulatory Submissions in Electronic Format – Standardized Study Data" was published. This guidance describes the requirements for an electronic submission of standardized clinical and nonclinical study data as per Section 745A(a) of the Federal Food, Drug, and Cosmetic Act.

A technical specification document, the "Study Data Technical Conformance Guide," is also published by the US FDA. This document contains nonbinding guidance for submission of both clinical and nonclinical electronic study data. The objective of this document is to communicate best industry practices that enable effective agency review of electronic data in a document that is regularly updated based on industry feedback and agency experiences. The original guidance was published in January, 2014; however, this document is updated more frequently than the binding guidance and contains information that is useful to companies creating or verifying SEND datasets. The current version (version 4.4) was published in October, 2019.

As with all submissions to the FDA, the SEND Study Submission Package must follow specific rules. These rules are defined and published by both the Clinical Data Interchange Standards Consortium (CDISC) and by the FDA. CDISC, as the standards development organization, defines the rules that SEND datasets must follow to be considered in conformance with a specific version of a standard, as the standards are updated often. The FDA publishes business rules, which focus on content that enables the FDA reviewers to use the FDA review software. In addition, the FDA publishes a "Technical Rejection for Study Data" as part of the eCTD validation criteria which would assist in automating a review of an eCTD-based submission for the presence of required electronic study data.

For details of the contents and layout of electronic submissions, the FDA requires the inclusion of the nonclinical Study Data Reviewers Guide (nSDRG) associated with study SEND datasets. The nSDRG will be discussed later in this chapter. The nSDRG is submitted as a PDF document. Any PDF documents that are included as part of an electronic submission, must adhere to must adhere to the FDA technical specification "Portable Document Format (PDF) Specifications", that FDA technical specification. Following this specification ensures that PDFs submitted to the agency are in a format that the receiving Center currently supports (the receiving FDA Center has established processes and technology to support the receipt, processing, reviewing, and archiving of files in the specified standard format).

The FDA Data Standards Catalog (Catalog) lists the data standards, format, and terminologies that FDA supports for use in regulatory submissions. This may be found at https://www.fda.gov/media/85137/download

In addition, the FDA currently has an active website with information on eCTD submission standards which may be accessed at https://www.fda.gov/media/93301/download. This webpage also includes a table containing a listing of the specifications and supportive information, current versions, and hyperlinks for eCTD submissions to both CDER and CBER.

It is important to remember that the guidance states that a study starting after December 17, 2016, which is included in an NDA, ANDA, or BLA, and a study starting after December 17, 2017, which is included in an IND, must be submitted with electronic study data.

STUDYID	DOMAIN	USUBJID	BWSEQ	BWTESTCD	BWTEST	BWORRES	BWORRESU	BWSTRESC	BWSTRESN	BWSTRESU	BWSTAT	BWREASND	BWBLFL	VISITDY	BWDTC	BWDY
ABC123	BW	ABC123-0193	1	BW	Body Weight	274	g	274	274	g				-4	2007-06-08T08:48:52	-4
ABC123	BW	ABC123-0193	2	BW	Body Weight	299	g	299	299	g				-1	2007-06-11T08:10:06	-1
ABC123	BW	ABC123-0193	3	BW	Body Weight	307	g	307	307	g			Y	1	2007-06-12T07:17:53	1
ABC123	BW	ABC123-0193	4	BW	Body Weight	348	g	348	348	g				8	2007-06-19T07:37:34	8
ABC123	BW	ABC123-0193	5	BW	Body Weight	377	g	377	377	g				15	2007-06-26T07:31:58	15
ABC123	BW	ABC123-0193	6	BW	Body Weight	400	g	400	400	g				22	2007-07-03T06:21:08	22
ABC123	BW	ABC123-0193	7	TERMBW	Terminal Body Weight	378	g	378	378	g				29	2007-07-10T11:32:14	29

Fig. 11.2 Example of SEND body weights

Study Identifier (STUDYID)	Domain Abbreviation (DOMAIN)	Unique Subject Identifier (USUBJID)	Sequence Number (BWSEQ)	Test Short Name (BWTESTCD)	Test Name (BWTEST)	Result or Findings as Collected (BWORRES)	Unit of the Original Result (BWORRESU)

Fig. 11.3 Example of SEND labels and descriptions

SEND Features

All SEND datasets are organized into a simple table with rows and column, where one row is a record of information from the study, and each column contains some distinct detail related to that information. Body weights, for example, are reported in a SEND dataset named BW. Each live-phase and terminal body weight collected on the study for each animal is reported in a separate row, and each column represents information about the collected body weight. The columns include identifiers for the study and the animal weighed, whether the weight is a live-phase or terminal body weight, the study day and date that the weighing was performed, as well as the weight collected and units of measure. The information included in this SEND BW dataset is equivalent to an individual animal body weight table included in an appendix to the study report. Figure 11.2 shows SEND body weight dataset rows for one study animal.

Other numeric results, including feed consumption, clinical pathology parameter values, etc. that are collected during a study, are similarly reported in other SEND datasets with additional information reported as needed for a clear and complete representation of the collected data.

Complex, non-numerical observational data such as clinical signs, gross observations, and histopathology findings are also included in SEND.

The files are organized so that they are fairly easy to understand. Columns in different datasets that contain the same type of information will either have the same column heading or will have a column header with the dataset name as a prefix to a common "stub" column name. For example, across all files for a study, the column STUDYID will contain the study ID, and the column

USUBJID will contain the unique identifier for the animal. The data will be reported in BWORRES column for the body weight file BW, in LBORRES column for the laboratory tests file LB, and in the MIORRES column for the microscopic observations file MI.

SENDIG will have descriptive labels for each dataset's column names. An abbreviated/short or full column header, or both, may be visible depending on how the files are displayed. Figure 11.3 illustrates the first eight column headers of the SEND body weight file showing both the short column name and the descriptive label when viewed using the SAS Viewer. A full description and examples of each file header can be found in the SEND Implementation Guide.

Study protocol information is separated from the study data and may be found in a collection of datasets called trial design datasets.

SEND datasets also will contain data from individual animal dosing. Dosing information are typically not reported in the study report. These are found in a dataset called Exposure (EX). Exposure is intended to report the dose administered per animal, with either one row per animal dose or one row to represent all doses administered over a defined period.

Table 11.1 shows the list of SEND datasets that can be created for a study using SEND Implementation Guide version 3.1 from CDISC. This version is intended to support data typically found in single-dose general toxicology, repeat-dose general toxicology, and carcinogenicity studies, as well as respiratory and cardiovascular testing done during safety pharmacology studies.

As mentioned above, the documentation of clinical observations is more complex than documentation of numerical values. A helpful component of SEND is the use of controlled terminology. To fully take advantage of what SEND has to offer, including for uses like data mining, observational data must be aligned into a standard format, and the terminology utilized must, therefore, also be standardized, so that the same concept is represented by the same term within a nonclinical study, across nonclinical studies, and across clinical and nonclinical studies. For example, for body weights (BW) "g" is used to represent grams as a unit of measure; any other representation such as "grams" or "G" cannot be used. Urinalysis test codes and names, as well as units of "mL," are standardized. For severity grades, a grade number is standardized ("grade 1"), may be reported as MINIMAL scoring. A tissue defined as "ADRENAL GLANDS" is reported as "GLAND, ADRENAL" and will have a modifier of "BILATERAL", for example, to indicate that both of the pair were observed. Tissues with no abnormalities observed reported as "NORMAL." These are all examples of SEND controlled terminology.

Table 11.1 SEND version 3.1 Implementation Guide list of standard domain models

The following standard domains with their respective domain codes are included in the document:

Special-purpose domains (data that do not conform to the three categories below)
  Demographics – DM
  Comments – CO
  Subject elements – SE

Interventions general observation class (dosing)
  Exposure – EX

Events general observation class (subject disposition)
  Disposition – DS

Findings general observation class (observations resulting from study activities)
  Body weight – BW
  Body weight gain – BG
  Clinical observations – CL
  Death diagnosis and details – DD
  Food and water consumption – FW
  Laboratory test results – LB
  Macroscopic findings – MA
  Microscopic findings – MI
  Organ measurements – OM
  Palpable masses – PM
  Pharmacokinetics concentrations – PC
  Pharmacokinetics parameters – PP
  Subject characteristics – SC
  Tumor findings – TF
  Vital signs – VS
  ECG test results – EG
  Cardiovascular test results – CV
  Respiratory test results – RE

Trial design domains
  Trial elements – TE
  Trial sets – TX
  Trial arms – TA
  Trial summary – TS

Relationship datasets
  Related records – RELREC
  Pool definition – POOLDEF
  Supplemental qualifiers – SUPP datasets

SEND Study Submission Package

Every nonclinical study for which SEND electronic data is required in the FDA submission, a specific collection of files must be included; this full collection of files is commonly called a study SEND Study Submission Package. This package contains:

- SEND datasets using a specified version of controlled terminology
- A define.xml file and associated stylesheet to enable viewing of define.xml with a browser
- A nonclinical Study Data Reviewers Guide (nSDRG)

The SEND datasets must be submitted to the US FDA in version 5 SAS Transport File format. Files in this format have an extension "xpt" and can only be viewed intact by software applications designed to read this format.

A define.xml file, or Data Definition file, must also be provided in a study submission. The define.xml file describes the SEND datasets in machine-readable format. It is considered the most important part of the electronic dataset submission, as it describes the "metadata" of the datasets. It describes what domains are included, with description of each, and it has a description of each variable in each domain, along with a description of entries in those variables. It also has any controlled terminologies and algorithms used, along with any other comments that describe the data.

The nSDRG, or nonclinical Study Data Reviewers Guide, as mentioned earlier in this chapter, is a document that also needs to be included in the submission. It helps the reviewer of the SEND datasets understand the study report and the content of the datasets. Again, this document must be submitted in a PDF format. Some of the information included in the nSDRG for a study is as follows:

- Study design overview or introduction, including a diagram of the study design in the SEND trial design datasets. It also needs to include study identification correspondence to link document with SEND datasets.
- The version of controlled terminology used in the SEND datasets, the rationale for selection of that version, and a list of any nonstandard terms used and definition of each.
- A description of how the SEND datasets were created and verified
- Reviewer a confirmation that SEND datasets accurately represent the study

report, or, if needed, a description of any differences between the SEND datasets and individual animal data tables that were in the final study report

- A list of any FDA rules that the submitted SEND datasets do not comply with and the rationale for noncompliance
- Where the SENDIG allows sponsor-defined entries, a definition of those entries
- Version of define.xml standard used when creating the define.xml file and the rationale for selection of that version

As mentioned earlier, the data included in a SEND Study Submission Package for each study is included in the submission alongside the study report in Module 4 of the eCTD. The location of the SEND Study Submission Package within the eCTD structure is described in the FDA Study Data Technical Conformance Guide, and it is also discussed above.

Determination of Studies that Need Data to Be Submitted as SEND Files

Based on the regulations and guidances, there are four aspects of a nonclinical study that determine whether or not a SEND dataset must be included with a submission to the agency. These would be (1) the FDA Center to which the application is submitted, (2) type of application, (3) study start date, and (4) study type.

FDA Center

SEND data standards requirements only apply to certain FDA Centers. However, currently, the SEND entry in the FDA Data Standards Catalog shows that out of all of the FDA Centers (e.g., CBER, CDER, CDRH, CSFAN, CVM, CTP, OC, ORA, and NCTR), SEND file standards are accepted only by the Center for Drug Evaluation and Research (CDER).

Type of Application

The following four types of applications require SEND for a submission (IND, NDA, ANDA, BLA); however, that requirement may be predicated on the study start date (see immediately below).

Study Start Date

The FDA has published two "on or after" dates for two categories for inclusion of SEND files: one for studies included in NDAs, ANDAs, and certain BLAs (studies starting on or after December 17, 2016) and one for studies included in INDs (studies starting on or after December 17, 2017). A start date is defined as the date that the study director signs the study protocol.

Study Type

The type of study that is required to be included in a SEND data package is still causing confusion and raises questions to regulators and those giving talks on SEND. The FDA uses study types as defined in the eCTD Module 4 sections to determine whether a study requires a SEND Study Submission Package or not. Note that currently, there are no exclusions for non-GLP studies or studies with just a draft report being submitted. Therefore, if the study is going into the FDA submission, and if the type of study falls into the above categories, whether it is GLP or non-GLP, draft or final report, there must be SEND data submitted for that study. The eCTD Module 4 Study Report Sections are discussed earlier in section "Module 4 Study Reports and Data" of this chapter.

The current Technical Rejection Criteria for Study Data document states that the nonclinical study data will apply to section 4.2 of the eCTD. Therefore, the studies listed in Table 11.2 require SEND datasets. This information can be generally correlated to the eCTD Module 4 sections 4.2.3.1, 4.2.3.2, and 4.2.3.4 (Table 11.2). It also lists studies where current study data is not required to be submitted in SEND format (Table 11.3).

For every report in Module 4, nonclinical data is submitted in Module 4 of the eCTD. This includes the demographic dataset and the define.xml files.

Table 11.2 Current nonclinical study types requiring SEND data

Module	Study type
4.2.3	Toxicology
4.2.3.1	Single-dose toxicity
4.2.3.2	Repeat-dose toxicity (including supportive toxicokinetics evaluations)
4.2.3.4	Carcinogenicity (including supportive toxicokinetics evaluations)
4.2.3.4.1	Long-term studies (including range-finding studies that cannot appropriately be included under repeat-dose toxicity or pharmacokinetics)
4.2.3.4.2	Short- or medium-term studies (including range-finding studies that cannot appropriately be included under repeat-dose toxicity or pharmacokinetics)
4.2.3.4.3	Other studies

Table 11.3 Current nonclinical study types not requiring SEND data

Module	Study type
4.2.1	Pharmacology
4.2.2	Pharmacokinetics
4.2.3.3	Genotoxicity
4.2.3.5	Reproductive and developmental toxicity
4.2.3.6	Local tolerance
4.2.3.7	Other toxicity studies

The eCTD sections where SEND is required for nonclinical studies are listed in the FDA Technical Rejection Criteria, as mentioned above; this requirement will change over time. The next version is scheduled to include some types of reproduction/developmental toxicology studies, so it is very important to watch the FDA Technical Rejection Criteria for these important updates.

SEND Responsibilities

Overall, the sponsor is responsible to the entire regulatory submission, which would include SEND files and activities. However, in most medium and large CROs, standard industry practice is that the test facility that is responsible for a study will also be responsible for creation and verification of the study SEND Study Submission Package. Note that the regulations are silent on who will prepare the electronic data package. Preparing for a study that will incorporate SEND data must be planned well in advance of the study start date, as there is a lot of planning to do, including ensuring that the terminology used on the study correlates with standard SEND terminology.

To prepare for SEND, the sponsor must determine upfront who will create the SEND Study Submission Packages. Contracting SEND substantially changes the pricing and may also change the scope of the work done. In addition, if the entire package is to be submitted simultaneously, it also may delay the timing of the final study report. There must be clear and established responsibilities assigned to each facility involved with SEND.

As with any outsourcing activity, potential SEND partners must be qualified to perform the activities. Unless SEND datasets are used to make study decisions, e.g., if the electronic SEND data are used to perform analyses that contribute to the study director's interpretation of the conclusions drawn in the study, then the datasets are not considered to be Good Laboratory Practice (GLP) quality data and are normally not audited by quality assurance. Normally, non-GLP activities are not audited; however, if the SEND data files are not correct in any study, the FDA may not accept the submission. If the study or entire submission is rejected due to SEND database issues, what happens next? Any type of recourse should be addressed in the contract with the supplier, as should be pricing, performance requirements, and data security provisions. Therefore, it is wise to properly, and thoroughly, qualify vendors or CROs who are preparing the SEND data for the submission. The following items may be useful to assist with discussions during qualifications in advance of hiring a company to prepare SEND data files:

- Assess their SEND knowledge and experience creating SEND from their own data sources.
- Pilot conversion study.
- Participation and keeping current with the SEND community.
- Do data packages (datasets and associated define.xml) and the nSDRG go through quality control procedures to ensure correctness and completeness?
- Is the lab using SEND controlled terminology during data collection?
- Has the lab moved all paper-based data collection to an electronic data capture system and ensured collection of additional metadata associated with the study results and observations?
- What are the lab's practices for receipt and management of electronic data from subcontracted test sites?
- Ensure that all CRO test facilities have detailed comprehension of the standards, e.g., SEND, define.xml, and controlled terminology, and also of regulatory expectations for SEND, and are prepared to address updates early.

Conformance Validation

Unless the sponsor contracts out the entire submission to a consultant or CRO, the sponsor will submit the data in SEND format. The study data files then get checked to ensure that they conform to the required, current standards. If they do not conform, the FDA sends an acknowledgement to the sponsor via the Gateway for an unsuccessful validation and processing. If the data do conform, the FDA sends an acknowledgement to the sponsor via the Gateway for a successful validation and processing. Concurrently, the data is sent to the Electronic Document Room.

Storage of Files at the FDA

After the validation, storage of the data takes place in FDA data repositories. These data may be accessed by FDA reviewers who may opt to use analytical tools to analyze the data. Using this system is a huge timesaver for FDA reviewers, since, in the past, the reviewers typically transcribed data to spreadsheets and created their own charts and tables to analyze the data.

Wrapping Up

Electronic submissions and their individual components, including SEND files, are regulatory driven. The FDA expects the sponsor to submit accurate documents that will be validated for compliance at the FDA. It is in the sponsor's best interest to ensure that the package is correct and complete. The most important thing to remember is that a sponsor can delegate all they want to a CRO or consultant to get the eCTD or SEND database files prepared. However, in the end, the sponsor is still responsible for the entire submission.

Acknowledgment I would like to sincerely thank Jennifer L. Feldmann, Epreda LLC, for her enormous and valuable contribution to the SEND portion of this chapter. I do appreciate it!

References

Note: all Internet links were last accessed in December 2019.

EMA. (2003a). ICH topic M4S common technical document for the registration of pharmaceuticals for human use – safety. Step 5. https://www.ema.europa.eu/en/documents/scientific-guideline/ich-m-4-s-common-technical-document-registration-pharmaceuticals-human-use-safety-step-5_en.pdf

EMA. (2003b). ICH topic M4S common technical document for the registration of pharmaceuticals for human use – safety. Step 5. Questions and answers. https://www.ema.europa.eu/en/documents/scientific-guideline/ich-m-4-s-common-technical-document-registration-pharmaceuticals-human-use-safety-questions-answers_en.pdf

FDA. (2017). FDA final guidance document: M4 organization of the common technical document for the registration of pharmaceuticals for human use. https://www.fda.gov/regulatory-information/search-fda-guidance-documents/m4-organization-common-technical-document-registration-pharmaceuticals-human-use-guidance-industry

Public Law. (1962). Public Law 87-781-.Oct. 10,1962 (S1552), p. 780. https://www.govinfo.gov/content/pkg/STATUTE-76/pdf/STATUTE-76-Pg780.pdf. Accessed 30 Nov 2019.

Resources

The FDA website has valuable information on the topics of eCTD and SEND. Note: all Internet links throughout this document, including the text and references, were last accessed in December 2019.

eCTD Web Page: http://www.fda.gov/ectd

Electronic Common Technical Document (eCTD) Course: https://www.accessdata.fda.gov/cder/eCTD/index.htm

Electronic Submissions Gateway: http://www.fda.gov/esg

Electronic Submissions Presentations: http://www.fda.gov/Drugs/DevelopmentApprovalProcess/FormsSubmissionRequirements/ElectronicSubmissions/ucm229642.htm

Questions about submitting electronically to CDER: ESUB@fda.hhs.gov

FDA Data Standards Resources: https://www.fda.gov/industry/fda-resources-data-standards/study-data-standards-resources

FDA eCTD Resources at: https://www.fda.gov/drugs/electronic-regulatory-submission-and-review/ectd-resources

CDISC Standard for Exchange of Nonclinical Data: https://www.cdisc.org/standards/foundational/send

FDA Data Standards Resources: https://www.fda.gov/ForIndustry/DataStandards/StudyDataStandards/ucm2005545.htm

Study and Project Monitoring

12

David G. Serota

The monitoring of studies conducted at preclinical contract research organizations (CROs) is an important and critical aspect of the use of outside laboratories in the performance of safety testing. In general, study monitoring refers to an active program of on-site review of an ongoing study that usually coincides with various critical study milestones. However, on-site qualification inspections for a previously unused CRO are necessary to ascertain if the CRO of interest has the necessary trained scientific and technical staff, facilities, instrumentation, processes, and compliance standards for consideration of the placement of future studies (often referred to as a facility inspection). Such qualification inspections may involve numerous key staff from the sponsoring organization (scientists, technical experts, quality assurance staff, veterinarians, etc.), with the inspections extending over a period of days. In addition, some large sponsoring organizations will conduct follow-up facility inspections every couple of years to ensure that any changes in the organizational structure or process are still consistent with their original expectations. The focus of this chapter, however, will be on study monitoring of ongoing studies

D. G. Serota
7th Inning Stretch Consulting LLC, Kalamazoo, MI, USA

© Springer Nature Switzerland AG 2020
S. C. Gad et al., *Contract Research and Development Organizations-Their History, Selection, and Utilization*, https://doi.org/10.1007/978-3-030-43073-3_12

although most of the points discussed in this chapter are also relevant for a facility inspection. When multiple studies testing the same experimental compound are being conducted at the CRO (many times simultaneously) to fulfill the needs for an investigational new drug filling (IND) or a New Drug Application (NDA), the opportunity exists for the study monitor to conduct inspections on multiple studies during a single site visit – this is referred to as project monitoring.

While it may seem obvious, it is important to ask and understand the question "why should studies being conducted at a CRO be monitored? From a historical perspective, up until the early 1990s, the vast majority of studies conducted at CROs were for either the chemical, agrichemical, food industries, or state and federal governmental agencies. The Toxic Substance Control Act (TSCA) requirements directed most of this activity for chemicals, while the Federal Insecticide, Fungicide, and Rodenticide Act (FIFRA) requirements directed most of this activity for agrichemicals. Big pharmaceutical companies (big pharma) had their own large in-house laboratories and outsourced very little, while the birth of the biotech industry was just in its infancy. While Good Laboratory Practice (GLP) procedures had been in place for approximately 40 (1979–2019) years, the frequency of study monitoring visits was much less than is occurring today. As we moved into the 1990s, the CRO industry experienced a dramatic growth through the opportunities offered by both big pharma and the rapidly growing biotech industry. Big pharma realized that it was more cost-effective to contract studies to CROs than it was to maintain their fixed-cost traditional and generally under-utilized in-house laboratories, while almost all the emerging biotech companies had neither the experienced staff nor the necessary facilities for conducting safety studies.

So in terms of answering the question as to why you should monitor studies at CROs, the answer is risk mitigation. The sponsoring organization can't afford to slow down and/or jeopardize its testing program because of problems or issues at the CRO. And since there is a real sense on the part of the sponsoring organization of not being in complete control of the studies being conducted, the monitoring of studies by either an experienced member of the sponsoring organization (company study monitor) or by an independent consultant (hired study monitor) contracted by the sponsoring organization to perform such responsibilities, serves that critical bridging role in providing the sponsoring organization's leadership with a level of confidence regarding the performance and quality of outsourced studies.

Therefore, the study monitor should be evaluating the following areas in the monitoring of outsourced studies: scientific integrity, technical/operational integrity, and compliance.

Scientific Integrity

The GLPs direct that the study director is the single point of control in the conduct of all regulated studies, so clearly the study director should be a focus point for the study monitor. However, the study director does not conduct studies in a vacuum, as most studies almost always also involve an anatomic and clinical pathologist, and a clinical veterinarian, and at times a toxicokineticist, an analytical chemist, a veterinary cardiologist, and a host of other potential specialists. Thus, the scientific integrity of all the involved professional staff must be evaluated. This should be accomplished through a review of their curriculum vitae (CV) and their in-house training records to have the confidence that their education, experience, and certifications exhibit the necessary and required scientific knowledge to not only contribute to the scientific excellence of the study but to also have the confidence and knowledge to provide guidance when unusual findings and observations or unexpected events occur. While an advanced educational degree might be thought to be critical, a better predictor of these abilities may well be a person's years of experience in conducting similar types of studies.

It is important to gauge how effectively the scientific staff interact with each other and how they work together in interpreting the study findings and writing the final report. A professionally written study report should present the study results in a clear, scientific manner and should have the flow and consistency of a good novel. Each of the various professionals that participate in the writing of that report all have a story to tell based on the data that they are directly involved with. It is the responsibility of the study director to ensure that the flow of interpretations and discussions demonstrate a consistency of findings throughout the report and present a clear and accurate description of the study findings. The study monitor should meet with these key professionals and ascertain their understanding of the study intent and learn of any concerns or recommendations that they might have regarding the study.

It is also critical that the study monitor establish the expected communications process during the life of the study and negotiate compliance with this process with the study director. The communications process should include such questions as: who makes the final study-related decisions at the sponsoring organization, does all information from the CRO go to the study monitor or are there others in the sponsoring organization that also need to be communicated with, and if significant issues or questions arise during off hours, weekends, or holidays, who does the CRO communicate with and what is the best method for doing this? However, it is important to remember that an effective communications process is a two-way process. The CRO will do everything possible to meet requirements, but they need to be provided with ample time and notification to accomplish these requirements. If there is a delay in receiving test compound, they need to know immediately so that they can better plan their resources and develop a new study schedule. If there is a need to perform an additional blood collection interval, they need time for scheduling of resources. If there is a need to receive the draft final report earlier, such requests are best made early in the reporting process.

Technical/Operational Integrity

The study monitor should evaluate the technical/operational integrity of the staff members that are conducting the various technical functions of the study. This includes both in-life functions, such as dose formulation, dose administration, blood collection, clinical signs, and body weight measurements, and post-life functions such as necropsy and histologic tissue processing. It is always appropriate to review the training records of technical staff to ensure that those conducting the critical study functions have the necessary knowledge and experience to successfully perform those functions and that such training and experience is fully documented. It is important to work with CROs that have well-organized and up-to-date training records. CROs that have a poorly designed and/or incomplete system of training documentation are much more likely to produce a lower-grade quality study as this can reflect on the quality philosophy of that organization's senior leadership. The study monitor should ask about the turnover rate within the technical staff and, if it is unusually high, inquire as to the reasons why and the actions being taken to correct it since a high turnover rate can result in significant quality problems in the conduct of the study. The study monitor should be aggressive in questioning any concerns that arise upon reviewing training records and present these concerns to both the study director and the operational leadership of the CRO.

The study monitor should review the organizational structure of the CRO and evaluate if it describes an organization that is consistent with good management practices. Are the staff in middle management roles competent, and do they have the training and experience to lead successfully? Are the organizational linkages clear and concise, and do they make sense? How many staff members are reporting to each management member, and does this number allow for adequate study oversight? Have there been any recent significant changes in the organizational structure that raise any concerns?

The study monitor should also ask questions about the CRO's training program and evaluate the effectiveness of the program to ascertain the corporate commitment to training. Is there a dedicated group of in-house training staff? Are there dedicated animal rooms and areas for training and dedicated training colonies for all commonly used species? How often does training occur, and what is the training process for new employees? How is training documented, are American Association of Laboratory Animal Science (AALAS) certification programs being utilized, and is there an active effort among the technical staff to receive such certifications? If there is a dedicated in-house training staff, the study monitor should meet with members of the training team to develop a firsthand impression of both their understanding of the importance of their role and their passion and commitment for imparting these skills to others.

Compliance

The study monitor should ascertain the philosophy, commitment, and procedures put into place by the CRO senior leadership for maintaining compliance with all regulatory guidelines, standards, and laws. An examination of all regulatory and certifying inspections conducted over the previous 5-year period should be reviewed and studied. Deficient finding, including those identified through the issuance of any FDA 483 findings, should be evaluated and discussed with CRO leadership, including the steps taken to correct and resolve such findings. The study monitor should ensure that the CRO has an active and engaged quality assurance (QA) unit, and they should meet with QA leadership to discuss expectations for QA to be actively involved in the study. In addition, the study monitor should ensure that they communicate with QA leadership their belief that QA is an important part of the team working on these studies and that they are being counted upon to assist in delivering a high-quality final report. The study monitor should review the internal QA inspection reports to ensure that critical in-life phase inspections have occurred accordingly to QA standard operating procedures (SOPs). The content of these reports should be evaluated as a means of ensuring adherence to both the study protocol and the SOPs in place at that time. The study monitor should also attempt to gauge the interaction between QA and the rest of the study teams to be confident that the relationship is one of cooperation and teamwork and not one of adversarial conflict.

Many CROs have implemented some form of internal process to evaluate and characterize study errors by employing some version of the CAPA (corrective and preventive action) process. This methodology allows for an overall evaluation of the type and frequency of errors to pinpoint and identify such errors as arising from a common event, whether it be person or process related. Once identified, then specific enhancements to either training or process can be implemented to improve quality. In general, those CROs that have initiated CAPA processes have committed to a quality culture and tend to offer a higher-quality performance. The study monitor should inquire as to whether the CRO has initiated CAPA processes, and if the answer is yes, they should ask to review some of the completed programs to ensure the ongoing commitment and success to these programs.

Over the past decade, the role and responsibilities of the Institutional Animal Care and Use Committee (IACUC) and staff veterinarians have taken on a much greater importance as animal welfare concerns and compliance with the 3Rs (replacement, reduction, refinement) have become a major focus for all animal testing facilities. The study monitor should ascertain that the CRO has an active and functioning IACUC and has a veterinary staff of sufficient size and experience to lead and manage animal welfare issues. In addition, the study monitor must develop a confidence that the veterinary staff have the full support of CRO senior leadership in carrying out their responsibilities in this area – which is a way to determine that senior leadership has an animal welfare philosophy and embrace its importance.

Monitoring Strategies

To ensure that the study monitor completes a successful monitoring visit at the CRO, the study monitor would be well served to pre-plan such visits by adopting a simple but critical monitoring strategy that should include preparing for the visit and deciding on when and what to monitor. When the study monitor does not prepare effectively before such a visit, the experience for both the study monitor and the CRO can be less than optimal.

In preparing for the visit, the study monitor should have a clear vision of what they want to accomplish during the visit, and they should share that information with the study director in a timely manner so that the study director can transmit that information internally to produce a seamless visit. The study monitor must be knowledgeable of both the intent of the study and the design of the study protocol. In addition, if specific technical study functions are to be observed or if study data are to be reviewed, the study monitor should have a basic understanding of the procedures being observed and the data being reviewed. The study monitor should project a sense of competence and professionalism at the CRO, including having a working knowledge of the CRO, the key staff involved on the study, and the procedures that will be utilized. Obviously, if the study monitor has made previous visits to the CRO, this information should already be known, but for a first-time visit, these aspects are vital to the success of the monitoring visit.

It is important to note that every CRO may conduct procedures differently than what might have been observed at other CROs or at the study monitor's own organization if animal facilities are present. This does not make it wrong, it only makes in different. The technical staff at the CRO is trained to perform procedures in a standard manner, based on their training protocols and training SOPs, and to suggest that they perform procedures in a manner more familiar to the study monitor could cause quality problems. If the study monitor has a concern about any procedures, this should be discussed with the study director and operational management.

In coordinating the visit to the CRO, the study monitor should provide a timely notification to the study director of the intent of the visit with proposed dates so that they can coordinate the visit with other internal areas associated with the study; studies to be reviewed and any specific study activities to be observed should be specified. If traveling to locations that have seasonal weather challenges, the study monitor should consider arriving a day earlier to allow for travel delays if a specific study function is to be observed. Most of the major CROs have internal sponsor services groups that can assist in hotel and ground transportation arrangements, and the study monitor should take advantage of those services. The study monitor can generally expect opportunities for socialization activities (i.e., dinners) with the study director and other key professionals to be offered at times during the visit, and they should be accepted. This presents a great opportunity to develop and deepen professional relationships and strengthen the partnership between organizations.

In terms of when study monitoring visits should occur, there are no specific rules to follow. Monitoring on the first day of study dosing is common as it provides the study monitor and the sponsoring organization with a comfort level that the study has been successfully initiated. Based on the size and difficulty of the study, monitoring on the first day of dosing also provides a mechanism to observe how organized and knowledgeable the CRO staff is of the study design, providing an even greater level of confidence in their ability to conduct the study successfully. If there are concerns regarding the successful initiation of the study, especially if it involves a difficult procedure, it is recommended that the study monitor arrive at the CRO at least a day prior to the study initiation to meet with the study director and the technical staff to discuss these concerns and suggest other options.

Depending on the study duration, study monitoring visits during other key study events, such as an interim or terminal necropsy, should be considered, as should visits to address any unexpected study findings and/or significant study omissions. In the latter case, the tone of the visit should be one of learning what occurred, how it occurred, how it will be corrected, and what effect it had on the integrity of the study. As in any organization, CROs are not infallible, and no matter the amount of training, education, SOPs, and quality procedures in place, errors can occur on studies. The experienced study monitor knows and accepts this reality and is able to work with the CRO in understanding the reasons behind the event and the correction process. While such events are never desirable, they do provide an opportunity to evaluate how the CRO responds which can tell much about its commitment to a quality culture.

What to monitor during a monitoring visit is a function of whether this will be a first-time visit or a continuing set of visits. Examples of a generalized audit checklist for both GLP and GMP studies are presented in Appendix J. The components of the monitoring function, however, are most often specific to each study and/or CRO so the information in the generalized audit checklist is best used as a starting point for monitoring considerations. If a first-time visit, the study monitor should spend time reviewing SOPs, training procedures and training files, and organizational charts, along with an inspection of the facilities (animal rooms, cage wash areas, feed and bedding storage areas; along with clinical pathology, necropsy, tissue processing, and archival areas). The study monitor should review the procedures in place at the CRO regarding animal receipt and quarantine and ensure that research animals are only purchased from reputable animal breeders. As part of this review, the role and opinions of the clinical veterinary staff in the selection of animal breeders should be confirmed as these are the in-house experts in this area. Additionally, the study monitor should ascertain that qualified veterinarian staff at the CRO have made periodic on-site inspections of the breeder sites to monitor their breeding and animal health programs.

In addition, the monitor should ask questions about ongoing quality programs, quality initiatives, and quality metrics – this is not a QA function but rather a means of learning about the quality culture at the CRO and its senior management. If the monitoring visit is part of a number of ongoing visits over time, the study monitor should generally focus on those areas most closely associated with the ongoing study. The study monitor should be aware that most CROs have specific requirements for entering certain areas of the facility, so they should understand that they will need to be escorted and that specific laboratory apparel and protective items (lab coats, scrubs, shoe covers, masks, ear plugs, safety glasses) may be required to be worn. To enter a primate area, submitted proof of a recent negative tuberculosis (TB) test may also be required.

At the end of the monitoring visit, the study monitoring team should hold an exit meeting with the study director and other key technical and support staff to discuss their findings during the visit. Even if there were no significant findings, this is a great way for the study monitor to thank and congratulate the CRO staff on their performance to date. If significant findings were detected, a representative from senior leadership should also be in attendance. The study monitor should be clear in their concerns and provide the CRO staff an opportunity to comment on such findings. In many cases, what might have been thought of as a significant finding might well be due to the study monitor not fully understanding, and this forum provides the opportunity for clarification. However, if findings were, indeed, significant, this is the time to hold open and frank discussions with the CRO staff, including the processes that are being considered to resolve and correct them and the anticipated timeline to accomplish this. While there is no hard and fast rule regarding the study monitor issuing a written report to the CRO regarding the monitoring visit, this is generally considered a good idea since it removes any ambiguity regarding the discussed topics and the timelines associated with the discussion. In addition, some study monitors provide the CRO with a draft for review and comment prior to finalization.

Interaction with the CRO Staff

Interactions with the staff members of the CRO are a most important and crucial part of any study monitoring visit. These are the individuals that are leading, performing, and/or auditing the study so an awareness of their strengths and abilities on the part of the study monitor can only enhance the monitor's confidence and expectation for a high-quality, well-conducted study. In addition, these interactions provide the study monitor with the opportunities for providing the CRO staff with important information regarding the test compound and its intended clinical use, which tends to "personalize" the study, especially among the technical staff.

The Study Director

In reference to the study director, the study monitor needs to develop a confidence in their experience and knowledge in conducting the types of studies that they are directing and to seek positive signs of active and ongoing study involvement. This can occur by reviewing the data files for active internal communications between the study director and the technical staff, along with any internal documentation that provides the reasons and number of times that the study director has been in the animal room. The study monitor needs to ascertain the scientific writing skills of the study director. While this is not always easy to perform, a review of previously published scientific papers and/or a review of previous technical reports for the sponsoring organization, if applicable, or a review of redacted reports for other sponsoring organizations is a good starting point. The study monitor should evaluate the communications skills and responsiveness of the study director for both internal correspondence and external correspondence. For external correspondence, especially associated with the study monitor and the sponsoring organization, the expectations need to be negotiated with the study director. Once both parties agree on the expectations, the study monitor must hold the study director accountable for meeting those requirements. However, it is important to note that communications represent a two-way process, and the sponsoring organization, especially the study monitor, must also be accountable for meeting any negotiated requirements, such as prompt review and approval of protocol amendments, on-time delivery of test compound, and reasonable reviewing time for draft reports.

The relationship between the study director and the study monitor is the most important relationship that occurs between the sponsoring organization and the CRO. Therefore, the bonding between these two individuals is key to the overall success of the study outcome. The relationship should be open and honest such that both professional and personal respect is created and maintained. Most CROs conduct a pre-initiation study meeting with all key professional and operational staff prior to study initiation to discuss the study protocol and any outstanding challenges or concerns. The study monitor should be an active participant in this meeting, either in person (the best option) or on the telephone. This is the opportunity for the study monitor to discuss the intent or the study, where it fits into the overall drug development process, the type of test compound and its intended clinical use, and any pertinent information regarding any anticipated toxicities and findings. This has tremendous value toward the overall scientific integrity and quality of the study since such information is not only critical in assisting the CRO staff in conducting the study; it also tends to personalize the study and make its intent even more important, especially for the technical and support staff.

The Technical Staff

The study monitor should have a good feeling about the experience and knowledge of the technical staff performing functions on their study, and this can occur through reviewing documented training records and spending time observing them conducting study functions. The study monitor should have direct interactions with the technical staff and ask questions about the study protocol to ascertain that they have read and understand their responsibility in the conduct of the study. It is also a good idea to ask them questions regarding the study intent and nature of the test compound to ensure that the study director had previously shared this information with them prior to the study initiation.

Since interactions with the technical staff performing the actual study functions in the animal room or supporting laboratory areas are a critical component of any monitoring visit, the study monitor should consider the best way to go about this since such interactions can go badly if not handled correctly. When meeting technicians, the study monitor should introduce themselves and their organization and title and explain why they are there. If observing a technician performing a specific technical function is required, it is best to always ask them if they mind since some technicians may become nervous and uncomfortable when strangers are observing them, which could result in a poor performance. If you were pleased and impressed with the performance of any observed technical function, compliment the staff for their efforts as such positive comments can create a sense of professional pride and impress upon them their importance in the overall drug development process. Following the successful completion of a difficult study, it is not uncommon for the study monitor and the sponsoring organization to show their appreciation for a job well done by recognizing the technical staff with an activity such as a pizza lunch or something similar. Such opportunities cost very little in terms of dollars but go a long way in establishing a sense of accomplishment and reward among the technical staff.

And finally, the study monitor can learn much about the culture of the organization and the positive outlook of its technical staff by just observing people as one moves around the facility. Do staff members lower their voices, refuse eye contact, or develop an almost defensive posture as you pass them by, or are they talking and smiling, greet you with eye contact, and speak to you with a hello or good morning? If the latter, then you can believe that staff feel that they are part of a quality organization and that its management has their best interests in mind. And because of that, the study monitor and the sponsoring organization should appreciate that this can also positively reflect in the quality of work that is being conducted. If the study is being conducted in a CRO outside of the United States, the study monitor should familiarize themselves with the culture and customs of the country the study is being conducted in.

The Quality Assurance Staff

The study monitor should develop a sense that the QA unit of the CRO has the experience and knowledge for conducting industry-expected auditing. This is determined by both reviewing documented training records and by conducting face-to-face conversations with the assigned study auditor and with QA management. It can also be important to learn if the QA staff is involved in the activities of the Society of Quality Assurance (SQA) and has SQA-certified auditors. It is critical to ascertain that the QA staff associated with your study have a study protocol awareness regarding the functions to be performed. Are they aware of any unusual or critical study functions, and have they planned/are they planning to audit the performance of these functions? Certain studies can have some special components in their design, so the QA function should not be operating on the "one-size-fits-all" philosophy in terms of their auditing plans.

The IACUC

As previously discussed, the role and responsibilities of the IACUC and staff veterinarians have taken on a more critical and active role within the CRO industry. The study monitor should spend time meeting with the IACUC chairperson and with other members of the IACUC to firmly gauge the commitment of the CRO to animal health and welfare issues and to the 3Rs. The composition of the IACUC should be reviewed to ensure that the representation is balanced and consistent, and questions regarding how members are selected and how long they serve should be asked. It is very important to inquire about the outside members of the IACUC and ascertain that they are taking an active role in the process of animal care and welfare issues. The study monitor should inquire about the review and approval processes, and on what issues the IACUC might deny a protocol approval. They should learn how often the IACUC meets and how difficult decisions are resolved. They should ask to review the results of any recent United States Department of Agriculture (USDA) inspections or Association for Assessment and Accreditation of Laboratory Animal Care International (AAALAC) site visit findings, and if there were deficiencies noted, the actions being taken by the CRO to correct them and when.

Information Technology

In today's world where most laboratory data are captured electronically and most study reports are prepared electronically, the study monitor should evaluate the strength and capabilities of the information technology (IT) leadership and staff of the CRO and ascertain that IT at the CRO is current in its understanding of regulatory requirements and has in place the necessary systems to protect the integrity and confidentially of the study raw data. If the study monitor does not feel qualified in conducting such investigations, the sponsoring organization should select a knowledgeable person (either from inside their organization or using an independent consultant with strong credentials in this area) to assist the study monitor in conducting this review. As part of this review, an evaluation of the commitment of the CRO senior leadership to support IT staffing and initiatives should be paramount since an understaffed or under supported IT function could lead to significant quality and/or timing issues associated with ongoing studies.

Security

In the unpredictable world that we live in today, it is critical that the CRO have systems and procedures in place to maintain the security of the staff and the entire facility, including study animals, study data, and study equipment and instrumentation. The study monitor should establish that the CRO has a strong focus on security and ascertain the security philosophy of the CRO. Is there a dedicated security staff, and what is their security background? How large is the security staff, and is the facility secured around the clock 7 days a week? What physical barriers are in place to deter a possible break in, such as a high fence around the perimeter of the site, and are entrances to the facility controlled? Are both external and internal areas monitored by security camera? Are certain areas in the facility, such as animal areas, considered limited access areas, and do they require some type of card reader to enter? Does the facility have an emergency action plan in case of a natural disaster, and are emergency drills conducted at reasonable intervals? Does the facility have a fire suppression system, and what type do they use? If the sponsoring organization is using the CRO for the first time, the study monitor should meet with security management at the CRO to ask these questions directly.

Senior Leadership

The study monitor should request an opportunity to meet with the senior leadership at the CRO, especially for a first-time visit. Organizations almost always function in a "top-down" manner when it comes to essential attributes such as company philosophy and quality commitment, and the experienced study monitor can learn much through conversations with senior leadership. Not all senior leadership members have a science background, and while it might be preferred, it is not critical to the success of the organization. What is critical, however, is for senior leadership at the CRO to be open and honest in the interactions with both outside sponsors and inside staff and to have a passion for the work that is being conducted by their staff. While leadership styles are dependent upon each individual, the study monitor should seek to identify the style of the CRO leadership as this could become important if difficulties arise with any ongoing study or relationship issues arise in working with members of the CRO staff, and the study monitor and the sponsoring organization need to reach out to senior leadership for a resolution.

Subcontracted Services

While most of the larger preclinical CROs describe themselves as "one-stop shopping" sites, there are numerous occasions when certain components of a safety study are required to be subcontracted to other organizations that specialize in those areas. This is more the rule than the exception for the smaller CROs. Examples of the type of functions that might be subcontracted would include histopathology, pharmacokinetic modeling, electrocardiography, and archiving. When it is the CRO's decision to subcontract, the sponsoring organization should be made aware of this decision as early in the study as possible and should have the right to disapprove and recommend an alternative laboratory. If the sponsoring organization selects the subcontracted laboratory, it should be their responsibility to ensure that that laboratory is fully able to conduct the work in terms of both technical and regulatory compliance, and in the time frame required. If the sponsoring organization wants the preclinical CRO staff to monitor and audit the subcontracted facility and its work output, they should expect that the CRO will need to include the cost of this in the study contract price.

Contracting, Pricing, and Cost of Works Performed by CROs

13

Once a source is selected to perform a body of work under contract, a great deal of effort still remains for the sponsor or sponsor's agent before work can be actually initiated, and more still before the desired product is in hand. At the front of this process is the development of a contract that ensures that desired work will be done and that the final product will meet your needs and expectations.

As a starting place, consider a few "rules" that any contractor should adhere to:

A vendor or consultant should:

1. Provide open, detailed, realistic costs, dates, and number estimates to the client or potential client.
2. Do whatever is possible to establish and maintain a positive, open, and honest relationship with each client.
3. Be proactive about providing information and suggestions to help a client enhance the quality or speed of their work.
4. Appoint a primary contact person to interact with each client. This needs to be a single person and not a group or multiple individuals.
5. Do whatever is necessary to meet one's time and cost commitments.
6. Provide the highest quality product possible given the time and cost constraints.

© Springer Nature Switzerland AG 2020
S. C. Gad et al., *Contract Research and Development Organizations-Their History, Selection, and Utilization*, https://doi.org/10.1007/978-3-030-43073-3_13

7. Provide all services required and be willing to go beyond the strict limits of the contract to ensure the client is pleased with the services and expectations are met.

At the same time, both parties must be particularly vigilant for scope creep – either the addition of expected work to a project with no explicit agreement to pay for some or the addition of costs and billing to a project without the client clearly being advised as to the fact and of totally new cost expectations.

With all this fresh in mind, careful consideration can now be given to key areas.

Costing/Pricing

Probably the first component of a contract to be addressed is the cost of the work. Indeed (as presented in Chap. 5) this is almost always a part of one's consideration in the process of vendor selection. But the need to be clear and precise in what is expected from a contractor does not end with the selection of same in the bidding process. From this point an agreement and/or contract must be developed. If a protocol is involved, it should also be considered as a significant part of the specifications of the work.

We live in a time when social concerns over the growing impact of technology on our environment and our ultimate well-being erupted into positive political action leading to a new array of laws and regulations. This of course is a bonanza for attorneys, who in customary unbeloved fashion have proceeded to establish themselves as indispensable participants in defining and resolving new fields of conflict, fields about which their knowledge and experience are significantly lacking. Quite obviously, it is also a bonanza for bureaucrats, who have inherited a Solomon's mine of new power and jurisdiction from which they have already produced considerable gold plated gobbledygook along with a veritable waste dump of semantic sludge.

But lawyers and bureaucrats have not been the only ones to find prosperity in these new laws. They have served to increase demand for well-educated toxicologists and other scientific professionals, to whom we must all look for answers to so many questions and whose services are therefore in such marked demand. The current (late 2010) economic situation aside, this will undoubtedly continue for the foreseeable future.

Some people continue to battle what they regard the "nonproductive nature" of all this activity and expense, even while reluctantly accepting it as a fact of contemporary business life. Certainly the impact of the environmental era is making it harder for some businesses to make money, at least in the short term. Certainly the additional costs of regulatory requirements ultimately add to the cost of goods and are aggravating our vexatious inflation problems. Certainly the social cost is compounded by the huge new bureaucracies that this movement has fostered. But a purely materialistic balance sheet concept of productivity seems far too narrow. If productivity is defined more generously to include the objective improvement of everyone's health and safety, then the great surge of concern over health and the potential hazards of drugs are very productive indeed.

In all events, it is clear that lawyers, investors, managers, and scientists must learn to deal productively with each other if the problems of the environmental era are to be resolved in a positive fashion for everyone involved. This means that they must communicate effectively and resultingly completely understand each other. In the interest of such understanding, and before passing to a discussion of some practical legal issues, it will be useful to mention one dichotomy that frequently gives rise to confusion, failure of communication, and sometimes outright antagonism between lawyers and scientists. We are referring to the difference between "scientific fact" and "legal fact."

This dichotomy arises from the different basic objectives of the two disciplines. The objective of science is the pursuit of knowledge about the physical world in all its attributes. The objective of law, however, is the minimization and resolution of disputes. To the scientist, a "fact" is a particular aspect of objective reality; to the lawyer, a "fact" is simply a state of knowledge that is adequate to support the interest of the client in a particular dispute. For example, toxicologists are typically extremely interested in the mechanism of genetic mutation as an element in understanding the biochemistry and molecular biology of carcinogenesis. They want to know objectively whether a single dose or a few doses of a new drug can induce a cancer or whether the mechanism requires some threshold of concentration or duration of exposure. The question has enormous practical consequences, but scientists are fundamentally interested in finding out the truth, regardless of the consequence. The lawyer is also interested in scientific truth, but will seldom be objective about it. If the business men and clients in or of a pharmaceutical manufacturer whose business would be wiped out by a "zero tolerance" rule, the lawyer will try to persuade the court or agency that there is in fact a "no-effect" level within which the client should be allowed to operate. Representing a "class" of possible injured patients who would like to see the specific drug or class of drugs taken off the market, the lawyer will argue that the single-molecule concept is in fact correct. If doubt must be conceded, the lawyer will still argue that the theory most congenial to his or her client's interest is the more likely. In short there would be no hesitation to build arguments in support of the clients desired conclusion and to ignore or explain away any contrary views, which is the very opposite of the scientific method. Furthermore, if the trend of objective scientific research seems to be running against the argument, the lawyer will often mount a rearguard action to postpone as long as possible the legal recognition and acceptance of this adverse scientific reality. To attorneys, the law and fact is what and how one can twist and contort it to leverage their own position. To scientists laws and facts are what they are, proven experimentally and only changing when errors are discovered.

Of course, this is possibly an unfair oversimplification of the lawyer's role. In practice there are ethical constraints on the lengths to which counsel may go in advocating the client's cause, and sophisticated clients will seldom want their lawyers to fight to the bitter end at the cost of adverse publicity and a poor public image. Nevertheless, the lawyer dealing with a scientific issue will frequently dispute the fact which a scientist regards as settled. Attorneys also will attempt to eradicate the value of a scientific fact with some trivial ancillary distraction that really bears no actual weight on the issue at hand. Attorneys and scientists should understand that their choices in career paths dictate differing roles may which compel differing views of reality, at least over the short run.

So much for philosophy and generalities on this topic. Let us pass now to some more important specific legal issues that toxicologists are likely to encounter in their work, first in relation to research contracts and second in relation to their regulatory responsibilities.

The Contract

The enormously increased demand for contract research and development has produced a corresponding increase in research contracts. Companies of small and medium size generally do not have the technical or financial resources to conduct in-house development efforts such as preclinical safety studies, while even the larger companies often elect to farm out at least a part of this work. By their nature such arrangements are likely to involve highly sensitive issues, which may have economic implications far beyond the cost of the research itself. Contracts of this kind should be negotiated by a team of lawyers and scientists who have a thorough understanding of the problems to be investigated, including both the scientific issues and the potential business implications. If the research is to pursue a specific, predefined problem, such as evaluating carcinogenicity, as distinguished from a general screening program, such an understanding is particularly important.

Contracts are promises that the law will enforce. The law provides remedies if a promise is breached or recognizes the performance of a promise as a duty. Conflicts arise when a duty does or may come into existence, because of a promise made by one of the parties. To be legally binding as a contract, a promise must be exchanged for adequate consideration. Adequate consideration is a benefit or detriment that a party receives that reasonable and fairly induces that party to make the promise/contract.

A point worth mentioning here is that for many people contracts are binding instruments of understanding governing behavior and conduct involved in a specific area of concern. However, there is a not insignificant number of individuals out there who view contracts merely as necessary hurdles to clear in the course of doing business. These special people have no intention of complying to any contract that they sign and will do what they will. Their attitude is that contracts are nothing more than feed or slop for the attorneys to banter over. Although not recommended, contracts are not truly necessary if dealing with completely and totally honest people. Contracts can be truly valuable instruments to document expectations of both sides. In the course of contract negotiation, try to assess the level of commitment of the "alternate" party, and if a sense of lack of long-term honoring of the agreement is not there, perhaps it is better to take a different approach to a solution.

Contracts are mainly governed by state statutory and common (judge-made) law and private law. Private law principally includes the terms of the agreement between the parties who are exchanging promises. This private law may override many of the rules otherwise established by state law. Statutory law may require some contracts be put in writing and executed with particular formalities. Otherwise, the parties may enter into a binding agreement without signing a formal written document.

In our experience, good contracting is a result of three components: legal expertise, subject matter expertise, and common sense. Assuming a modicum of common sense and a substantial understanding of the subject area of the contract, presumably contract law is the only area for which the RA (regulatory affairs) professional needs knowledgeable guidance. Most of the principles of the common law of contracts are outlined in a compilation entitled *Restatement Second of the Law of Contracts* published by the American Law Institute. The restatements are an attempt to organize (restate) common-law rules in selected broad areas (e.g., agency, contracts, conflicts of law, etc.). Restatements do not reflect statutes, which can alter common-law rules and principles. Restatements are secondary authority, not law, but they are drafted by respected scholars, attorneys, and jurists. They are useful as research tools and study aids.

Of greater importance is the Uniform Commercial Code (UCC), whose original articles have been adopted in nearly every US state. The UCC represents a body of statutory law that governs important categories of contracts, so it should be consulted whenever an issue arises. The UCC Article 2 regulates every phase of a transaction for the sale of goods and provides remedies for problems that may arise. It provides for implied warranties of merchantability and fitness. There is also a duty of good faith in the UCC that is applicable to all the sections.

The RA (regulatory affairs) and product safety professionals routinely enter into the contracts themselves as well as their negotiation, or review draft contract proposals, related to a wide range of goods and services necessary to develop and commercialize a regulated product. These include confidentiality agreements and service agreements (e.g., contract manufacturing, raw material purchases, consulting agreements, clinical research organizations, clinical investigator agreements, etc.). It is essential that the RA and toxicology professionals understand the essential elements of contract law (offer, acceptance, consideration, breach, remedies, etc.) as they relate to the technical aspects of their particular industry and the specific scope of the contract. The effort these professionals should invest in properly drafting or reviewing a contract is directly proportional to the criticality of the product or service to be provided. Like regulatory submissions, poorly drafted contracts can significantly affect the regulatory timetable and delay product commercialization resulting in lost market opportunity. In particular, pay close attention when specifying the goods or services expected from the vendor. Whenever possible, tie deliverables to well-recognized and ascertainable standards (GLP compliance, cGMP compliance, GCP compliance, etc.). Vague, unspecified, or imprecisely defined standards often result in a legally binding agreement that is hard to enforce and totally unsatisfactory deliverables.

Part of the job is to educate the lawyer about the nature of the work, including its limitations. The lawyer needs to know, for example, the extent of which test instruments and procedures are reliable and must have a grasp of the statistical presumptions and methods so that the contract can be approached with these parameters in mind. Do not assume that your attorneys are incapable of assimilating a good knowledge and understanding of the scientific issues. Their job requires them to become experts pro tem in such matters whenever they have legal relevance. Any competent lawyer should be able to understand and talk the language of toxicology and research with appropriate instruction. Many companies have sought out lawyers with appropriate technical backgrounds to make this process easier and more dependable.

Armed with this technical understanding, the attorneys can then proceed to develop a contract that is relevant to the situation. For a low-risk, uncomplicated job, they may suggest a relatively simple letter agreement with a minimum of verbiage. They might even be willing to go along with an oral understanding if the issues are very simple, but this will be rare and depends upon the parties involved. For a more extensive project on which substantial economic interests are riding, they will undoubtedly propose a very thorough and definitive agreement. Much of the language will be routine or "boiler plate," the type commonly found in agreements of various kinds. Other clauses may be addressed specifically to the special situations of research contracts. What are some of these special problems?

Purpose and Description of Work

The basic purpose and end goals of the project should be described carefully in the contract with sufficient breadth and detail as to ensure that the researchers do not overlook something because of an inadequate understanding of the context. While some contracts may call for "pure research" and be concerned only with the objective development of new data or information, most projects, particularly from the private sector, will have one or more very pragmatic objectives that are specific to the business purposes of the sponsor. These purposes may well affect the design and scope of the research project. For example, a pharmaceutical company may be looking for a more effective antiviral agent for use in the HIV therapeutic market. By this the company may mean that the new agent must be biologically effective for a broader range of patients, be effective in a smaller dose than the current agent, have a longer shelf-life when combined with the other ingredients of the product, or have a lower incidence of side effects. Any one of these factors might justify the use of a new antiviral and could be the objective of contracted research, but it is obvious that an antiviral with more than one of these qualities would be even better. Researchers should know about these advantages so that their work can be designed for maximum usefulness and synergy with other research on the same general problem.

Of course, the sponsor may be concerned about confidentiality and may therefore want to limit the extent of the research's knowledge and involvement. A producer might be aware of some emerging side-effect problem with the drugs currently on the market. Obviously, this kind of balancing is for the sponsors to decide, but they should remember that researchers working with blinders on may overlook some collateral problems and opportunities if their efforts are too constrained.

In addition to identifying the purpose, the contract should also identify the research methods that are to be employed. In some cases the method itself may be a subject for research, but in most situations there will be at least a general understanding of the work to be done. This should be spelled out, along with any limitations or variations from normal practice. Specific research protocols found in the literature may be adopted by reference, or the sponsor and the researcher may jointly work out a protocol of their own. There must be absolutely no ambiguity about what the researcher is called on to do as well as the anticipated results.

Time Frame

Much development research is mandated by various regulatory agencies such as the FDA, and marketing of a product or reaching a milestone associated with payments from partners or investors may have to await the results. Thus, companies will frequently insist that time is of the essence, that the researcher must meet the stipulated timetable or be liable for damages or forfeiture of fees. Faced with such a clause, the researcher will want to be sure that he or she can in fact meet the deadlines.

Regulatory and Judicial Proceedings

Toxicological research data and results will often be of key importance as evidence in regulatory proceedings or in lawsuits. Hence, it is important that the work product, or at least key parts of it, be reflected in documents and records (written and/or electronic), which will be useful for this purpose. A brief overview of the applicable rules of evidence may help one understand this. These are procedural rules that are applied quite strictly in the courtroom and somewhat less strictly in administrative hearings. Basically, a document that purports to contain information that is relevant to the issue at hand cannot be admitted as evidence without first being authenticated. This means that a live witness must testify from personal knowledge that the document is genuine and that the information is in fact what it purports to be. The live witness might be the research scientist who actually produced the report, or it might be a higher-echelon person under whose supervision the work was done. Whoever he or she is, the live witness can expect to be the subject of intensive cross-examination, first in an attempt to show that the document is not admissible as evidence and then, if this fails, in an attempt to discredit the methods, the results, the conclusions, and indeed the competence of the researcher.

Needless to say, this can be a very stressful and unpleasant business, particularly if the document is ambiguous or incomplete or if the witness has not done the necessary homework. It can also be very time-consuming. Hence, the research contract should spell out the understanding with regard to the use of researchers as potential witnesses. Typically, the contract will require the research institution to supply an appropriate person or persons to testify for the purpose of authenticating and defending documents reflecting the work done. Such appearances are usually made at the expense of the interested party, including a reasonable per diem or other fee and the reimbursement of expenses. If special preparation for the appearance is anticipated, the contract should indicate whether this time is subject to special reimbursement.

Incidentally, the courts and agencies are not limited to final reports to the client in their search for relevant documentary information. It is entirely possible that research notebooks, reports of internal meetings, diaries, emails (personal and company), and even informal scratch notes may be requested and scrutinized. CROs, like business corporations, should therefore develop carefully designed record management programs to control the creation and maintenance of formal and informal paperwork. The destruction of relevant documentation for the purpose of keeping it out of court can be a criminal offense (ask ENRON or Arthur D. Anderson). Consequently, it is important to limit the information that becomes part of the written record and to establish and observe a general record retention and destruction policy and schedule that will justify the routine weeding out of nonessential records.

For similar though not identical reasons, the contract will usually require the researcher to retain samples of testing materials, feed samples, histological specimens, and the like. These do not usually find their way into the court-room, but may be critically important in confirming the accuracy of challenged data, rebutting allegations of misfeasance or faulty diagnosis, or accomplishing similarly constructive purposes.

As to retention period, it is almost impossible to be too conservative. The longer the better, not only to satisfy regulatory agencies and requirements but also to help establish a solid defense against future damage claims. Unfortunately for manufacturers, the statutes of limitation on claims for breach of warranty and negligence often do not begin to run until the damage or injury occurs. Thus, companies have been held liable for asserted defects in drug taken to market decades before the damage or injury is discovered. Since both drugs and devices are an easy target of such claims, proof of adequate toxicological research can be of great defensive importance. Generally, the sponsor of a project should want samples retained for a substantial time (10 years or more), and researchers will generally share this desire in order to minimize their own potential exposure.

The long-term retention of documents and samples creates obvious storage problems and their associated costs. Document retention can be minimized by the disciplined use of microfilming or PDF techniques. For almost all legal purposes, a properly made and authenticated microfilm copy is equivalent to a paper original. Sample storage is a more difficult matter. The main legal problem is to be absolutely sure that each sample can be properly identified and authenticated for possible future use. Procedures for cataloging and retaining samples should be carefully worked out and scrupulously followed. This is not a mere clerical or managerial responsibility; it calls for careful and continuing management attention. Storage conditions (environmental) themselves cannot be ignored as well as security.

Reports

Depending on the nature and extent of the research, the contract will include provisions for reports of various kinds. Progress reports will usually be appropriate if the work is complex and extended, and a final report is routine. The parties may or may not wish such reports to include editorial matter or commentary on the results.

This raises a very difficult and potentially sensitive problem area, namely, the extent to which the sponsor should be entitled to review, comment on, and edit proposed reports before they are issued. Sponsors will generally require a review of a draft report, and will often react with questions, comments, and suggestions for change. They may also want the opportunity for informal discussion of the draft report and the data and results on which it is based. There is nothing inherently wrong with this, but if the work relates to product safety and is being performed in the context of present or anticipated regulatory involvement, the parties should be extremely careful to preserve the fundamental integrity of the final report. The right to review and offer comments should never be constructed as a right to censor or suppress. This has become quite the area of concern with the FDA of late. It appears that the FDA's position is that subcontractor reports (veterinary cardiologist, veterinary ophthalmologist, bioanalytical, etc.) are to be finalized with no input from the sponsor nor the study director. The study director then writes the final report with all of this information with no input from the sponsor. This is foolish, because the true expert in any research or development project is the sponsor. SO with this approach good science is the true loser. Until this matter is completely resolved, one needs to make sure that EACH AND EVERY step along the way to the production of the final report is heavily documented showing changes made, when they were made, by whom they were made, and for what reason they were made to demonstrate to the agency that no collusion or misrepresentation of facts has occurred.

It is easy to believe and affirm that no ethical businessman, attorney, or scientist would tolerate or encourage the suppression or distortion of research results. It is less easy to apply this faith in a specific situation, which may involve large gray areas concerning the reliability of test methods, the adequacy of samples, the significance of an occasional anomalous result, and the subjective assessment of results as a whole, not to mention the semantic nuances that can arise in the process of articulating all these issues. Because we are human, we tend to see what we want to see and to find what we want to find, if there is any room at all for doubt or more favorable alternate interpretation. The legal danger lurks in the possibility that editorial changes in a research report may be influenced, at least subliminally, by considerations of self-interest.

There are several ways to minimize this problem. First, and perhaps most obvious, the contract may simply provide that the sponsor shall have no right of prior review. Unhappily, this deprives both parties of the opportunity for legitimate synergy and may simply be unacceptable to the sponsor. Second, the contract might provide expressly for review and comment by the sponsor but affirm the researcher's right to control the form and content of the report. This is a good approach, provided the parties do in fact observe the contract.

A third technique is to apply what might be called the "future appearance" test to the editorial process and its end result. The test can be posed as two questions:

1. Do any of the editorial changes involve a matter that, with the benefit of future hindsight, could be viewed as having material significance in the context of any presently applicable health or safety law or regulation or reasonably foreseeable health or safety problem?
2. If so, do the changes tend to lean toward avoiding or obscuring a potentially adverse condition?

If the answers to both questions are "yes," the changes that produced these answers are vulnerable to future criticism and should probably be omitted or modified.

Note that the first question calls for a deliberate effort to view present events from a future perspective, because that is the way our present judgments are being judged in the context of health and safety regulation.

An example may help to clarify this concept. Suppose you are engaged in some rabbit feeding studies to determine the oral toxicity of a submitted compound. At a certain point in the studies, several test animals die. Autopsy discloses gross liver damage, which is not encountered in the remaining test animal, all of which live considerably longer. You discover that an inexperienced technician may have inadvertently contaminated some of the feedstock given to the animal that died early, but you cannot prove this. There is no other obvious explanation for the early deaths. The size of the study is such that the anomalous deaths are of minimal statistical importance. Nevertheless, you decide to mention the early deaths and the liver damage in your final draft report and to include the deaths in the statistical data base. Your sponsor then suggests that since the early deaths are clearly anomalous and do not affect the general conclusions of the study, it would be preferable that they be omitted from the report.

Applying the future appearances test, it seems clear that if other studies were later to confirm that liver damage is a potential side effect of the ingestion of this compound (perhaps in animals other than rabbits), it might be said, with benefit of hindsight, that your anomalous results were in fact significant. It is also clear that the requested deletion of these results would tend to minimize or discount their importance. Hence, both questions are answered affirmatively. One should reject the proposed deletion. The anomalous results should be included for what they may be worth.

If, on the other hand, the sponsor had simply requested the addition of a footnote explaining your suspicions concerning contaminated feed, this would not tend to avoid or obscure a potentially adverse conclusion. Hence, your answer to the second question would be "no," and the requested addition would be acceptable.

Innocent Mistakes and Culpable Tampering

A related issue, though not strictly a contract matter, is what to do when it is discovered that someone has made a significant mistake in the course of the study or has perhaps even fabricated or tampered with the results. If the work is not yet public and is not part of a submitted or approved regulatory program, it may be possible to make corrections without announcement or publicity, provided a complete record of the situation is maintained. However, if the study is part of a submitted record or an established compliance program, the best course will be to "fess up" promptly and completely candidly, with an offer of full collaboration in any resultant investigation or necessary follow-up. This is embarrassing and could have serious legal consequences, but delay and/ or cover-up can only make things worse. Remember, one typically in situations has only one chance at saving their integrity and credibility, so behave accordingly.

Communications

One of the most important problems to be addressed in a research contract is communications. No matter how competent and sophisticated the work, its value will be reduced or even lost if its significance is not properly communicated to and understood by the sponsor. This is particularly true with projects whose shape and direction involve some subjective judgment or "art" on the part of the researcher. If the implications of a judgmental decision are not made known, the sponsor may be deprived of important information for the evaluation and utilization of the results.

Therefore, the contract should specify the frequency, method or methods of communication, the timing (if there are to be interim reports), the circumstances, if any, in which a special report may be appropriate, and the channels through which communications are to be made. Specific contact points should be well-defined. Each project will have its own specific needs, but generally speaking, the broader or more loosely defined the methods and objectives, the greater the need for ongoing close communication between the parties.

Since scientific issues and judgments will invariably be involved, the sponsor should designate specific scientific personnel in its organization as the initial recipients of reports. It is not uncommon to designate a manager for each project, with responsibility to receive all reports, communicate as appropriate with the researcher, and distribute the reports within an organization.

The communication of new information can have important legal implications for both parties. The researcher will have a duty to report any significant adverse results or effects as promptly as possible, because actual knowledge of such things may trigger a reporting responsibility on the part of the sponsor, either under FDA or under some other regulatory body's requirements on a common-law duty. For this reason it is critically important to maintain a good record of all communications on ALL matters and especially those of potential significance. In addition to copies of written reports, it may be appropriate to maintain copies of all emails, a log of telephone or other oral communications, and a record of any meetings between the parties. The phone log can simply be a record of calls made, giving date, time, and names of the communicants or participants. If the project is likely to produce sensitive interim information, it may be wise to go further and include a brief synopsis of the conversation. The same options apply to meeting records.

This raises a difficult policy question for both parties. If they elect to keep separate records, there is always the chance that the two records may be inconsistent in some important respect. This could produce embarrassment in the future. One needs to work in such a way as to think of themselves being in court at some point and use that perspective to decide how to handle a given situation. On the other hand, if the parties decide to maintain a single record of their communications, the editorial dangers discussed earlier will obviously be raised.

Whatever the record-keeping protocol, it is a good idea to be consistent when following the agreed procedure. Variations from a customary pattern are favorite clues for hostile lawyers to find evidence of malfeasance, nonfeasance, or cover-up. Nothing is more intriguing and suspicious than a hole in a file at some critically important time.

The problem of communication also embraces some very difficult judgmental questions for the researcher whose work uncovers some new and perhaps significant information. What constitutes a reportable event, and when should it be reported? The basic standard is one of reasonableness and good faith. For our purpose, reasonableness will be judged in relation to your scientific expertise and sophistication or the "reasonable scientist" test. If it would be reasonable for a competent scientist to believe that the development is materially significant in relation to the regulatory purpose or some other legal issue, it should be reported to the sponsor, even though you yourself might not share this belief. If, in good faith, that scientist does not believe that the development is significant in this sense, it need not be reported immediately, although it may become a part of some later routine report. However, relationships are best maintained if full disclosure is maintained on a timely basis.

Proprietary Rights

If the research is of such nature that original methods, techniques, or equipment may have to be developed, the contract should deal with the problem of ownership and right of use. Generally, parties who pay for the research will want to own any resultant inventions, although they may be willing to give shop rights to the researcher for applications that are not adverse to their particular interests. A research company may be reluctant to surrender the right to further use of its own inventions. Obviously these situations should be addressed in the contract. The final result will depend on the negotiation itself. Even with a well-drawn contract, difficult problems can sometimes arise in the problem area.

Confidentiality

Every research contract should include a clause dealing with the use and disclosure of proprietary information. The first, often difficult step is to define what is meant by proprietary information. Although many judicial decisions attempt to define this term, the peculiar nature of research will often justify a carefully drafted contractual definition based on the specific situation. The clause should cover both information supplied to the researchers by the sponsoring party and information developed by the researchers in the course of their work. The party supplying data will want the broadest possible definition, usually one that attempts to cover all submitted information regardless of whether it is actually proprietary or a trade secret. Researchers, on the other hand, should be careful not to accept an excessively broad clause that might seriously hamper their legal or ethical responsibilities.

A very common traditional approach is to restrict the use and disclosure of all submitted information except in three specific categories: (1) information known to disclose prior to disclosure, (2) information properly available to disclose from another source and without restriction, and (3) information in the public domain.

Despite its popularity, this approach can pose problems for parties involved in research because the traditional language does not adequately protect a party's rights with respect to the future fruits of ongoing or incipient projects. For example, if a research organization has begun a line of inquiry that may lead to valuable new information or methodology, the receipt of related data from another party under conditions that restrict its use may restrict the freedom of researchers to pursue their preexisting inquiry along its logical path. For this reason, each party to a proposed research agreement should carefully review his or her then-current activities to determine whether the confidential receipt of information would be likely to cause any problems with other projects. If a problem is foreseen, the lawyer may be able to draft contract language to reduce or avoid the difficulty. The confidentiality clause should also cover such questions as mandatory disclosure to government agencies, limitations on the persons within the contracting organizations who will be allowed access (frequently limited to those who have a "need to know"), and limitations on publication rights, if any. If there are to be subcontracts, the confidentiality clause should be extended to cover the subcontractors.

In conclusion, it should be clear that there is almost no such thing as a routine research contract and that an adequate contract demands close cooperation and mutual understanding between the attorneys and the scientists involved and any other ancillary personnel (e.g., management, marketing, etc.). The contract may end up looking simple and commonplace, but its underlying homework should always be thorough.

Ethical and Legal Problems of Regulatory Disclosure

It should be obvious by now that many scientists involved in research may need help in understanding the legal aspects of their position. There is nothing wrong with using a company's law department or legal counsel as a first recourse, but bear in mind that they represent the employer, not the individual researcher. While such an option is possibly financially attractive, it may not provide the best outcome. These points remain, ultimately, personal ethical issues to resolve.

Consultants and Their Role

14

Shayne C. Gad and Charles B. Spainhour

Consultants are individual organizations that are independent of the companies developing and marketing drugs and devices as well as the regulatory agencies that govern the processes serving to provide specific knowledge and expertise to the organizations (particularly the commercial side) attempting to put a product on the market, be it a drug, biologic, radiopharmaceutical, or medical device. They have been in existence since modern industries started appearing and since the origin of the modern pharmaceutical industry during the Second World War. Until the late 1980s, most individuals or groups of individuals elected to become consultants either as a transition between jobs or as a "sunset cruise" that marked a means of transition from leaving full-time employment and full-time retirement.

There are currently ~350 independent or small organization toxicology consultants globally. Most are located in the United States, but the vocation is becoming more globalized. The largest organization of such consultants is the Roundtable of Toxicology Consultants (www.toxconsultants.com), currently with 147 members. Its website provides a directory of its members and their

S. C. Gad
Gad Consulting, Cary, NC, USA
e-mail: scgad@gadconsulting.com

C. B. Spainhour
Scott Technology Park, Calvert Laboratories, Scott Township, PA, USA

© Springer Nature Switzerland AG 2020
S. C. Gad et al., *Contract Research and Development Organizations-Their History, Selection, and Utilization*, https://doi.org/10.1007/978-3-030-43073-3_14

areas of expertise and is a good place to find consulting help in the field. It is an organization of independents, so large (more than two member) firms cannot belong and are thus have to be found elsewhere.

However, as these industries (particularly the pharma industry) have consistently and continually been reducing their internal capabilities and human resources, consultants and consultancies have evolved to a form of "gig economy," paying for the services of consultants only as they need them. Such a move reduces the "fixed costs" (helping the appearance of financial spreadsheets) for any company needing and utilizing the services of a consultant. Here we will focus on the areas of toxicology and pathology (drug and device safety assessment consultants), with some discussion of consultants in the related disciplines of pharmacokinetics and chemistry, manufacturing, and controls (CMC) and regulatory consultants. One of the authors has been a consultant since 1993, first as an individual and then as the head of a consulting firm, which at the present time has 13 employees. During this time, this author has tracked the number of practicing independent toxicology-pathology consultants. The number of individuals was stable at about 250 for the period of 1993 until 2008. Since 2008, as large firms have sourced increasingly more (most) of their needs, the number of consultants and the areas for which consulting services are sought has increased substantially. Since about the year 2000, such independent consulting has become a legitimate long-term career in and of itself.

The scope of services that a consultant or consultancy provides is generally a reflection of the experience of the individual(s) involved.

Basics

A consultant is a temporary or part-time employee of one or (more often) more companies. Generally, there are at least two sets of documents that govern the interaction, responsibilities, and duties of the involved parties. The first is entitled either a confidentiality or nondisclosure agreement, which protects the intellectual property and often confidential information shared and discussed between the involved parties. The second is an agreement governing compensation for the consultant for his/her/their services. The latter may take a shape in a number of forms, a simple letter agreement, a purchase order issued in response to a written or verbal request/quotation, a contract covering services over a longer period of time (usually a year with a provision of scheduled renewal), or a master service agreement under which multiple invoices can be submitted. Payment may be for either a specific piece of work, expenses, and services in general or just a regularly scheduled retainer. Type and timing of payment is specified as due within a set period of time with 30 days being most common. Most businesses usually pay around 42 days, but large companies have recently been seeking longer payment periods up to 90 days and even longer. It is extremely one-sided and unfair to drag the payment for services out to such extraordinary time periods. People have financial responsibilities, and payments should be made as requested in the agreements made.

Part of these agreements are specifications of the range or scope of services that are to be provided with limitations on doing work for other clients with competing interests. The principal traits that a consultant brings to the table are experience, knowledge, training, the ability of problem-solving, and most importantly the ability to provide the weight of their professional reputation.

By definition, then, a consultant's most valuable assets are his/her/their reputation and level of knowledge in staying current on relevant science, technology, and regulations. There are now well-recognized professional certifications for toxicologists (Diplomate American Board of Toxicology, DABT), veterinary pathologists (Diplomate American Board of Veterinary Pathology, DABVP), and regulatory affairs specialists (Regulatory Affairs Certification, RAC). There is a plethora of other relevant certifications established by specialty societies or groups (e.g., safety pharmacology, European Registered Toxicologists, etc.) that seem to be more "guild-type memberships" at this time.

Types of Toxicology Consultants

There are two orthogonal ways of defining the various types of toxicology consultants. The first is by the field of expertise: forensic, environmental, occupational, agrochemical, consumer product, pharmaceutical, and medical device. In these cases, here we will limit ourselves to pharmaceutical, industrial chemical, and medical device.

The second approach is based on type of consulting. The usual categories are investigational, technical, regulatory, and litigation support. In this volume, for interactions with CRPs, we will be focusing on technical and regulatory, with the most common type being regulatory.

Necessary Attributes for a Consultant

When a consultant is retained, a choice is made between multiple candidates identified by a search or reference from a relevant, trusted colleague. The search could be performed by reviewing a listing of consultants in the technical and regulatory arenas, such as that which is available on the RTC site (Roundtable of Toxicology Consultants – www.toxconsultants.com). A general search on Google is another option in each case; factors point to be considered should be:

- The education of the consultant.
- The relevant experience of the consultant.
- The personal reputation of the consultant.
- The professional technical reputation of the consultant.
- The consultants reputation working with regulators.
- The interpersonal skill of the consultant.
- The communication skills of the consultant.
- The location (time zone) of the consultant.
- The personality of the consultant: does it clash with yours?
- General philosophy of the consultant with regard to drug development.
- The reputation of the consultant among his or her peers.
- The familiarity of the consultant in working with the agencies.
- The history of attendance of the consultant at relevant scientific meetings and participation in continuing education opportunities.

To be productive, generally, the selection of a toxicology consultant should involve the discussion of confidential information. Therefore a confidential disclosure agreement (CDA) or non-disclosure agreement (NDA) should be put in place early in any interaction. If the selected individual is not already known to the sponsor, a teleconference or face-to-face meeting is certainly strongly recommended.

Once a consultant has been selected, a consulting agreement should be set in place to establish what work is to be done, how it is to be assigned, proposed timelines, rates and terms of payment, confidentiality, and process for termination of the agreement. An example of such an agreement is provided at the end of this chapter.

The duties and responsibilities of the consultant vary with the needs of the sponsor organization, but commonly they could include:

1. Planning nonclinical programs and studies.
2. Identifying and eliciting proposals from identified qualified CROs (it is generally the case that proposals should be sought from three qualified organizations). Some individuals press the consultant to get as many as 14 different proposals, which is more information than one can reasonably and fairly manage. So the upper limit should be four proposals for consideration.
3. Recommending or selecting specific CROs. It is not currently unlikely that more than one CRO will be needed to execute a CRO program.
4. Protocol design/modification.
5. Study monitoring and directing. Ensuring proper study conduct and reporting as well as adhering to an agreed timeline. Ensuring study completion and reporting, including production of a SEND suitable form from submitted to FDA.
6. Resolution of any problems that may arise in the conduct of the program.
7. Arrangement and coordination of meetings and interactions with regulatory organizations.
8. Preparation and submission of briefing documents for regulatory meetings.
9. Preparation, submission, and maintenance of product regulatory submissions such as INDs, 510(k)S, IDEs, CE Mark Applications, and annual reports.

Scope Creep

This chapter would not be complete if the concept of "scope creep" was not at least mentioned. The problem of scope creep exists in various forms present across the entire CRO universe of operations. So what is "scope creep"? For purposes here are the two relevant versions. The first is that the consultant expands the range (and billing for) of his or her work beyond what is originally authorized (or requested) by the client. The second is that the sponsor requests the addition to previously agreed deliverables (with no match offer or intent to pay for additional work beyond that originally quoted or agreed to by the consultant. Accordingly, one can see the importance of spending an adequate amount of time fleshing out the details of the financial and technical aspects of the working relationship. Working hard to define the limits of the working relationship can significantly reduce or eliminate the changes of ambiguity and the development of bad feelings later in the relationship.

Topics for Discussion with Prospective Consultants for a Potential Project

Again – Establish Early What Each Side Needs and Wants!

- State up front what is important to you.
- Expectations as regards venues of communication.
- Guidelines for verbal/voicemail communication.
- Guidelines for email communication.
- Define accessibility and relevant contact information.
- Define frequency of communication.
- How is data to be handled.
- How are team members to be involved in the communication process.
- How are subcontractors to be communicated with in the process.
- Understand the role of the veterinarian in the project and at the CRO.
- Understand and appreciate the role of IACUC in the project and at the CRO.
- Clearly understand as best as possible the techniques in the performance of all aspects of the study, and make any recommendations or express concerns up front.
- Understand the protocol generation process and the times required for IACUC approval, the ordering of animals, periods of time for quarantine and acclimation, etc.
- Clearly state the reasonable expectations with regard to performance/quality.
- Make available any preferred document templates and formats.
- Understand up front fully the report generation process.
- Understand the test article completely.
- Characteristics of the test article.
- Adequately discuss projected required amounts of test article.

- Make it understood what the test article is going to be used for (indication).
- Clarify when the test article is supposed to or needs to arrive.
- Define guidelines or a protocol for interaction.

Bibliography

Amon. (2009, June 6). Challenges in contract strategy and operations for pharmaceutical manufactures. *Pharmaceutical Comments*.

EHTRA. (2018). *Report on survey of worldwide CRO's: Costs and practicalities of two new OECD guidelines for testing chemical substances*.

Gad, S. C. (2009). Marketing yourself as an expert witness and consultant in toxicology. *Comments on Toxicology, 7*, 139–150.

Kwasny, M. J. (2019, September). Why be a statistical consultant? *Amstat News*.

Kwok, S. K. (2019, September). Career opportunities at contract research organizations: CRO's present opportunities in scientific, technical and business and commercial development. *AAPS News Magazine*.

Messmer-Blust, A. (2016, January 29). From scientist to toxicology consultant. *Crosstalk*. http://crosstalk.cell.com/blog/from-scientist-to-toxicology-consultant.com. Accessed 4 Sept 2019.

Moore, N. (2008). Workforce shortage. *Science, 365*, 6456.

Optimizing Your Experience and Relationship with Your Preclinical CRO

15

David G. Serota

In theory, optimizing the success of your experience and relationship with your preclinical CRO would seem relatively simple since the sponsor organization has the need for certain testing to be conducted that will meet both scientific and regulatory scrutiny, while the preclinical CRO has the technical ability and knowledge to conduct these studies with high quality and acceptance. However, a variety of issues can develop that cause roadblocks that can impede that relationship. In many cases, these roadblocks emanate from the absence of clear and concise communication and processes that need to be developed and followed between both parties to ensure that both parties are on the same path.

Experience has shown that these processes can be categorized as:

Developing a Communications Strategy
Managing Expectations
Building a Team
Celebrating Success
Integrity and Honestly Come First

Developing a Communications Strategy involves establishing a chain of command, sharing of information, and negotiating the expected requirements.

D. G. Serota
7th Inning Stretch Consulting LLC, Kalamazoo, MI, USA

© Springer Nature Switzerland AG 2020
S. C. Gad et al., *Contract Research and Development Organizations-Their History, Selection, and Utilization*, https://doi.org/10.1007/978-3-030-43073-3_15

Establishing a chain of command is absolutely critical for the success of the relationship since all parties in the relationship must understand who the key decision-makers are. From the preclinical CRO side, this is straightforward since the Good Laboratory Practice standards (GLPs) clearly designate the study director at the preclinical CRO as the single point of control of the study. This, however, does not mean that the study director is denied the opportunity to seek out opinions from other professionals or from test facility management at the preclinical CRO because this occurs fairly routinely. However, the ultimate decision-making responsibilities still reside with the study director. Things, however, are not always as clear from the sponsor organization side. Ideally, the sponsor organization should assign a single person to serve as the contact person that the study director will be working with, and that person should have both the ability and knowledge to answer questions posed by the study director and have the authority to make decisions. Usually this individual is designated as the sponsor representative and is the person that handles all communications from the study director, including those requiring actions involving both the conduct of the study and the completion of the final report. Unfortunately, this does not always occur, especially when the sponsor is a large organization where multiple opinions and approvals may be required for a decision to be reached or when an independent consultant is utilized by the sponsor as the sponsor representative and the consultant must pass final decisions through the sponsor organizations' hierarchy. There are times over the course of a study when decisions must be made immediately, such as those involving the welfare of a study animal or with an issue that could affect the integrity of the study. In the absence of such real-time decisions, there exists the possibility that the study could become compromised, and all parties should be cognizant of this fact. Therefore, the importance of establishing the chain of command becomes obvious as the study director must have confidence that the sponsor representative is the decision-maker that they go to for any necessary instructions and approvals.

Sharing of information is an absolute necessity on the part of both parties. The study director must keep the sponsor organization fully up to date on all aspects of the study and with the status of all timelines and milestone dates. The sponsor organization must be willing to share all current information regarding the test compound (such as availability, certificate of analysis, storage conditions, and analytical methodology), anticipated toxicity and/or results from studies conducted previously, intended clinical use, and critical milestone dates with the

CRO. This allows the study director and CRO staff to timely review this information so as to plan for the success of the study and to make useful recommendations that the sponsor organization may not have considered. This includes an early review of the proposed study protocol to ascertain that the study design is in compliance with animal health and welfare requirements regarding such things as dose volumes, blood sample volumes, pain production and avoidance, and housing requirements. In all likelihood, the CRO has more experience in these areas than the sponsor organization, so it is very important to identify any concerns very early and prior to receipt of test animals. The sponsor organization also needs to understand that in today's regulated world, the Institutional Anima Care and Use Committee (IACUC) at the CRO wields great power and authority over any proposed study design and can halt or delay the initiation of the study if certain requirements are not met in the study design.

Negotiating the expected requirements is a key component of the communications strategy and one that is often overlooked in the partnership. Requirements such as the type and frequency of communications, interim data reporting, and scheduling of monitoring visits need to be considered and agreed upon early in the relationship. Surprises are not a good thing to deal with as such events generally impede both the conduct of the testing program and the relationship between organizations. All expectations must be discussed and negotiated early in the relationship so that the CRO can meet the sponsor's requirements. In most cases, the CRO can "work its magic" to accommodate the sponsor's requests but only if they are given the time and ability to consider how to handle such requests. Depending on the scope of these requests, the sponsor organization should understand and accept that significant changes beyond which those included in the original scope of work will be accompanied by a cost increase and may require a renegotiation of milestone timelines for the study.

Managing Expectations involves clear communication, trusting your CRO, effective study monitoring, and dealing with unexpected events.

Trusting your CRO is perhaps one of the most misunderstood components for the relationship with your CRO to be successful. While it might seem obvious that the sponsor organization trusts the CRO since why would one choose to place their critical studies with that organization, they can also be highly critical of the CRO's ability, experience, and knowledge in conducting these studies, especially if they have their own in-house capabilities for conducting similar studies. Most preclinical CROs have conducted a vast number of different types of studies over the years which involved many different animal species, routes of administration, and compound classes. They have had to deal with and explain a large variety of challenges relating to toxicity that were both expected and unexpected. Thus, most preclinical CROs have more experience in conducting these studies than does the sponsor organization, and, as such, a high level of trust between the parties should be a hallmark of the successful relationship.

A key component of building this trust is an acknowledgment that every CRO probably conducts certain technical procedures a little differently from other CROs and differently from the sponsor organization if it has its own in-house facilities. This does not make it wrong; it only makes it different. The technical staff at the CRO is trained to perform procedures in a certain manner, and for the sponsor organization to request that they do things differently will only create quality problems. Unless there is an overriding concern that the procedure in place will not accomplish its designed function, the sponsor organization should allow the technical function to be performed per the standard operating procedures (SOPs) of the CRO unless there is a specific reason associated with the test material in question.

Study monitoring is a critical part of the relationship between the sponsor organization and the CRO, but it needs to be handled properly and professionally by both parties. It is important to understand that the purpose of monitoring studies at CROs is risk mitigation since the sponsor organization needs assurance that the studies are progressing as planned with no quality or timing issues. Study monitoring should include an evaluation of both the scientific and operational integrity of the studies, along with the necessary compliance to study protocol and regulatory expectations. The timing and frequency of study monitoring visits should be agreed upon between the sponsor representative and the study director. These visits should be of such a frequency and duration to provide the sponsor organization with a confidence that all is going well. However, the sponsor organization should understand that while such visits are strongly welcomed by the CRO, they do involve time and effort on the part of the CRO to schedule and host, especially on the part of the study director and other key professional staff involved in the study conduct. Thus, it is best that such visits be discussed and planned as far in the future as possible to allow the CRO the time to schedule resources and to make the necessary preparations to ensure that sponsor expectations are achieved. In addition, if specific data or information will need to be available, timely instructions need to be provided to allow the CRO the time to prepare this information. The individual conducting the monitoring visit for the sponsor organization should prepare for the visit prior to arriving at the CRO. They should have a clear strategy of what they want to accomplish during the visit, and they need to share that information with the CRO prior to the visit so that the CRO can facilitate that information internally to produce a seamless visit. The monitor must be knowledgeable of both the intent of the study and the study protocol design. If technical functions are to be observed or study data reviewed, the monitor needs at least a basic understanding of what they are observing or reviewing.

Dealing with unexpected results can be a challenge for both the sponsor organization and the CRO. Unexpected results can be considered as either study findings that were not expected or performance issues that occurred during the conduct of the study. Unexpected study findings that are not the result of any performance issue on the part of the CRO need to be fully shared in a timely manner with the sponsor organization and evaluated together. All possible theories for the unexpected findings should be considered, and, if appropriate, additional test parameters should be considered that might assist to achieving an identifying and verifying. The nature of scientific testing can always bring the unexpected, so a total team approach to evaluating the findings and proposing an explanation is the best course of action.

Performance issues can and do occur on outsourced studies no matter the amount of training, education, SOPs, and quality procedures put into place at the CRO. No CRO is pleased that a mistake occurred, but the tone of the sponsor reaction should be in accord with the way that the CRO is responding to and handling the mistake. It is worth noting that very few mistakes can actually invalidate the integrity of a study, so the sponsor organization should not overreact when they occur because in all likelihood, the CRO is already embarrassed and hard enough on itself and its staff. Nothing positive will occur if the sponsor chooses to create a negative interaction. The CRO should notify the sponsor organization as soon as possible regarding the mistake, and it should be prepared to state what happened, how it happened, how it will be fixed, and what effect it had on the study. The sponsor organization should evaluate this information, and if the course of action is unacceptable, they should communicate any concerns in a timely manner and recommend an alternative course of action. In the rare case that an issue arises that is due to willful action on the part of CRO personnel, CRO management responsible sponsor personnel should seek to handle the issue professionally.

Building a Team involves the study director and sponsor representative bonding and a physical presence of the sponsor representative at the CRO.

The bonding of the study director at the CRO and the sponsor representative is another key component in maximizing the CRO/sponsor organization relationship. Clearly the absence of a strong relationship between these two key performers does not bode well for a successful study outcome if they are not able to function together as a unified team. For many sponsor organizations, once they find a study director that is easy to work with and scientifically strong and demonstrates great communications skills, they will continue to place their studies at that CRO if the CRO will assign that individual to serve as the study director on any future studies. Over time, a strong relationship develops with that study director at both the professional and personal level, and that relationship becomes invaluable over the course of a study, especially if any difficult situations occur later. This same relationship can also occur between the study director and any consultant that the sponsor organization might choose to utilize in support of their studies. However, when selecting a consultant for such a purpose, the sponsor organization should only use those consultants that understand their role in the study relationship and have a strong foundation and knowledge of both the study design and of the CRO industry. Consultants that do not meet these specifications usually bring little value to the conduct of the study and in some cases create friction and confusion in the CRO/sponsor organization relationship.

The physical presence of the sponsor representative at the CRO is an often overlooked characteristic of team building not only for the study director but also for the entire technical team involved in the conduct of a study. One of the most important meetings conducted by the CRO regarding a study is the study pre-initiation meeting where the study director discusses the details of the study with the entire technical staff to ensure that everyone understands their role in the study and where any final concerns or issues with the study protocol are discussed and resolved prior to study initiation. The sponsor representative's physical presence at this meeting is extremely important since this augments team building by personalizing the intent of the study with the technical staff. If the sponsor representative is unable to be physically present for this meeting, they should participate over the telephone. It is here that the sponsor representative can discuss the intended therapeutic uses of the test compound, the patient population that would benefit if the test compound reaches the marketplace, and what effects the technical staff might expect to be observed during the study. Thus, instead of just being a study with compound X, the technical staff tends to become more interested in the study outcome where a successful test compound could change the quality of life for thousands of people suffering from a certain condition, including themselves or someone that they know and love. Knowing this information can't help but cause the technical staff to conduct the study with a bit more enthusiasm and focus to ensure a quality study performance. When the sponsor representative is at the CRO to monitor interim milestone phases over the course of the study, they should always endeavor to meet and interact with the technical staff involved with their study to update them on the current progress of the overall testing program and to provide them with positive comments regarding their contributions to its success.

While at the CRO, the sponsor representative should not be resistant to the opportunities offered by the CRO, especially by the study director, to dine and socialize together. Such opportunities are a strong point in building solid relationships and provide a conduit away from the laboratory where people can be themselves to learn and laugh, and either to begin or to cement the bonds of friendship and respect that can be important in the future.

Celebrating Success involves a basic human emotion to share a positive outcome with those that played a significant role in ensuring the successful complete of an activity.

Celebrating success is a logical outcome at the end of the completion of a successful study or a successful testing program. While the CRO will have processes in place internally to congratulate and reward staff for the successful completion of a study, what is being referred to here is an active effort on the part of the sponsor organization to celebrate and acknowledge this success. Sadly, however, this involvement by the sponsor organization, which does not need to be elaborate or costly, only occurs rarely. Events such as a luncheon pizza party or an afternoon cookie and soda break or the distribution of sponsor organization hats or coffee mugs have a tremendous effect on staff morale, job satisfaction, and sense of worth and contribution, especially among the technical staff. Such appreciation not only is perceived by the staff as a clear recognition on the part of the sponsor organization of both the effort and commitment put forward by them to deliver a study conducted with high quality but also serves as an acknowledgment of their role in the overall test compound development process.

Honesty and Integrity Come First must be the tenets of any relationship between parties no matter what the outcome of that relationship displays.

While it might seem obvious in today's world that integrity and honesty always come first in the relationship between the sponsor organization and the CRO, this is, unfortunately, not always the case. While the rank dishonesty that was displayed by some organizations in the mid-1970s does not seem to exist anymore, there are still people and organizations today that can feel the need to pressure and bully their CRO and its professional staff, especially over reported study findings that are not beneficial to the sponsor organization. For the CRO, its staff is committed to providing the sponsor organization with its best performance in both conducting studies in the highest quality manner possible and in accurately interpreting and reporting the study findings in a highly scientific manner. The CRO understands that it is neither the bricks and mortar of the facility nor the equipment and instruments contained within that influence sponsor organizations to place studies with them; it is the honesty and integrity of the CRO and its scientists, technicians, and senior management. They understand that once you lose your honesty and integrity, you can never get it back, and the industry that it supports will never have trust in them again. While recognizing that honest differences in scientific interpretation can occur, pressuring the CRO to change an interpretation is not the best way to handle these differences. There have been cases where the sponsor organization may not have shared some additional information with the CRO regarding the test compound which might have helped clarify the interpretation, and there have been cases where what were assumed to be minor differences in the study design resulted in significant and unexpected outcomes. In many cases, the disagreement between the sponsor organization and the CRO is the result of differences in the interpretation of histopathologic findings. In such cases, it is recommended that a pathology peer review be conducted as an attempt to reach a consensus regarding the findings. If that is unsuccessful, a pathology working group (PWG) can be assembled to review the findings. The PWG consists of a panel of expert pathologists who are charged with providing an independent unbiased assessment of the findings, with both parties agreeing to abide by the eventual interpretations. While generally not commonplace, the use of a PWG is a powerful tool in reaching a consensus of the findings and is highly accepted as a useful process in resolving such issues by the various regulatory agencies.

In summary, the successful partnership between the sponsor organization and the CRO is not overly difficult to achieve, but it does require a clear and concise set of processes that need to be considered and managed by both parties. In essence, the ultimate success of this relationship requires a common-sense approach in working together to achieve the desired end results that benefit both parties. The outcome of achieving this success will be rewarding to all involved and not only will allow for the successful completion of the ongoing testing program but will also create the confidence and environment where the sponsoring organization will continue the relationship with the CRO for future projects and opportunities for years to come.

Common Problems and Solutions

16

Despite the best efforts and intentions of all involved, there will always be an incidence of problems involved in even successful subcontracting (many if not all of these problems are also present when work is performed using internal resources, but such are not the subject of this volume). What can be done is to be aware of the potential of such problems and to be prepared to solve them if they arise. Preferably the initial step to a solution is knowledge of how others have previously solved similar problems so that one can only de novo solve the new ones.

In each of the cases that follow, a first step might well be to avoid the situations in the advance place. So for each of the common problems that are considered, a history of how some arose is provided.

Changes in Key Personnel Part of the initial selection process for a contractor should be based on the experience and qualifications of their staff, particularly the study director, has increased. Unfortunately, such assumptions may not hold true in at least two cases.

In the first case, key personnel may leave the organization through changing jobs, disability, or death. In the second situation, a key individual (such as a study director in a toxicology study) may prove to look better on paper than in reality and not be up to the task at hand (this is not uncommon) particularly as

© Springer Nature Switzerland AG 2020
S. C. Gad et al., *Contract Research and Development Organizations-Their History, Selection, and Utilization*, https://doi.org/10.1007/978-3-030-43073-3_16

demands on study director. In either of these cases, a central figure involved in the completion of desired work is no longer present or involved.

Avoiding the occurrence of this problem is difficult, as there is really no advance warning in the situations cited as examples. Solution options here are limited. Other than the provision of the highest degree of assurance by the CRO that the on-the-job (as opposed to on paper) competence of replacement key individuals will not reduce the quality of the study, there are a few options.

When faced with this situation, there are three potential solutions. The first is to have the vendor reassign another suitable individual to fill the vacancy – should such a person be available. Unfortunately, it is uncommon that this is possible due to limited human resource redundancy within the vendor (or now of days, any) organizations.

The second approach is to hire (or, rather, have the vendor organization hire) a suitable person for the completion of the task. The vendor may know such individuals, or a search of the appropriate website (www.toxconsultants. com for a toxicologist or www.chemconsultants.com for a chemist), as examples. This is the more common approach, with the effective subcontract being limited to the period of need. The third approach (generally viable if a project has not yet actually been initiated) is to delay the start or completion of a project until a full-time replacement or adequate substitute is hired.

Client Signing Protocols and Amendments When work is contracted out, there is a tendency in many organizations to maintain (and even delimit) control and authority even though technical skills are not present. This is most commonly experienced by sponsors as well as contracted experts (consultants/ monitors) being signatories for protocols, amendments, and other documents. This leads to (at best) a lack of clarity in lines of authority and responsibility for decisions, and perhaps much worse. In such a situation, most contractors will take no action until there is consensus or clarity, which in nonclinical and clinical studies many times becomes an (unintended) decision itself.

The means of avoiding this problem are clear, having only a single technical signatory from the sponsor regardless of whether said individual is internal to the sponsor or a consultant at project initiation. The worst case, by the way, is rare in the pharmaceutical industry but common in other industries (such as chemicals) – a committee in charge. Enough said. If, however, this problem cannot be avoided, then ensuring open and continuous communications through a well-understood line of authority with clarified responsibilities is essential.

Time Slippage The most valuable asset in the development of new products in the industries that we are concerned with is not money but rather time. This leads to most activities being precisely scheduled with the shaky assumption that no problems or natural disasters will occur (to ensure either the quickest time to overall project completion or the optimal use of resources such as money). As was made clear earlier, a clean set of expectations for project completion must be part of the contracting process. However, the nature and the course of human events may preclude on-time completion. Any extra time available between the initiation of an activity and its scheduled or required completion (delivery of a report or drug substance or for alternate dosage form) constitutes "float" in the terminology of project management and must be carefully monitored and controlled. Small delays which on their own seem trivial all too often accumulate over the course of a program to produce a painful protraction in completion. A frequent admonition to clients and contractors is "don't eat my float and I won't eat yours."

Delays can arise from a vast number of causes, but usually these translate to a shortage of a resource (availability of equipment, test animals, or manpower) or the lack of an essential skill set such as expertise with using a specific instrument or the performance of a necropsy on test animals or delivery of materials (especially test article and/or vehicle). When such are identified, their impact is commonly significantly underestimated. The key to avoiding or minimizing the impact of these is to ensure that causative factors and events are identified as soon as they occur and that corrective actions are initiated as rapidly as possible. A second step is to allow some level of redundancy of resources to be included in plans. Extra starting material for synthesis or a few extra animals on hand over the minimal requirements are cheap insurance for on-time completion of the projects in question.

If such events still come to pass, then the best means of minimizing their impact is to provide a supplement or replacement for the limiting (critical path) resource in the completion of the entire project (i.e., drug or device approval). One should over engineer to avoid disappointment.

Regulatory Noncompliance The industries with which we are concerned with here are heavily regulated in virtually all aspects. Small occurrences of noncompliance with such regulation (such as not taking samples of dosing solutions for analysis or not following quality assurance procedures) can invalidate entire studies or activities, leading at best to a need for the repeat of same or performance of additional work, costing money and time.

All such regulated activities now must have some form of quality system (QS) in place. Regulatory noncompliance in such situations can occur only if the QS was incomplete (overlooked in the initial system set up) or failed. Procedures to avoid such occurrences are best discussed in the pre-award phase of a contract work. Initially, insure that necessary systems are in place as evidenced by SOPs, validation reports, operative QAU – quality assurance unit – and the existence of a quality program effective for the critical points/activities involved in the work to be performed. Subsequent to these, there should be a program for monitoring any ongoing work. Consider having a full system (GLP/GMP/GCP) audit performed on any facility, which either is doing a large, critical project or is providing services on a number of separate projects.

If a noncompliance issue is identified, the solution is to document both the problem and corrective action in a timely manner: What happened? Why did it happen? What steps have been taken to prevent it from happening again?

Quality Control/Assurance Failures Again there are several aspects of this topic. The first is if quality assurance and control procedures are not followed. An example is when plasma samples from a group of volunteers, subjects, or animals are analyzed and samples demonstrate erroneously high or low reported levels of the agent of interest. The second is when the understanding of regulatory quality assurance or study design requirements on the part of contractor personnel is different than those of the sponsor. Such differences of opinion can be legitimate, but the impacts on cost, quality, and timing are potentially enormous.

This issue has some degree of overlap with regulatory noncompliance. Here we wish to focus on aspects not covered under that other topic (1) that there is a significant disagreement between the contractor's quality assurance and the client's professional opinion (experience) or (2) that a QC/QA failure caused actions to be taken which cannot be solved simply by documenting the event and taking post action.

The first of these can take several forms: that a quality problem has or has not occurred or, in some contract organizations, what is or is not presented in a final report. For these, both the client and vendor management must work to arrive at a mutually acceptable solution.

The second case is harder. If an erroneous finding has caused an irreversible action to be taken (such as shutting down a clinical trial or making a regulatory filing which was incorrect), fixing the matter has two separate aspects. First, all involved must be notified in writing of the error. Second a legal issue of restitution of damages will need to be resolved between the client and vendor.

Inappropriate Technology This may be due to decisions by the sponsor or the contractor (or both). The former may have an existing analytical method which served them well during earlier work on a project (such as an RIA method for measuring drug levels instead of a more sensitive LC/MS/MS method) and do not want to spend the money or delay progress on work while a better method is developed.

Contractors, on the other hand, usually play to their strength. If they have certain equipment and methods on hand, such are likely to constitute the recommended means of addressing a problem. An example here might be using a mass balance approach with a limited number of organs to evaluate the distribution of a drug and its metabolites throughout the body as opposed to using whole body autoradiography.

It behooves both the client and vendor to ensure that technologies involved in project conduct are either, according to the current industry norm, that the data from such work will provide answers to the desired questions or that there is a well-documented reason for otherwise to be the case.

If it is found that the methodology employed does not meet current regulatory expectations (despite the rationale behind their use being good), then the performance of a bridging study establishing that results comparable to those from the desired method (or animal species) is advisable.

Facility Shutdown Sometimes a facility will cease operations while work on a study or projects are still ongoing. Causes of such situations in the best of circumstances have included financial failure, death of essential personnel, and an acquisition of the facility by new management. The performance of thorough due diligence before the award of the contract is the best means to avoid this problem. Make sure the financial stability and other factors cited here are evaluated before an award.

Such an occurrence, if detected in a timely manner, can be addressed in one of two manners: either the means may be acquired or negotiated (in the case of an acquisition) to resume operations and continue then until the contracted task is completed, or the work can be moved to another facility for completion. The past has documented the relocation of entire colonies of laboratory animals in just such circumstances.

Acts of Nature Natural disasters do happen. Floods, hurricanes (wiping out animal colonies, remember Houston, Texas, in the late 1990s), fires, and earthquakes are all possibilities that can disrupt or totally discontinue the conduct of development activities. The occurrence of these cannot be either predicted or avoided, but the ability of a facility to withstand such occurrences and continue operations can and must be evaluated as a part of pre-award considerations.

CROs May Stretch the Truth While in our experience this has become much less of a problem than it once was, it still occurs that contractors may represent that they have capabilities that they don't or can meet timelines, which have more of a spiritual than managerial basis. Avoidance of this problem is best pursued by careful review of past performance. While asking for and checking with provided reference clients is a useful step, a sponsor should also seek to use their professional contacts to seek out and query a broader range of prior clients. Alternatively, a strict financial penalty clause can be included in the contract with regard to the achievement of timed milestones.

The degree of the problem dictates the appropriate response. If the contractor has been overly optimistic about their ability to provide timely results, this can be addressed as previously discussed under time slippage. But if an actual untruth is detected, the problem is much more serious. Impact and corrective actions after such a breach of faith must be carefully considered.

Silent Subcontractors Just as sponsors subcontract, so do contractors. Very common cases for toxicology labs, for example, include pathology, cardiology, ophthalmology, bioanalytical and analytical chemistry, and statistical analysis. It may not be made clear to the client that such is the case before a project is initiated. It is thus essential that documents such as protocols clearly disclose any subcontractors and their specific responsibilities, as well as providing sufficient contract information to allow independent sponsor contract and follow-up. This problem has increased in occurrence in recent years. When in doubt, ask.

Alliances Again just as with client organizations, informal or formal arrangements may exist between contractors which can influence, complicate, or impede progress on a project. Examples include (1) a data entry analysis CRO which will not provide support to phase I studies initiated at other than their "partner" clinical facility once work has been done at that facility and (2) a GMP synthesis facility which has an arrangement with specific formulation and CTM manufacturing organizations.

Such arrangements do not inherently cause any harm but also should be disclosed at the beginning of the study or project and in no way bind the sponsor to use (or even consider) the contractor's related organizations. Any "alliance" organizations must be evaluated on its own independent merits.

Sponsors must insist on full and timely disclosure of any such arrangements and evaluate any resulting impact.

Too Many Eggs in a Basket While there are both good reasons and a natural tendency to "reward" a vendor or consultant that performs well with additional work, it is always a sound practice to have more than a single contractor available to conduct a particular type of work (if at all possible). There are several reasons for this.

Even the best of contract service providers have limits on how much work they can do and also will be subject to circumstances beyond their control from time to time.

These occurrences can easily lead to (1) having to accept delays or compromises in study or task performance or (2) in some cases finding that you are (in effect) competing against yourself for resources on different projects.

The essential solution to this problem is to be aware of viable alternative providers and if possible to have the necessary preparation work (site visits, confidentiality agreements, and such) completed and set in place in advance. It is even well advised to split work loads between two separate vendors – while the cost of operations may be modestly increased in the short run, such an arrangement can be managed in such a fashion as to actually better control the project and even decrease costs in the long run.

Extraneous Event
Ranging from technique-associated animal deaths to sample loss to finding test article in the plasma of control animals, into every study, stuff happens. The best solutions are to rapidly identify such events, investigate causes, insure sound and effective communication, and document all the facts.

Appendix A: Nonmedical Device Toxicology Lab List

© Springer Nature Switzerland AG 2020
S. C. Gad et al., *Contract Research and Development Organizations-Their History, Selection, and Utilization*, https://doi.org/10.1007/978-3-030-43073-3

	Address/location	Phone #	Website	Labs acquired by this lab	Specialty/additional services	Rat	Rabbits	Dog	Carcinogenicity	DART	Inhalation	Primate	Pig	IV infusion	Genotoxic	Metabolism	Analytical	Special studies	Receptor panels
Absorption Systems	PA, CA, Sapporo, Hokkaido, Japan	(610) 280–7300 (p) (610) 280–9667 (f) +81–11–223–7456	www.absorption.com	TGA Bioservices LLC (Cambridge, MA), Perry Scientific	"GLP & GMP compliant in vitro cell based. In vivo animal models." Express ADME assays, custom ADME assays, BCS toxicology, preclinical transporter studies, formulation assessment, vivarium rooms, hERG	X		X					X			X	X		
	Perry Scientific (now part of Absorption Systems) San Diego, CA	858–560–9000			Large animals	X	X	X	X	X			X	X		X		X	
Accelera	Viale Pasteur 10 – CP11	+39 0331 1984 444	www.accelera.org		Developmental, bioanalysis, PK											X	X		
Altasciences	Laval, Quebec, Canada; Montreal, Quebec, Canada; Kansas City, KS, USA; Seattle, WA, USA	Laval, 450–973–6077; Montreal, 513–381–2546; Kansas City, 913–696–1601; Seattle, 425–407–0121	https://www.altasciences.com/	SNBL USA, Skeletech	Preclinical (small and large molecule), clinical (first-in-man through phase II), bioanalysis	X	X	X				X	X	X		X			
APS (American Preclinical Services)	8945 Evergreen Blvd NW, Minneapolis, MN 55433	763–717–7990 877–717–7997	www.americanpreclinical.com			X	X	X			X		X	X			X		
Aurigon-Toxicoop Research	Germany	+49(0)8158–2597-30	www.atrc.eu		Ames, HPRT, chromosome, aberration	X	X	X		X		X				X			
Austrian Research Center	Kramergasse 1, A- 1010 Wein, Seibersdorf, Austria	+43 50550–4400 +43 50550–4450	www.ait.ac.at/en			X	X		X		X								
Batelle	505 King Avenue Columbus, Ohio 43 201	800–201-2011	www.battelle.org		Yes	X				X								X	
Bertin Bioreagent (formerly SPI-bio, aka Bertin Pharma)	Parc d'Activités du Pas du Lac, 10 bis avenue ampère, F-78180 Montigny-le-Bretonneux, France	+33 (0)139 306 036	www.spibio.com		Clinical	X X	X	X		X	X	X	X		X	X X	X		

Company	Address	Phone	Website	Services										
BioDuro	Beijing, China.. + 11011 Torreyana Rd. San Diego, CA 92121	86–1080768000 + 1858–529-6600 (908)647–5012 (855)779–9260 (781)237–6688	www.bioduro.com	GLP		X	X	X	X	X		X	X	X
BioReliance	14920 Broschart Road, Rockville, Maryland 20850–3349	800-756-5658	www.bioreliance.com	Microbiological Associates	Biologics safety, toxicology services, assays	X					X			
BioMed PreClinical Solutions	52 Maze St. 65789 Tel-Aviv Israel	972–3–560-21-02	www. biomedpreclinical.com	GLP, DRF, MTD, CNS behavior, teratological studies	X	X	X	X		X		X	X	X
Bioneeds India Pvt. Ltd.	Devarahosahalli, Sompura Hobli, NH-4, Nelamangala Tz. Bangalore Rural District-562211, Karnataka	91-816–2243751-54 (P) 91-816–2243755 (F)	www.bioneeds.in	Physical-chemical testing (5-batch analysis), toxicity studies (acute and subacute, chronic, acute inhalation, reproductive, and developmental), mutagenicity studies (Ames assay, micronucleus test in vivo and in vitro, chromosomal aberration test in vivo and in vitro, NRU phototoxicity test), environmental toxicity studies on aquatic and terrestrial organisms (acute toxicity, acute immobilization test, alga growth inhibition test, honey bee toxicity test), GLP, PK/PD, safety, efficacy, bioassays	X	X	X	X		X		X		X
BioSafety Research Center (BSRC)	Shizuoka, Japan	+0538-58-1266, +81 538–58-3572	https://www.anpyo. co.jp/		X									
BioTest	Biotest AG Landsteinerstraße 5 63303 Dreieich (or mail to) P.O. Box 10 20 40 D-63266 Dreieich	+496 10/38 01–0 (P) +496 10/38 01–150 (F)	www.biotest.de https://www.biotest. com/de/en/index.cfm	GLP Genetox, Ames test, chromosome aberration in vitro (human lymphocytes), in vivo micronucleus test	X	X	X		X			X		

(continued)

	Address/location	Phone #	Website	Labs acquired by this lab	Specialty/additional services	Rat	Rabbits	Dog	Carcinogenicity	DART	Inhalation	Primate	Pig	IV infusion	Genotoxic	Metabolism	Analytical	Special studies	Receptor panels
BRI	101–8898 Heather Street, Vancouver, BC, V6P 3S8	604-432-9237	www.bripharm.com		Pharmaceutical development	X									X	X	X		
BRT (Burleson Research Technologies)	120 First Flight Ln., Morrisville, NC 27560	919-851-4499 and 919-719-2500	www.brt-labs.com		Specialty immunotox	X	X												
BTS Research (BioTox Sciences)	P.O. Box 910418 San Diego, CA 92191 (or) 10665 Sacramento Valley Rd. San Diego, CA	858-605-5882	www.btsresearch.com	Bio-Quant	ISO 10993, transgenic mice, CA disease model	X	X	X	X			X	X	X		X			
Calvert	Corporate: 1225 Crescent Green Suite 115 Cary, NC 27518 Laboratory address: 100 Discovery Drive, Olyphant, PA 18447	570-586-2411	www.calvertlabs.com	Pharmakon, Phoenix, Crysallis, MDS (France)	Yes, Radioactivity Telemetry, mouse tumor Model, +	X	X	X	X	X		X	X	X		X	X	X	
Care Research, LLC	Ft. Collins, CO	970-493-2660	www.careresearchllc.com			X	X	X		X			X			X	X	X	
CBSET	500 Shire Way Lexington, MA 02421 USA	+44(0)1625 505 100 (UK) 1-888-297-7683 (US)	www.cbset.org		GLP, disease models, pharmacokinetics, ADME, ISO 10993, chronic and surgical							X	X						
Cyprotex (an evotec company)	HQ No.24 Mereside, Alderley Park Nether Alderley Cheshire SK10 4TG, United Kingdom (or) 313 Pleasant St., Watertown, MA 02472, USA	781-541-5555	http://www.cyprotex.com	ADMETRx, CeeTox	Chemistry, in vitro, cell culture											X	X	X	
Center for Drug Safety Evaluation and Research, Shanghai Institute of Materia Medica	555 Zu Chong Zhi Road, Zhang Jiang Hi-Tech Park, Pudong, Shanghai, 201203	86-21-5080-6600	http://english.simm.cas.cn/rd/dsdp/cdser/		Guinea pig	X	X		X					X		X	X	X	

	Address	Phone	Website	Collaborators/Sites	Notes											SP
Charles River	MSL, 54943 North Main Street, Mattawan, MI 49071-9399 USA	(269)668-3336	www.criver.com	Argus (PA), CTBR (Montana), Inveresk (Scotland), Redfield (AZ), Springborn (OH), TS Mason (MA), WIL (OH), MPI, Biotechnics LLC, Citoxlabs, Xenometrix, Celsis International Ltd.	Safety pharm., transgenic mouse CA Radioactivity	X	X	X	X	X	X	X	X	X	X	SP
	Elphinstone Research Centre, Tranent, EH33 2NE, UK, & 87 Senneville Road, Senneville-Montreal, Quebec, Canada, H9X 3R3	44 (0) 1875 614555 (514) 630-8200			Clinical, ferret emesis	X	X	X	X	X		X	X	X	X	SP
	Celsis International Ltd. 6200 S. Lindbergh Blvd., St. Louis, MO 63123 & 165 Fieldcrest Avenue, Edison, NJ 08837	314-487-6776		CharTest, MPI, Agilux, CIT, MSL, Scantox	Stability, methods	X	X	X	X	X	X	X	X	X	X	X
	Biotechnics, 310 Millstone Drive, Hillsborough, NC 27278	919-245-3114				X	X				X	X		X		
	251 Ballardvale St., Wilmington, MA 01887-1000 (this is the original)	508-925-6000			Clinical, ferret emesis, surgical	X	X	X	X	X	X	X	X	X	X	X
	Reno, NV	775-331-2201				X	X	X		X	X		X	X		
	Malvern Horsham, PA	215-443-8710			Photoxicity, ferret emesis	X	X	X		X		X				
	Spencerville, OH	419-647-4196			Photoxicity, ferret emesis											
					Chronic and surgical											
	54943 N. Main Street, Mattawan, MI	269-668-3336			Clinical, ferret emesis	X	X	X	X	X	X	X	X	X	X	X
	Tranent, Scotland	44-0-1875-614555				X	X	X	X	X		X	X	X	X	X
	Piedmont, Morrisville, NC	919-206-7000			Tumor models, implant studies	X	X	X	X	X	X	X	X	X	X	X
	Montreal, QU	514-630-8200			Clinical, ferret emesis	X	X	X	X	X	X	X	X	X	X	X
	1407 George Rd. Ashland, OH 44805	(419)289-8700 (p) (419)289-3650 (f)			Radioactivity	X	X	X	X	X	X	X	X	X	X	X
	S'Hertogenbosch, the Netherlands (Previously NOTOX)	31073 640 67 00(p) 31073 640 67 99(f)			Birds, +			X	X	X	X	X	X			
	Skokie, IL				Gene Tox	X	X	X	X	X	X	X	X	X	X	X
	L'Arbresle, France	514-333-0033			Clinical, ferret emesis, surgical	X	X	X	X	X	X	X	X	X	X	X

(continued)

	Address/location	Phone #	Website	Labs acquired by this lab	Specialty/additional services	Rat	Rabbits	Dog	Carcinogenicity	DART	Inhalation	Primate	Pig	IV infusion	Genotoxic	Metabolism	Analytical	Special studies	Receptor panels
	Minato-ku, Tokyo, Japan	81 33 454 7571	www.mpiresearch.com		Safety pharm, transgenic mouse CA Radioactivity				X			X				X			
	Worcester, MA	508-762-4402	www.agiluxlab.com		Melanin binding, bioanalyzed, GLP												X		
	CI Fox Lab, Cedex, France Laval, Canada Veszprem, HU	+33 2 32 292626 (p) +33 2 32 678705 (f) (450)973-2240 (416)815-0700	www.criver.com			X	X	X	X	X		X	X	X		X	X	X	
	MPI (formerly Exygen) 3058 Research Drive, State College, PA 16801	(800)281-3219 (p) (800)272-1019 (f)			Methods, development											X	X		
SCANTOX	Hestehavevej 36a, DK-4623 Lille Skensved, Denmark	+45 56 82 12 02 (f) +45 56 86 15 00 (p)				X	X	X	X	X	X	X	X	X	X				
ChemPartner	ChemPartner Co., Ltd., No. 5 Building, 998 Halei Road, Zhangjiang Hi-Tech Park Pudong New Area, Shanghai China, 201203	86 215 132 0088	www.chempartner.com		Oncology, pathology, immunology, neuroscience, cell biology; in vitro biology; epigenetics, DMPK, biomarkers	X				X	X	X	X	X	X	X			
Cirion	2121 Rue Berlier, Laval, (QC), Canada H7L 3 M9	450-688-6445	www.cirion.ca		Clinical	X	X	X				X	X	X	X				
Cliantha Research	Opposite Pushpraj Towers, Near Judges Bungalows, Bodakdev, Ahmedabad-380 054. + St. Petersburg Florida, South Africa, Canada, and Turkey	+91 7 926853088 info@cliantha.com	www.cliantha.com	Inflamax Research, Hilltop Research, Karmic Life Sciences	Early phase, late phase, respiratory, dermatology, consumer research, IVRD, biometrics, pharmacovigilance, PK, immunogenicity	X				X						X			
Clintox Bioservices	Hyderabad, India	91(40)55153222 91(40)24480666	http://www.clintoxbio.com/contactus.html		Phototoxicity, hamsters	X	X	X	X										
Colorado Histo-Prep & CARE Research LLC	Fort Collins, CO	(970) 493-2660 (970) 493-8834 (Fax)	www.histoprep.com		PK, TK, implants, neurotoxicity, neurosurgical, in-house clinic chemistry and histopathology	X		X	X					X	X		X	X	
Comparative Ophthalmic Research Lab (CORL)	Madison, WI University of Wisconsin, 2828 Marshall Court, Suite 200, Madison, WI, 53705	(608) 206-3614 (alternative) (608) 206-9441	www.vetmed.wisc.edu/research/corl/		Ocular toxicity												X	X	

Company	Address	Phone	Website	Special
Comparative Biosciences	786 Lucerne Drive, Sunnyvale, CA 94085	(408)504-8871, (408)738-9278	www.compbio.com	Special discovery, models
CorDynamics	2242 W. Harrison St. Chicago, IL 60612-3552	312-421-8876, 817-644-3142	www.cordynamics.com	CV safety only
Covance	9200 Leesburg Pike, Vienna, VA 22182 & 309 West Washington Ave, Madison, WI 53703 + Harrogate, UK, + Muenster, FRG	(888)COVANCE (888)541-LABS	www.covance.com	Clinical, consulting, chronic and surgical. Hazelton (AZ) (Greenfield), Raltech, Warf (Formerly Harlan, then envigo), Biodynamics, Harlan, LSR (Scotland), RCC
	East Millstone, NJ	(732) 873-2550		
	Cambridgeshire, UK	44 (0) 1480 892000		(Switzerland), Huntington Life Sciences (HLS), Raltech
	Zelgliweg 1, CH-4452 Itegen, Switzerland (Previously Safety Pharm)	(410) 385-1666- US sales office +41 619 751 111(p)		
	Germany	34-937-190361		
	Spain			
	Madison, WI	(317)806-6080 x2922		
	Indianapolis, IN	(317)806-6080 x2922		
	Derby, UK	00 44 (0) 1332 792896		
CPTC (Consumer Product Testing Company)	70 New Dutch Lane, Fairfield, NJ 07004	973-988-2223	www.cptclabs.com	Clinical
CTI (Clinical Trial & Consulting)	100 E. RiverCenter Blvd., Covington, KY 41011	513-598-9290	www.ctifacts.com	Eurotrials, CRS Clinical Research Services, S2 Statistical Solutions, Community Research. Humanized mouse models, ISO 1993
Crown CRO	Vaisalantie 4, FI-02130 Espoo, Finland	+358 98 870 0500	http://crowncro.fi/	Consulting, device, pharmacovigilance

(continued)

	Address/location	Phone #	Website	Labs acquired by this lab	Specialty/additional services	Rat	Rabbits	Dog	Carcinogenicity	DART	Inhalation	Primate	Pig	IV infusion	Genotoxic	Metabolism	Analytical	Special studies	Receptor panels
CSIR-IITR (Council of Scientific & Industrial Research-Indian Institute of Toxicology Research)	Main Campus: CSIR-Indian Institute of Toxicology Research, Vishvigyan Bhawan 31, Mahatma Gandhi Marg, Lucknow–226 001, Uttar Pradesh, India Gheru Campus: CSIR-Indian Institute of Toxicology Research, Sarojini Nagar Industrial Area, Lucknow–226 008, Uttar Pradesh, India	Phone (Main Campus): +91–522-2 217 497 Phone (Gheru Campus): +91–522-2 476 227, 2 476 228 Fax: +91–522-2 628 227 Email: director[at] iitrindia[dot]org	www.iitrindia.org		Irritation, behavioral	X	X		X	X	X				X		X		
Dermitech	11099 N. Torrey Pines Road, Suite 100, La Jolla, CA 92037	(860)450-4223 (858)450-4222	www.dermitech.com		Drug discovery and development focused on cancers and inflammatory diseases. Phases IIII	X	X	X											
Drik	865 Research Parkway, Suite 415, Oklahoma City, OK 73104	405-384-8580 405-202-0117	www.atdrik.com		Pharmacology, toxicology, ADME, blood chem, histopathology, bioanalytical, assays	X	X									X	X		
EKG Labs	EKG Life Science Solutions 4633 World Parkway Circle, Saint Louis, MO 63134	810-EKG-LABS	www.ekglabs.com		Chicken, cattle, food animals												X	X	

Company	Address	Phone	Website	Description	Services
Eurofins	Evans Labs, Missouri, IA. N. Ireland, UK. Columbia, MO	(573)474-8579 44 (0) 2870 320 639 (800)538-5227	www.eurofins.com	Consumer products lab, Lancaster, Pan Labs, Product Safety Labs, ABC Labs, Cerep, Evans Labs	Bioanalysis, methods development, radioactivity
	Le Bois l'Evêque, 86600 Celle L'Evescault, France Cerep–15318 N.E 95th street, Redmond, WA, 98052	+33-(0)5 49 89 30 00 (alternate) 425–895-8666			Chemistry, in vitro
	EAG Laboratories Columbia, MD	Phone: 573–777-6168 Fax: +1 573 777 6033			Respiratory devices
	Dayton, NJ + Taiwan	732-438-5100 ext. 270 Fax 732–355-3275 Cel 732–744-6579US: 515–280-8378			Bioanalysis, CMC, radiolabeling, manufacture
	Advinus Therapeutics Ltd. Plot No. 21 & 22, Phase-II, Post Box No. 5813, Peenya Industrial Area, Bangalore–560 058, India	91–80-28394959, 28397338 (p) 91–80-28394015, 28396023 (F)	www.advinustherapeutics.com		Physical-chemical testing Environmental toxicity on aquatic and terrestrial organisms. Studies on behavior in water, soil, and air, bioaccumulation Residue studies Safety pharmacology GLP
Evotec AG	Evotec ID (Lyon) SAS Campus Mérieux, 1541 Avenue Marcel Mérieux, 69 280 Marcy l'Etoile,, Evotec (US) Inc., 303B College Road East, Princeton, NJ 08540, USA, Lenbury, India, UK, US	1–732-329-2355, +44 (0) 131 451 2560 916–767-3900 (US) 44(0) 131 451 2451 (EU) +33-437-668-400	http://www.evotec.com	Aptuit	Clinical development
Experimur	4045 South Morgan Street, Chicago, Illinois 60609–2514	773-254-2700	www.experimur.com		PK, TK, implants, neurotoxicity, neurosurgical, in-house clinic chemistry and histopathology
Fraunhofer ITEM	Nikolai-Fuchs Str. D- 30625 Hannover, Germany	+495 115 350 169 +495 115 350 8100	www.item.fraunhofer.de		
Frontage Labs	HQ: 700 Pennsylvania Drive, Exton PA 19341	610–232-0100	http://www.frontagelab.com/		Chronic and surgical

(continued)

	Address/location	Phone #	Website	Labs acquired by this lab	Specialty/additional services	Rat	Rabbits	Dog	Carcinogenicity	DART	Inhalation	Primate	Pig	IV infusion	Genotoxic	Metabolism	Analytical	Special studies	Receptor panels
Frontier Biotechnologies Inc.	China	US Office (301)251-0231	www.frontierbiotech.com/en/	Diamond, Shamrock, Sumitomo		X	X	X	X	X		X	X		X	X	X	X	
GLP Compliant Laboratory, Jubilant Biosys Ltd	96, Industrial Suburb, second Stage, Yeshwanthpur, Bangalore – 560 022 (Karnataka)	91-80-66628400 or 91-80-66628333	www.jubilantbiosys.com		Toxicity studies (acute and subacute) Mutagenicity studies (Ames assay, chromosomal aberration test in vitro, micronucleus assay in vivo) Analytical and clinical chemistry testing GLP	X		X	X			X		X			X		
HemoGenix	Colorado Springs, CO	719-264-6250	www.hemogenix.com		In vitro tox/PK			X				X							
Hurley Consulting Associates LTD	25 De Forest Avenue, Summit, NJ 07901	Phone: (908) 273-8490 Fax: (908) 273-2670	www.hurleyconsulting.com		Statistical analysis, study design, preclinical assessments, data management, QA, regulatory affairs, pharmacovigilance, training, etc.						X	X				X	X		
Ibex Preclinical Research, Inc.	1072 West RSI Drive, Logan, Utah 84321	435-752-4448	www.ibexpreclinical.com		Cardio telem.	X	X	X		X		X			X				
ICP Firefly	ICP Firefly Pty Ltd. P.O. Box 6198 Alexandria NSW 2015 Sydney, Australia	Phone: + 61-2 9310 3899 Fax:+ 61-2 9310 4889	http://www.icpfirefly.com.au/00_home.html		ISO 1993, chronic and surgical	X	X	X	X	X				X					
IIBAT (International Institute of Biotechnology and Toxicology)	Test Facility, Padappai–601 301, Kancheepuram Dist., Tamil Nadu, India. Administrative Office, Old No:12, New No:62, Kilpauk, Chennai, Tamil Nadu, India.	Phone: +91-044-27174 24666 Fax: +91-044-27174455 E-Mail: director@iibat.com	www.iibat.com		Ecotox	X		X	X	X		X	X	X		X	X		
IITRI (Illinois Institute of Technology Research Institute)	IIT Research Institute 10 West 35th Street, Chicago, IL 60616	(312)567-4487 (703)918-4480	www.iitri.org			X	X	X	X	X				X	X	X			

Company	Address	Contact	Website	Partners	Services
Invetus	Palmerston North 4442, New Zealand	Armidale Research Centre: +61 (0)2 6770 3200 Wongalburra Research Centre: +61 (0)2 6663 7255 Invetus NZ: +64 (0)7 857 0710	http://www.invetus.com		Veterinary Research, ISO 1993, cattle, horses, chicken, sheep, goat, alpaca
ILS (Integrated Laboratory Systems)	PO Box 13501 RTP, NC 27709	(919)544-5857 44(0) 1332-793000	www.ils-limited.co.uk	Estandan Limited/ Massey University	Data analysis, ecotoxicology
INA (Ina Research Inc.)	2148-188 Nishiminowa, Ina-shi, Nagano-ken 399-4501 Japan	Phone +81-265-72-6616 / Fax +81-265-72-6657	http://www.ina-research.co.jp/en/		
Innostar Bio-Tech, NCDSER (National Shanghai Center for New Drug Safety Evaluation and Research)	199 Guoshoujing Road, Pilot FreeTrade Zone, Shanghai, China, 201203	NCDSER, 199 Guoshoujing Road, Pilot FreeTrade Zone, Shanghai, China, 201203 — Tel:+86-21-60211999 Fax:+86-21-50801259 E-mail:services@ncdser.com	www.innostarsh.com; www.ncdser.com		Biomedicine, gene-technology; hERG, Safety Pharma
IIT (Indian Institute of Toxicology)	32 A/1, Hadapsar Industrial Estate, Pune (Maharashtra)- 411 013, India	Tel: + 91 20 26819962 Fax: + 91 20 26819962 E mail: iitoxicology@gmail.com Cell: +919822011159	http://www.iitoxicology.com		Toxicity studies (acute studies – oral, parenteral, dermal, inhalation, dermal irritation/corrosion, eye irritation/corrosion, skin sensitization – subacute studies, chronic studies) Mutagenicity studies (Ames assay, mammalian erythrocyte micronucleus test, in vivo and in vitro Mammalian Chromosome Aberration Test) GLP
Inotiv Co.	2701 Kent Avenue, West Lafayette, IN 47906, Europe	(800)845-4246 44(0) 247 663 9574 (EU)	http://www.basinc.com/	Seventh Wave Laboratories, Smithers Avanza Toxicology Services, MicaGenix	Histology Image analysis Non-GLP mice and rats
MicaGenix, Greenfield, IN		(888)-779-5500 (317)468-1760	www.micagenix.com	MicaGenix	

(continued)

	Address/location	Phone #	Website	Labs acquired by this lab	Specialty/additional services	Rat	Rabbits	Dog	Carcinogenicity	DART	Inhalation	Primate	Pig	IV infusion	Genotoxic	Metabolism	Analytical	Special studies	Receptor panels
Intox (Intox PVT. LTD.)	375, Urawade, Tal. Mulshi, Dist. Pune, Maharashtra, 412 115, INDIA.	Tel: +91–20-66548700 Fax: +91–20-66548799 Email: info@intoxlab. com	www.intoxlab.com		Physical-chemical testing Toxicity studies (Acute toxicity– oral, dermal, inhalation, parenteral routes - skin irritation/ sensitization, eye irritation, subacute, chronic, reproductive) Mutagenicity studies (Ames assay, chromosomal aberration test in vivo and in vitro, micronucleus assay in vivo and in vitro, in vitro sister chromatid exchange, in vitro mammalian cell gene mutation test) Environmental toxicity studies on aquatic and terrestrial organisms. Analytical and clinical chemistry Irritation, Farm animals GLP	X	X		X	X	X				X		X		
IonsGate Preclinical Services	222-2176 Health Sciences Mall, Vancouver, British Columbia, Canada, V6T 1Z3 2350 Health Sciences Mall, Vancouver Canada, V6T1Z3	604-827-1733	www.ionsgate.com		Rat CV safety, Rat CNS toxicity, ion channels	X				X							X		
Intl. Inst. Of Biotech and Toxicology (IIBAT)	Padappai, Kancheepuram District, Tamil Nadu, Chennai 603 301, India	91-44-27174246, 27174266 (P) 91-44-27174455 (F)	www.iibat.com		Physical-chemical testing Toxicity studies Mutagenicity studies Environmental toxicity studies on aquatic and terrestrial organisms Studies on behavior in water, soil, and air; bioaccumulation Residue studies Studies on effects on mesocosms and natural ecosystems Analytical and clinical chemistry testing Studies on natural enemies and predators GLP														

Company	Address	Website	Services										
iuvo BioSciences	iuvo BioScience 7500 W. Henrietta Road, Rush, NY 14543	800-836-4850 585-533-1672 info@iuvobioscience. com	https://www. iuvobioscience.com	Mice, guinea pig, hamsters, rats, po.im ip, sc, im, dermal, intratracheal, ocular/ intraocular, intranasal, rectal, intravaginal	X				X				X
IPS Therapeutics	3035 Boulevard Industriel, Sherbrooke, Quebec, J1L 2E9, Canada	Ph: (819)820-1515 Fax: (819)-820-6831 Email: info@ ipstherapeutique.com	www.ipstherapeutique. com/	Sheep, guinea pig.	X	X				X		X	
ITR (International Toxicology Research) Laboratories Canada	19 601 Clark Graham, Baie d'Urfé (Montréal), Quebec Canada, H9X 3 T1	Tel: 514457-7400 Fax: 514457-7303	http://www.itrlab.com		X	X	X		X	X	X	X	SP
Jai Research Foundation International	JRF India NH-48, Near Daman Ganga Bridge Valvada-396 105 (Old: 396108), Gujarat, INDIA JRF America 2650 Eisenhower, Suite C Audubon, PA-19403, Pennsylvania, USA.	India: +919909900950, 9998022968, America: +18779375732	www.jrfglobal.com		X		X		X	X	X		
JOINN Laboratories	Building C, 2600 Hilltop Drive, Richmond, CA 94806, USA, Germantown, MD Beijing China	1(510)408–7722 (301)540–5988 86–10–67869966	www.joinn-lab.com	Pharmacokinetics, toxicokinetics, Ames test, micronucleus test, chromosome aberration test	X	X	X	X					X
Korean Institute of Toxicology (KIT)	141 Gajeong-ro, Yuseong-gu, Daejeon 34114, Republic of Korea	+82–42–610-8204 Fax: +82–42–610-8085; global@kitox.re.kr	http://www.kitox.re.kr/ kitox_eng/main.php		X	X	X	X		X			
Krish Biotech Research Pvt. Ltd.	Krish Biotech Research Pvt. Ltd. 29, Lala lajpat Rai Sarani(Elgin Road), Kolkata-700 020, West Bengal, India Krish Biotech Research Pvt. Ltd. T-1, QK-17 (Part) WBIIDC, Kalyani, Phase III, Nadia, West Bengal-741 235, India	Phone: +91 33–7108 1010/1011 Lab Phone: +91 33–2582 4472/88499850 Email Id: bd@ krishbiotech.com	www.krishbiotech.com	Physical chemical testing Toxicity studies (acute) Mutagenicity studies (micronucleus assay in vitro and in vivo, Ames assay in vitro & in vivo) Environmental toxicity studies on aquatic and terrestrial organisms using fish, honeybees, alga, daphnia, and earthworms. Analytical and clinical chemistry testing. GLP	X	X					X		

(continued)

	Address/location	Phone #	Website	Labs acquired by this lab	Specialty/additional services	Rat	Rabbits	Dog	Carcinogenicity	DART	Inhalation	Primate	Pig	IV infusion	Genotoxic	Metabolism	Analytical	Special studies	Receptor panels
Litron Laboratories	3500 Winton Place, Rochester, NY 14623, USA	Phone: 585-442-0930, Toll Free: 877-4-LITRON Fax: 585-442-0934 info@LitronLabs.com	www.litronlabs.com											X	X		X		
Lovelace	2425 Ridgecrest Dr. SE, Albuquerque, NM 87108-5127	Phone: 505-348-9400 Fax: 505-348-8567	www.lovelacebiomedical.org		Clinical, ferret, guinea pig	X	X				X	X	X	X	X	X	X		
LPT (Laboratory of Pharmacology and Toxicology GmbH & Co. KG, Redderweg 8, 21147 Hamburg KG)	LPT Laboratory of Pharmacology and Toxicology GmbH & Co. KG, Redderweg 8, 21147 Hamburg	Phone: +49 40-70-20-20 Fax: +49 40-70-20-22-99 Email: lpt@lpt-hamburg.de	www.LPT-pharm-tox.de			X	X	X	X	X	X	X	X	X	X	X	X	X	
MB Research	PO Box 178, Spinnerstown, PA 18968	215-536-4110	www.mbresearch.com		In vitro and alternative models	X	X												
Mediction	Shanghai, China	US office: Dr. Mingzhu Zhang Tel: +1-(858) 504-1256 8621-51-320228 8621-5859-1500	http://www.mediction.com			X	X			X		X	X		X	X	X		
Merieux NutriSciences	Piracicaba, Campinas and Sao Paulo- BRAZIL, Lost Angeles, CA	626-810-2823 +55-19-3429-7720	https://www.merieuxnutrisciences.com/br/en	Used to be tied to BioAgri somehow		X	X	X					X	X	X	X	X		
MWRI (Magee-womens Research Institute)	204 Craft Avenue, Pittsburgh, PA 15213	412-641-8977	http://www.mageewomens.org		Women's research	X		X								X	X		
Nia Life Sciences Inc.	Libertyville, IL 60048	847-573-1852	www.nialifesciences.com		Pharmacokinetics, GLP and non-GLP, bioanalytical, fungal, and tumor model	X													
Nitto Avecia Pharma Services, Inc.	10 Vanderbilt, Irvine, CA 92618	TOLL FREE: (877) 445-6554	TEL: (949) 951-4425	FAX: (949) 951-4909	https://www.aveciapharma.com/	Irvine Analytical Labs, Inc.- Avrio Biopharmaceuticals (Avrio)	Extractables and leachables					X						X			
NAMSA	NAMSA World Headquarters 6750 Wales Road, Northwood, Ohio, USA 43619	+1-866-666-9455 (toll free) +1-419-666-9455 (outside of USA) +1-419-662-4386 (fax)	www.namsa.com		ISO 1993, Chronic and surgical												X		

Company	Address	Phone	Website/Email	Specialties	ISO 10993											
Nelson Labs	6750 Wales Road, Northwood, Ohio 43 619 USA. + Salt Lake City, UT	800-826-2088	www.nelsonlabs.com			X	X		X			X		X		X
Gibraltar Laboratories, Inc.	122 FAIRFIELD ROAD, FAIRFIELD, NJ 07004–2405	(973)227–6882(p) (973)227–0812(0)	www.gibraltarlabsinc.com	Microbiology		X	X				X		X			X
Noble Life Sciences	NOBLE LIFE SCIENCES PO BOX 242, WOODBINE, MD, 21797	PHONE: 800.864.1839 LOCAL: 410.795.2222 INFO@ NOBLELIFESCI.COM	www.noblelifesci.com	Sheep, goat, guinea pig, hamster, mice, Ferrets		X	X		X							
	Spring Valley Lab. PO Box 242, Woodbine, MD 21797	800–864–1839						X		X						
Northern Biomedical Research	1210 Fontaluna Road, Spring Lake, Michigan, 49 456	Phone: 231.759.2333 Email: info@ northernbiomedical.com	http://www. northernbiomedical.com			X	X		X			X	X	X		X
NOTOX	NOTOX CH Wallisellweg 2, CH-4704 Niederbipp P.O. Box 3476, 5203 DL 's-Hertogenbosch, The Netherlands	T: +41-(0)32-633-0015 F: +41-(0)32-633-2802	http://www. vogel-gmbh.ch/notox	General toxicology, ecotox, immunotox, reproductive, pharmacology								X		X		X
NSF	NSF International, P.O. Box 130 140, 789 N. Dixboro Road, Ann Arbor, MI 48105, USA	734-769-8010, 800 NSF MARK	www.nsf.org	GLP, REACH, GHS		X			X							
	Bioensaios analyses consultoria ambiental Ltda. Rua Palermo, 257-Viamão – RS, BRASIL–CEP 94480–775 Bairro Vila Santa Isabel	Phone 55 (51) 3493.6888 Fax 55 (51) 3493.6885														
Nucro-Technics	2000 Ellesmere Road, Unit 16, Scarborough, Ontario, Canada M1H 2 W4	(416438–6727 (p) (416438–3463 (f)	www.nucro-technics.com	Microbiology		X	X	X	X					X		X

(continued)

	Address/location	Phone #	Website	Labs acquired by this lab	Specialty/additional services	Rat	Rabbits	Dog	Carcinogenicity	DART	Inhalation	Primate	Pig	IV infusion	Genotoxic	Metabolism	Analytical	Special studies	Receptor panels
Olon Ricerca Bioscience	7528 Auburn Road, P.O. Box 1000, Concord, OH 44077–1000	888–742-3722 or 440–357-3300	www.ricerca.com		Synthesis, product development, radioactivity	X	X		X	X		X				X	X		
Pacific Biolabs	551 Linus Pauling Drive, Hercules, CA 94547	Phone: 510.964.9000 Fax: 510.964.0551	http://www.pacificbiolabs.com		Yes, ISO 10993, chronic and surgical	X	X	X	X	X	X		X		X	X	X		
Palamur biosciences Pvt. Ltd	Palamur Biosciences Pvt. Ltd. AIKYA, Flat: 401, H. No. 10-3-329/23 fourth Floor, East Marredpally, Tukaram Gate Road, Opposite Faust High School, Secunderabad-500 026, Telangana State, India	+91 8542231166 040–40122418 +91 9000411835	www.palamurbio.com		GLP	X	X	X									X		
Pharma Advance Inc.	Jiangyin, China	+86–510-8641-7090	www.pharmaadvance.com		Pharmacology, chemistry	X													
Pharma Hungary	Pharmahungary Group, Graphisoft Park, 7 Záhony street, Budapest, H-1031, Hungary	http://www. businessdevelopment@pharmahungary.com	www.pharmahungary.com			X	X					X				X			
Pharmaron	Pharmaron (US) 6 Venture, Suite 250, Irvine, CA 92618 USA Pharmaron Beijing Co., Ltd. (China) 6 Taihe Road, BDA, Beijing, 100 176, P.R. China	+650-859-3853, 408-739-1572 bd@pharmaron.com	http://www.pharmaron.com/			X	X			X	X	X		X		X	X		
Pharmaseed Pre-clinical CRO	Pharmaseed Ltd. 9 Hamazmera St. Ness Ziona 74 047, Israel	Tel: 972–8-930-2771 Fax: 972–8-930-2773	www.pharmaseedltd.com		Histopathology, biocompatibility			X						X					
Porsolt & Partners	Boulogne-Billancourt, France	33146109990	www.porsolt.com			X	X					X	X			X			
Powered Research	Research Triangle Park, NC	919-213-6035 info@poweredresearch.com	www.poweredresearch.com		Opthalmic studies, implant evaluation	X	X									X			
PreLabs	PreLabs P.O. Box 118 Hines, IL 60141	(708)613-6000 Fax: 708-613-6100	www.prelabs.com		Transgenic mouse CA studies	X	X	X		X		X							

Company	Address	Phone/Contact	Website	Services
Product Safety Labs (PSL)	2394 Highway 130, Dayton, NJ 08810	(732)438–5100 (732)254–9200	www.productsafetylabs.com	Environmental, ferret emesis studies, radioactivity, ISO 10993
QPS	Delaware Technology Park. 3 Innovation Way, Suite 240, Newark, DE 19711 + 11 locations worldwide	512 350 2827 302 369 5602 info@qps.com	www.qps-usa.com	Yes, radioactivity
JSW Research	JSW Research, Austria		JSW Research	
Quest Pharma	Ctra Cartagena to Alhama km23, 30120-Fuente Alamo de Murcia Spain	Tel and Fax 968 – 15 14 48	http://www.questpharma.com/	
Raj Biotech	Raj Biotech India Pvt. Ltd. 33/A Ganesh Krupa Society, Ram Krishna Pramahansa Nagar, Poud Road, Kothrud, PunePune, MH 411 038IN	091453 39356	https://rajbiotech.in/	Ames, chromosomal aberration, PK
Rallis Research Center	Rallis India Limited, second Floor, Sharda Terraces, Plot No. 65,Sector 11 CBD Belapur, Navi Mumbai 400 614	Offices: +91 – 022 – 6776 1700 +91 – 022 – 6776 1634 Research & Development: +91 – 080 – 67292600 +91- 080-67292601	www.rallis.co.in	Yes
RCC Laboratories India Private Ltd.	RCC LABORATORIES INDIA PRIVATE LIMITED Genome Valley, Hyderabad Post Code: 500078, Andhra Pradesh, India.	Tel: +91 40 2348 0421/ 422/ 423/ 424; +91 966 618 0422 Fax: +91 40 2348 0420	www.rccltd.com	Physical-chemical testing, Toxicity studies (acute, subacute, chronic, subchronic, reproductive, inhalation, carcinogenicity) Mutagenicity studies (Ames assay, chromosome aberration in vitro and in vivo, micronucleus assay in vitro and in vivo, mouse lymphoma assay) Environmental toxicity studies

(continued)

	Address/location	Phone #	Website	Labs acquired by this lab	Specialty/additional services	Rat	Rabbits	Dog	Carcinogenicity	DART	Inhalation	Primate	Pig	IV infusion	Genotoxic	Metabolism	Analytical	Special studies	Receptor panels
RIL (Reliance Life Sciences)	Dhirubhai Ambani Life Sciences Centre, R 282, Thane-Belapur Road, Rabale,NaviMumbai-400 701, U24239MH2001 PTC130654	+91 2235338000, +91-22-391 8500-05 (P), 0091-22-391 18099 (F)	www.rellife.com		Toxicity studies (acute studies – oral, dermal, eye irritation, skin irritation, skin sensitization, subacute, subchronic) Mutagenicity studies (Ames assay) Analytical and clinical chemistry GLP				X								X		
RTC S.p.A.	Research Toxicology Centre S.p.A., Via Tito Speri, 12, 00040 Pomezia RM, Italy	Tel +39 06 91095263-, Fax +39 06 9105737	www.rtc.it		Yes, consulting, regulatory	X	X		X	X		X	X		X		X	X	
RTI	PO Box 12194, Research Triangle Park, NC 27709	919-541-6000, webteam@rti.org	www.rti.org		Yes, consulting, regulatory	X			X	X				X		X	X		
Sa-Ford, Taloji, District, Raigad, Maharashtra	Sa Ford (office address) 601, PROXIMA, PLOT NO 19 sector 30 A, Vashi 400 705 Navi Mumbai, Maharashtra, India (Lab address) Plot No. V-10, MIDC Industrial Area, Taloja Distt. Raigad,Maharashtra-410 208, India	office Phone: +91 22 6794 4000, FAX:+91 22 6794 4001, Lab. Phone: 919152011590, 9152011591, 9152011592, 9152011593, Email:lab@sa-ford.com	www.sa-ford.com		Physical-chemical testing (5-batch analysis) Toxicity studies (acute, subacute, chronic, reproductive, carcinogenicity, inhalation, skin sensitization) Mutagenicity studies (Ames assay, micronucleus assay in vivo, chromosome aberration test in vitro and in vivo), analytical and clinical chemistry GLP	X					X								
SciMetrika	1420 Spring Hill Road, Suite 600, McLean, VA 22102	703-917-6623	http://www.scimetrika.com/	Hamner Institute		X		X	X	X					X	X			
Sekisui XenoTech LLC	Sekisui XenoTech, LLC, 1101 West Cambridge Circle Dr, Kansas City, KS 66103	(913)438-7450/877-	http://www.xenotech.com/		Yes	X	X					X			X	X			
Sequani Limited	Bromyard Road, Herefordshire HR8 1LH, Ledbury, UK	+44 1531 634121 (p), +44 1531 634753 (f)	www.sequani.com			X		X	X			X	X	X	X	X			

(continued)

Company	Contact	Website	Northview	Services / Notes											
SGS		http://www.sgs.com							X			X	X		X
	SGS Life Sciences Division, Fairfield, NJ	(800)747-8782 (800)777-8378		Implant, combustion, fish, industrial, consumer products	X	X	X		X			X	X	X	
	SGS Headquarters, 1 Place des Alpes, P.O. Box 2152, 1211 Geneva 1, Switzerland US Office: North Chicago, Illinois, + Northbrook, IL, + Sparta, SC	T + 41 22 739 91 11 F + 41 22 739 98 86 US: 847–564–8181, 864–574–7728		Yes			X					X			
Sinclair	562 State Road DD, Auxvasse, MO 65231	INFO@SINCLAIRRESEARCH.COM (573) 387-4400	www.sinclairresearch.com	Radiolabeled; cats; other, chronic and surgical	X	X	X	X	X	X	X	X	X	X	
Smithers (formerly Smithers Viscient)	121 S. Main Street, Suite 300, Akron, OH 44308	+1330–762-7441	http://www.smithers.com/	Toxigenics, molecular toxicology, investigative toxicology, toxicogenomics, toxicoinformatics, and biomarker qualification	X				X	X		X			X
SNBL Japan	Street address: St Luke's Tower 28F, 8-1 Akashi-cho, Chuo-ku, Tokyo,104–0044, Japan	Japan Phone: +81 3 5565 5001 Fax: +81 3 5565 6160 Email: info@snbl.co.jp	http://www.snbljapan.com/	Yes, clinical, irritation	X	X	X	X	X	X	X	X	X	X	X
	SNBL USA 6605 Merrill Creek Parkway, Everett, WA 98203	USA: 1–425–322-1687 E-mail: info@snbl.co.jp									X			X	
SoBran	Exec office: SoBran, Inc. 3110 Fairview Park Dr., Suite 250, Falls Church, VA 22042 Corporate office: SoBran, Inc. 4401 Dayton-Xenia Road, Dayton, OH 45432	exec: Ph: 703.352.9511 Fax: 703.352.9513 e-mail: info@sobran-inc.com Corporate: Ph: 937.426.0696 Fax: 937.426.4609	www.sobranbioscience.com	Formulation; Regulatory and accreditation assistance, dose range finding, toxicokinetics	X	X	X		X		X			X	X
Southern RI (Southern Research Institute)	HQ: 2000 Ninth Avenue South Birmingham, Alabama 35205 Mail: P.O. 55305, Birmingham, AL 35255–5305	205–581-2000 800–967-6774	www.southernresearch.org	Yes, formulation, development, tumor models, chronic and surgical	X	X	X	X	X	X	X	X	X	X	

	Address/location	Phone #	Website	Labs acquired by this lab	Specialty/additional services	Rat	Rabbits	Dog	Carcinogenicity	DART	Inhalation	Primate	Pig	IV infusion	Genotoxic	Metabolism	Analytical	Special studies	Receptor panels
SRI International	333 Ravenswood Ave. Menlo Park, CA 94025-3493	(650)859-2000 (866)451-5998	www.sri.com		Formulation, CTM, chronic and surgical	X	X		X	X			X		X	X	X		
Stillmeadow	12852 Park One Drive, Sugar Land, TX 77478	281-240-8828	www.stillmeadow.com		Companion animal studies	X	X	X			X		X			X	X		
Surpass, Inc	Greater twin cities, MN	(651) 303-3552	www.surpassinc.com	LyChron	Pig device implant studies, sheep, goats	X	X			X			X			X	X	X	
Synecor LLC	1340 Environ Way, Chapel Hill, NC 27517	919-883-3220	www.synecor.com		Surgical		X	X					X	X				X	
TECAM (technologia ambiental Ltda.	Rua Fabia, 59- Vila Romana- CEP 05051-030- Sao Paulo, SP	+55 11 3677 2553 +55 11 3677 2555	WWW.TECAM.COM.BR/US		Yes	X			X					X			X		
TNO Pharma	Utrechtseweg 48, NL-3700AJ Zeist 3704 HE, Netherlands	+31 30 694 4806 (p) +31 30 694 4845 (f) +31 30 694 4144	http://www.tno.nl/en/		Yes, packaging, food, nutrition, clinical	X	X	X	X	X	X	X	X	X	X	X	X	X	
Torrent Pharmaceuticals Ltd.	Torrent House, Off. Ashram Road, Ahmedabad- 380 009. Gujarat, India	Phone No.: +91-79-26599000 Fax No.: +91-79-26582100	www.torrentpharma.com			X	X		X	X		X			X	X	X		
Toxi-Coop	"Toxi-Coop" Toxicological Research Center Zrt., H-1122 Budapest, Magyar Jakobinusok Tere 4/B 5. em. 2. H-8230 Balatonfüred, Ifjusåg út 9/A	+36 30 846-2664	http://www.toxicoop.com		Guinea pigs, ecotox	X	X	X	X	X	X	X	X	X	X	X			
Toxikon Corp.	15 Wiggins Ave, Bedford, MA 01730	(781)275-3330 (p) (781)271-1136 (f)	www.toxikon.com		Yes, ISO 10993, chronic and surgical	X	X	X	X	X		X	X		X	X	X		
UIC Tox Research Lab	The University of Illinois at Chicago, College of Medicine, Dept of Pharmacology (MC 868), 1940 W. Taylor Street, Chicago, IL 60612-7353	312-996-9185	www.uic.edu/labs/tox/trlt.html		Pharmacokinetics, GLP	X	X									X			

Company	Address	Phone/Fax	Website	Services								
Vanta Bioscience	K2, 11th Cross street, SPICOT Industries Estate, Gummidipundi, Tamil Nadu – 601 201	91-44-67 910-300, 329, 306, 303 (P) 91-44-4220-2810 (F)	www.vantabio.com	Toxicity studies (acute, subacute, chronic, reproductive, in vitro skin corrosion and irritation using EpiSkin model) Mutagenicity studies (Ames assay, micronucleus test, chromosome aberration test in vitro and in vivo) Analytical and clinical chemistry GLP	X	X		X		X	X	X
Vimta Labs Ltd.	142, IDA, Phase II, Cherlapally, Hyderabad – 500 051 India. US office 6414 Fairways Road, Niwot, CO. 80 503	91-40-67404040 (P) 91-40-39847708 (F)	www.vimta.com	Clinical toxicity studies (acute, subacute, chronic, reproductive, carcinogenicity) Mutagenicity studies (Ames assay, chromosome aberration test in vivo and in vitro, mouse lymphoma assay, micronucleus test in vitro and in vivo), analytical and clinical chemistry testing Bioanalytical, pharmacokinetics, safety pharmacology GLP	X	X	X			X		X
Vivo Biotech Ltd.	central lab Sy #: 349/A, 350/A, 351, 356/3A, Pregmapur Village – 502 311, Gejwal Mandal, Medak District, Telangana	US phone: +1803–526–7267 central lab 91–845-4210411 (P) 91-40-27803612 (F)	www.vivobio.com	Toxicity studies (acute, subacute, reproductive) Mutagenicity studies (Ames assay, micronucleus assay in vivo) Analytical and Clinical chemistry GLP Immuno-deficient mice	X	X	X			X	X	
VivoPharm Pty. Ltd.	VivoPharm HQ Level 3 Office 29, 240 Plenty Road Bundoora VIC 3083 Australia	61-3-9088-1800 (p) 61-3-9923-6188 (f) email: info@vivopharm.com/au	www.vivopharm.com.au/	VivoPharm RDDT Mouse, tumor models	X	X	X	X		X	X	X
WestChina-Frontier PharmaTech	28 Gaopeng Avenue, Chengdu, Sichuan, China 610041	+86 (28) 85154334 ext. 502 (p) +86 (28) 85173043 (f)	www.glpcd.com	Guinea pig	X	X	X	X		X		X

(continued)

	Address/location	Phone #	Website	Labs acquired by this lab	Specialty/additional services	Rat	Rabbits	Dog	Carcinogenicity	DART	Inhalation	Primate	Pig	IV infusion	Genotoxic	Metabolism	Analytical	Special studies	Receptor panels
WuXi AppTec	St. Paul, Minn., Philadelphia, PA, Marietta, GA	(888)794-0077 (800)622-8820 (888)847-6633	www.wuxiapptec.com	Apptech, WuXi, XenoBiotics	Biotech, biocomp/med devices, microbiology, ISO 10993, chronic and surgical	X	X	X				X		X	X	X	X		
	WuXi Pharmatech 288 FuTe ZhongLu WaiGaoQiao Shanghai 200131, P.R. China	+82(21)-5046-1111			Rodent toxicity (oral, iv, and PK)	X	X	X				X		X	X	X	X		
	XenoBiotics 107 Morgan Lane, Plainsboro, NJ 08536	(609)799-2295 (609)799-7497			Formulation radioactivity	X	X	X				X				X			
Additional resources	http://www.contractresearchmap.com/places/north-carolina																		

Appendix B: Medical Device Biocompatibility CROs

© Springer Nature Switzerland AG 2020
S. C. Gad et al., *Contract Research and Development Organizations-Their History, Selection, and Utilization*, https://doi.org/10.1007/978-3-030-43073-3

Lab name (affiliated labs/past names)	Location(s)	Phone #(s)	Website	Additional services	Metabolism	Analytical (L&E)	ISO-10993 "Big Three"	Surgical Studies	Contract Sterilization	Physical Testing
American Preclinical and Devices	Minneapolis, MN	(763) 717–7990	www.americanpreclinical.com	Full range cardiovascular testing	X	X	X	X	X	X
ANPRO	Haw River, NC	(800) 523–1276	www.anpro.com							
Applied Tech	Calhoun, GA	(706) 629–4624	www.applied-technologies.com						X	X
BASI	West Lafayette, IN Europe	(800) 845–4246 (765) 463–4527 44(0) 247663 9574 (EU)	www.basinc.com	Method validation, stability, toxicology lab	X	X				X
BD Biosciences	San Jose, CA	(408) 432–9475	www.bdbiosciences.com	ADME	X		X			
Biopharmaceutical Research Inc.	Vancouver, Canada	(604) 432–9237	www.bripharm.com	Stability, label, QA, QC	X					
BioReliance (Sigma Aldrich)	Rockville, MD UK, India, Japan	(800)738–1000 (800)553–5372	www.bioreliance.com	*Full range Genotoxicity, Transgenic mouse CA models, (p53)	X	X				
BioSafety Research Center (BSRC)	Shizuoka, Japan	+81 538 58 3572	www.anpyo.or.jp	Immunotoxicity studies	X	X	X			
BTS	10 665 Sacramento Valley Rd. San Diego, CA	(858) 605–5882	www.btsresearch.com	Development, manufacturing, stability	X	X	X	X		
Calvert Preclinical	Olyphant, PA	(570) 586–2411	www.calvertlabs.com	Radioactivity Telemetry, Mouse Tumor Model, +, Pharmacokinetics, QA, ADME	X			X		
Case Medical	South Hackensack, NJ	(888) 227-CASE	www.casemed.com	Validation, product development, manufacture				X		

Company	Address	Phone/Fax	Website	Services	Range animal and cardiovascular testing						
CBSET	500 Shire Way Lexington, MA	(781) 541–5555	www.cbset.org		X	X	X	X		X	X
Cecon Consulting Group	Wilmington, DE	(302) 994–8000	www.cecon.com		X				X		
Charles River Labs	54943 N. Main Street Mattawan, MI	(269) 668–3336	www.criver.com	Imagery	X				X		
Covance	Princeton, NJ	(888) COVANCE	www.covance.com	Stability, clinical design and management, consulting	X	X	X		X		
CXR Biosciences	Dundee, UK Scotland, UK	+44 (0)-1382–432 163	www.cxrbiosciences.com	Development, consulting	X	X	X				
Dalton Chemical Laboratories, Inc.	Toronto, ON	(800) 567–5060	www.dalton.com	Scale up, development	X	X					
DEKA Research and Development Corporation	Manchester, NH	(603) 669–5139	www.dekaresearch.com	Design							
EAG Laboratories	Columbia, MD	(573) 474–8579	www.abclabs.com	Manufacture, stability, validation	X	X	X				
Eurofins	Multiple sites		www.eurofins.com		X	X	X				
Frontage	Concord, OH	(888) 763–4797	www.ricerca.com	Development, manufacture	X	X	X			X	
Geneva Laboratories	Elkhorn, WI	(262) 753–9955	www.genevalabs.com		X						
Gibraltar Laboratories, Inc.	Fairfield, NJ	(973)227–6882(p) (973)227–0812(f)	www.gibraltarlabsinc.com	Microbiology, method development, validation		X	X				
Gwathmey, Inc	Cambridge, MA	(617)491–0022 (p) (617)492–5545 (f)	www.gwathmey.com	Consulting, biology	X				X		
ICP Firefly	P.O. Box 6198 Alexandria NSW Sydney, Australia	91-2-9310-3899	www.icpfirefly.com		X	X			X		

(continued)

Lab name (affiliated labs/past names)	Location(s)	Phone #(s)	Website	Additional services	Metabolism	Analytical (L&E)	ISO-10993 "Big Three"	Surgical Studies	Contract Sterilization	Physical Testing
In Vitro Technologies	Baltimore, MD	(410) 455-1245	www.invitrotech.com	Validation	X		X			
INA (Int. Non-clinical Assessment)	Nagano-ken, Japan Philippines	0265-72-6616	www.ina-research.co.jp	Validation, consulting, pediatric toxicity				X		
ITR Laboratories Canada Inc.	Montreal, QU	(514)457-7400	www.itrlab.com	Method validation, development	X	X	SP			
MB Research	Spinnerstown, PA	(215) 536-4110	www.mbresearch.com				X		X	
Meridian Medical Technologies, Inc.	Columbia, MD	(800) 638-8093	www.meridianmeds.com	Validation, development			X		X	
Microbac	Pittsburg, PA	(412) 459-1060	www.microbac.com	Manufacture						
Micro-Med Inc.	Tustin, CA	(714) 731-6803	www.micro-med.com	Packaging						X
Midwest Research Institute	Kansas City, MO	(816) 753-7600	www.mriresearch.org	Method validation	X		X			
NAMSA	Toledo, OH Northwood, OH France Irvine, CA Kennesaw, GA	(419)666-9455 (866)666-9455 33-4-78-07-92-34 (949)951-3110 (770)427-3101	www.namsa.com	Packaging	X	X	X	X	X	
NASP	Franklin, NJ	(800) 392-6310	www.naspco.com	Packaging						
Nelson Labs	Salt Lake City, UT	(800)826-2088	www.nelsonlabs.com	Validation		X			X	
Nucro-Technics	Scarborough, Canada	(416)438-6727 (p) (416)438-3463 (f)	www.nucro-technics.com	Microbiology, phase II, III, IV, method validation		X		X		
OSG Norwich Pharmaceuticals	Norwich, NY	(607) 335-3100	www.norwichpharma.com	Package, QA, stability, validation						

Company	Location	Phone	Website	Services					
Pacific Biolabs	Hercules, CA	(510) 565–9000	www.pacificbiolabs.com		X	X	X		
Pathology Associates	Frederick, MD Durham, NC	(301) 663–1644 (919) 544–5257	www.paicriver.com	Software	X		X		X
Pharma Quality Control Testing	Geneva, Switzerland	+41 22 739 91 11	www.pharmardqc.sgs.com			X	X		
Product Safety Lab (PSL)	Dayton, NJ	(732) 438–5100	www.productsafetylabs.com		X	X	X		
QTI	Whitehouse, NJ	(908) 534–4455	www.QTIonline.com	Validation, stability, consulting			X	X	
Ruhof	Mineola, NY	(516) 294–5888	www.ruhof.com	Manufacture	X		X		
Southern Research Institute	Birmingham, AL	(888)322–1166 (205) 211–7472	www.southernresearch.com	Yes, formulation, development, tumor models. Cancer phases II and III					
SRI International	Menlo Park, CA	(650)859–2000 (866)451–5998	www.sri.com	Formulation, CTM, QA, QC	X	X	X	X	
Sterile Technologies	Queensbury, NY	(518) 793–7077	www.steriletech.com	Manufacture					
STS duo TEK, Inc.	Rush, NY	(800) 836–4850	www.stsduotek.com	Stability, microbiology package	X	X		X	
TOXIKON Corp.	15 Wiggins Ave. Bedford, MA 01730	(781)275–3330 (p) (781)271–1136 (f)	www.toxikon.com	Packaging, ADME, Pharmacokinetics/toxicokinetics	X		X		
Vetter	Ranesburg, Germany	49–751–3700–0	www.vetter-group.com	Aseptically pre-filled applications, package, stable, valid		X			
Wickham Labs	Oau, UK	44–01–1329–226 600	www.wickhamlabs.com		X				
Wuxi-Apptech	Oakville, ON	(866) 337–4500	www.wellspringpharma.com	Manufacture	X		X		

Reference

Gad, S. C., & Spainhour, C. B. (2011). *Contract research and development organizations: Their role in global product development* (p. 137). New York: Springer.

Appendix C: Phase 1 Labs

© Springer Nature Switzerland AG 2020
S. C. Gad et al., *Contract Research and Development Organizations-Their History, Selection, and Utilization*, https://doi.org/10.1007/978-3-030-43073-3

Lab	Location	Phone	Website	Specialties
AAI international	2320 Scientific Park Dr. Wilmington, NC 28405	800–575-4224	http://www.alcaminow.com/	Biologics
ACE pharmaceuticals	Ace Pharmaceuticals BV Schepenveld 41, 3891 ZK Zeewolde, Netherlands	+31–36-5 227 201	http://www.ace-pharm.nl/	
ACM Global Laboratories	160 Elmgrove Park Rochester, NY 14624	**866–405-0400**	http://www.acmlab.com/	Pathology
Alta Sciences	1200 Beaumont Ave Montreal, Quebec H3P 3P1 Canada	514–381-2546	http://www.algopharm.com/	
Aptuit – an Evotec Company	303B College Road East Princeton, NJ 08540	**855–427-8848** 732–329-2355	http://www.almedica.com/	
Agenus	3 Forbes Road Lexington, MA 02421	781.674.4400	http://www.agenusbio.com/	Vaccines
ARUP Labs	500 Chipeta Way Salt Lake City, UT 84108	800–522-2787	http://www.aruplab.com/	
BioSkin	Burchardstraße 17 · 20 095 Hamburg, Germany	+49–040–606 897-14	http://www.bioskin.de/	Dermatological testing
Bourn Hall Clinic	High St., Bourn, Cambridge CB23 2TN, UK	+44-0-1954-717 210	http://www.bournhall.co.uk/	Fertility
CATO	Westpark Corporate Center 4364 South Alston Ave. Durham, NC 27713	919–361- 2286	http://www.cato.com	

(continued)

Lab	Location	Phone	Website	Specialties
Cirion	3150 Delaunay Laval, QC H7L 5E1, Canada	450–682-2231	http://www.cirion.com	
Charles River	Global	877–274-8371	http://www.criver.com/	Dermatological testing
Chiltern – a Covance company	Raleigh, NC	888–268-2623	http://www.chiltern.com/	
Covance	100 Perimeter Park Drive, suite C Morrisville, NC 27560	(888) 268–2623	www.covance.com	
CRL Global Services (Clinical Reference Laboratory)	8433 Quivira Road, Lenexa, KS 66215	800–445-6917	http://www.crlcorp.com/	
DP Clinical	9201 Corporate Boulevard, suite 350 Rockville, MD 20850	301–294-6226	http://www.dpclinical.com/	
Envigo	Indianapolis, IN	800–793-7287 317–806-6060	http://www.Envigo.com	
Esoterix	4509 Freidrich Lane Building 1 Suite 100 Austin, Texas 78 744	800–444-9111	http://www.esoterix.com/	
Frontage	700 Pennsylvania Drive, Exton, PA 19341	610–232-0100	https://www.frontagelab.com/service/early-phase-clinical/	
ICON	South County Business Park Leopardstown Dublin 18, Ireland	+353–1–291–2000	https://www.iconplc.com	
Lambda	460 Comstock Road Toronto, Ontario, M1L 4S4 Canada	**416–752-3636**	http://www.lambdacanada-cro.com	

(continued)

Lab	Location	Phone	Website	Specialties
MDSPS	2420 West Baseline Rd. Tempe, AZ 85283 USA	602–437-0097	http://www.mdsps.com	
Medfiles	Volttikatu 5, P.O. Box 1450 Fl-70 700 Kuopio, Finland	+358–20–7446-800	http://www.medfiles.eu	
Northwest Clinical Trials of Denver	4495 Hale Parkway #101 Denver, CO 80220	(303)399–4067	http://www.horizonscrc.com/index.html	
Parexel	2520 Meridian Parkway Research Triangle Park, Suite 200 Durham, NC 27713	919–544-3170	http://www.parexel.com	
Patheon	4815 Emperor Blvd, Durham, NC 27703	919–226-3200	http://www.patheon.com	
Quotient Sciences	Mere Way, Ruddington Nottingham, NG11 6JS	+44–0–115-974-9000	https://www.quotientsciences.com/	
Philip Johnson Research Laboratory	Department of Biology University of Maryland 1210 Biology-Psychology Building 4094 Campus Drive, College Park, MD 20742	301–405-6176	http://science.umd.edu/biology/plfj/	
PPD	929 North Front St., Wilmington, NC 28401–3331	910–251-0081	http://www.ppdi.com	

(continued)

Lab	Location	Phone	Website	Specialties
PRA Health Sciences	4130 Parklake Ave, Suite 400 Raleigh, NC 27612	919–786-8200	http://www.prahs.com	
ProMedica	2801 Bay Park Drive, Oregon, OH 43616	419–690-7900	http://www.promedica.org	
PSI	Baarerstrasse 113a 6300 Zug Switzerland	+41–41–228-10-00	http://www.psi-cro.com	
Quantum	991 Discovery Drive, Huntsville, AL 35806–2811	(256) 971–1800	http://www.quantum-intl.com	
Sanofi Genzyme	Bridgewater, NJ	800–981-2491	http://www.sanofigenzyme.com	Rare diseases, blood disorders, MS, immunology, oncology
Schiff and Co.	583 Mountain Ave, North Caldwell, NJ 07006	973–227-1830	http://www.schiffandcompany.com	
SciAn	2150 Islington Ave. #200 M9P 3 V4 Toronto, ON, Canada	416–231-8008	http://www.scian.com	
Simbec	Merthyr Tydfil Industrial Park, Merthyr Rd. Pentrebach, Merthyr Tydfil CF48 4DR, UK	0–800–69-1995	http://www.simbec.co.uk	
Syneos Health	1030 Sync Street Morrisville, NC 27560	919–876-9300	https://www.syneoshealth.com	
Synteract	5909 Sea Otter Place, Suite 100 Carlsbad, CA 92010	760-268-8200	http://www.synteract.com	

(continued)

Lab	Location	Phone	Website	Specialties
Bibra	Cantium House Railway Approach Wallington Surrey SM6 0DZ, UK	+44 (0)208652 1040	http://www. bibra- information.co.uk	
Watson Clinic LLP	Watson Clinic Center for Research 1600 Lakeland Hills Blvd Lakeland, FL 33805	863–688-6826	www. watsonclinic.com	
West	530 Herman O. West Drive Exton, PA 19341	800–345-9800	http://www. westpharma.com/	
Worldwide Clinical Trials	3800 Paramount Parkway Suite 400 Morrisville, NC 27560	610–632-8151	http://www. wwctrials.com	

Appendix D: Analytical Labs

Vendor	Location	Phone #	Website	Analytical	Bioanalytical	Additional services
Abbott	Abbott Park, IL	(847) 935–0945	www.abbottcontractmfg.com	X		Delivery, biologics
ABC Laboratories	Columbia, MD	(573) 474–8579	www.abslabs.com	X	X	Manufacturing, stability
Alturas Analytics Inc.	Moscow, ID	(208) 883–3400	www.alturasanalytics.com	X	X	Pharmacokinetics, validation
BASi	W. Lafayette, IN	(800) 845–4246 (765) 463–4527	www.basinc.com	X	X	Method validation, toxicology lab,
Battelle	Columbus, OH	(800) 201–2011	www.battelle.org	X		Toxicology lab
Baxter	Bloomington, IN	(800) 422–9837	www.baxter.com	X		Stability, packaging, biological
Bertin Pharma	Montigny-le-Bretonneux, France	+33 (0)1 39 30 62 60	www.bertinpharma.com	X	X	Formulation, manufacturing, packaging, toxicology lab
Biopharmaceutical Research Inc.	Vancouver, Canada	(604) 432–9237	www.bripharm.com	X	X	Stability, pharmacokinetics, ADME
BioReliance Corp.	Rockville, MD	(301) 738–1000	www.bioreliance.com	X	X	Manufacturing, stability, biologics
Boston Analytical Inc.	Salem, NH	(603) 893–3758	www.bostonanalytical.com	X		Method validation, stability
BTC	Irvine, CA	(949) 660–3185	www.biologicaltestcenter.com	X		Toxicology Lab, pharmacokinetics, ADME
Calvert Preclinical	Olyphant, PA	(570) 586–2411	www.calvertlabs.com	X		Toxicology Lab, QA, pharmacokinetics, ADME
Catalent	Somerset, NJ	(877) 587–1835	www.catalent.com	X	X	Method development, manufacturing

Celsis Lab Group	St. Louis, MO	www.celsis.com	X	Method validation,, stability, safety, efficacy, pharmacokinetics
Charles River Laboratories	Wilmington, MA	(800) 523–5227 (312) 476–1200	X	Manufacturing
Chemir Analytical Services	Maryland Heights, MO	(877) 274–8371	X	Development, validation, stability
CIT	Evreux, France	www.chemir.com	X	Toxicology Lab, validation
Covance	Princeton, NJ	(800) 659–7659	X	Stability, clinical design, consulting, toxicology lab
		+33 2 32 292626 (888) COVANCE	X	
CPT Co.	Fairfield, NJ	www.citox.com www.covance.com	X	Method validation, stability, product testing, toxicology lab
CTBR	Quebec, Canada	(973) 808–7111	X	Method validation, analysis
Dow Chemical (parent corp.)	Midland, MI Smithfield, RI	www.cptclabs.com	X	Excipients, manufacturing
		(514) 630–8200 (800) 258–2436 (parent corp.)	X	
DPT	San Antonio, TX	www.ctbr.com www.dow.com (parent corp.)	X	Management, production, compounding, packaging, formulation
Elite labs	Northvale, NJ	(866) CALL DPT	X	Manufacturing
Fraunhofer ITA	Hannover, Germany	www.dptlabs.com	X	Toxicology lab
Galbraith Labs, Inc	Knoxville, TN	(201) 750–2646	X	Environmental, method validation
		+49 511 5353 0		
GEA Process Engineering	Hudson, WI	www.elitepharma. com www.item.fraunhofer. de/	X	Validation, equipment
		(877) 449–8797	X	
		www.galbraith.com		
		(715) 386–9371	X	
		www.niroinc.com		

(continued)

Vendor	Location	Phone #	Website	Analytical	Bioanalytical	Additional services
Glatt Contract Services	Ramsey, NJ	07621–664 319	www.glattair.com	X		Validation
Harlan Laboratories	Indianapolis, IN	(888) 265–2953	www.harlan.com	X	X	Microbiology, monoclonals
Hollister-Stier	Spokane, WA	(800) 655–5329	www.hollister-stier.com	X		Labeling, packaging, validation, manufacturing
Integrated Laboratory Services (ILS)	RTP, NC	(919) 544–5857	www.ils-inc.com	X	X	QA, toxicology lab
In Vitro Technologies	Baltimore, MD	(888) 4683400.	www.invitrotech.com		X	Validation, stability
Irvine Pharmaceutical Services	Irvine, CA	(877) 445–6554	www.ialab.com	X		Validation, inhalation, QC, environmental, formulation
Irisys	San Diego, CA	(858) 623–1520	www.irisys.com	X	X	Liquid-filled capsules, peptides, organics, formulation
Kendle Intl. Inc.	Cincinnati, OH	(513) 381–5550	www.kendle.com		X	Software, validation, project management
LabCorp	Burlington, NC	(336) 538–6595	www.labcorp.com	X	X	Phase I-III, DNA testing
Lancaster Labs	Lancaster, PA	(717) 656–2300	www.lancasterlabs.com	X	X	Stability, validation, microbiology, cell bank
Lyne Labs	Brockton, MA	(800) 525–0450	www.lyne.com	X		Manufacturing, stability, packaging
Magellan Labs	RTP, NC	(919) 481–4855	www.magellanlabs.com	X	X	Stability, validation
Maxxam Analytics Inc.	Mississauga, ON	(866) 611–1118	www.maxxam.ca	X	X	Method development
McKesson Bioservices	Rockville, MD	(888) 4-MBS-BIO	www.mckesson.com	X		Clinical management, package, label, store

	Location	Phone	Website		Biomarkers	Management
MDS (parent: Nordion)	Quebec, Canada	(613) 592–2790	www.mdsps.com	X	X	
Medtox Laboratories Inc.	St. Paul, MN	(800) 832–3244	www.medtox.com	X	X	Biomarkers
Metrics, Inc.	Greenville, NC	(252) 752–3800	www.metricsinc.com	X		Validation, stability, manufacturing, formulation
Microbac Laboratories	Pittsburgh, PA	(412) 459–1060	www.microbac.com www.southerntesting.com	X		Method development, specification, stability
Micron Tech	Exton, PA	(610) 425–5100	www.microntech.com	X		Validation, stability
Midwest Research Institute	Kansas City, MO	(816) 753–7600	www.mriresearch.org	X	X	Method validation, pharmacokinetics
MiKart	Atlanta, GA	(404) 351–4510	www.mikart.com	X		Validation, stability, package, formulation
MPI Research	Mattawan, MI	(269) 668–3336	www.mpiresearch.com	X	X	Toxicology testing, formulation
Nucro Technics	Scarborough, Ontario	(416) 438–6727	www.nucro.com	X	X	Method validation, stability
OSG Norwich	Norwich, NY	(888) 674–7979	www.norwichpharma.com	X	X	Manufacturing, package, QC, validation
Patheon	RTP, NC	(919) 226–3200	www.patheon.com	X	X	Manufacturing, method development, validation
Pharma Medica	Mississauga, Ontario	(905) 624–9115 (888) PHARMA1	www.pharmamedica.com	X	X	Phase II, III, IV, development, validation
Pharmatek	San Diego, CA	(858) 350–8789	www.pharmatek.com	X	X	Formulation, manufacturing, stability
Pion	Woburn, MA	(781) 935–8939	www.pion-inc.com	X		Permeability
Pisgah Labs Inc.	Pisgah Forest, NC	(828) 884–2789	www.pisgahlabs.com	X		Validation, manufacturing

(continued)

Vendor	Location	Phone #	Website	Analytical	Bioanalytical	Additional services
PPD, Inc.	Wilmington, NC	(910) 251–0081	www.ppdi.com	X	X	Phase I–III, pharmacokinetics
Product Safety Labs	Dayton, NJ	(732) 438–5100	www.productsafetylabs.com	X	X	Method development, toxicology lab
QTI	Whitehouse, NJ	(908) 534–1054	www.QTIonline.com	X	X	Validation, stability, extractables/leachables
Quality Chemical Laboratories	Wilmington, NC	(910) 796–3441	www.qualitychemlabs.com	X		Development, validation, stability, microbiology, metals testing
Quest Pharmaceutical Services, L.L.C.	Newark, DE	(800) 237–1970	www.qps-usa.com	X	X	Validation, phase I–II, pharmacokinetics
Quintiles	RTP, NC	(919) 998–2000	www.quintiles.com	X	X	Package, manufacturing, phase I–III
Ricerca	Concord, OH	(888) 763–4797	www.ricerca.com	X	X	Development, manufacturing
RTI	RTP, NC	(919) 541–6000	www.rti.org	X	X	Pharmacokinetics, biostatistics
Sequani	Ledbury, United Kingdom	+44 (0) 1531 634121	www.sequani.com	X	X	Program management, toxicology lab, pharmacokinetics
SGS	Rutherford, NJ	(877) 677–2667	www.sgs.com	X	X	Toxicology lab, phases I–III
Siegfried	Zofingen, Switzerland	+41 62 746 1212	www.siegfried.ch	X		Development, manufacturing
SL Pharma Labs	Wilmington, DE	(302) 636–0202	www.slpharmalabs.com	X		Method validation, stability, development, microbiology
SNBL USA Ltd.	Everett, WA	(425) 407–0121	www.snblusa.com	X	X	Toxicology lab, pathology

Lab	Location	Phone	Website			Services
Source Precision Medicine	Boulder, CO	(303) 385-2700	www.sourcemdx.com		X	Genomics outsourcing
Southern Research Institute	Birmingham, AL	(800) 967-6774	www.southernresearch.com	X	X	Cancer, phases II–III, medicinal chemistry
SRI International	Menlo Park, CA	(650) 859-2000	www.sri.com	X		QC, QA
Stiefel Laboratories	RTP, NC	(888) STIEFEL	www.stiefel.com	X	X	Topicals
Stillmeadow Incorporated	Sugar Land, TX	(281) 240-8828	www.stillmeadow.com	X	X	Inhalation, stability, pharmacokinetics, radio-tracing
STS duoTEK, Inc.	Rush, NY	(800) 836-4850	www.stsduotek.com	X		Stability, microbiology, package
Syngenta Central Tox. Labs.	UK	(302) 425-2000 (parent corp.)	www2.syngenta.com (parent)	X	X	Toxicology lab
TNO Pharma	Netherlands	+31 88 866 00 00 (parent corp.)	www..tno.nl (parent)	X		Toxicology lab
Toxicology Research Laboratory	Chicago, IL	(312) 996-9185	www.uic.edu/labs/tox/trlt.html	X	X	Toxicology lab
U. Pharmaceuticals of Maryland, Inc.	St. Baltimore, MD	(410) 843-3700	www.upm-inc.com	X		Formulation, manufacturing
Viromed Laboratories	Minnetonka, MN	(952) 563-3300	www.viromed.com	X	X	IVF testing, tissue (donor) testing
West Pharmaceutical Service	Lionville, PA	(800) 345-9800	www.westpharma.com	X		Device components, packaging, extractables/ leachables

Appendix E: GMP Contract Facilities

© Springer Nature Switzerland AG 2020
S. C. Gad et al., *Contract Research and Development Organizations-Their History, Selection, and Utilization*, https://doi.org/10.1007/978-3-030-43073-3

Vendor	Location	Phone #	Website	CGMP synthesis	Synthesis of radiolabeled Compound	Biologic product manufacture	Additional services
ABC Laboratories	Columbia, MD	(888) 222–4431	www.abclabs.com	X	X		Manufacture, stability, analytical, extractable, leachable
Accucaps	Ontario, Canada	(800) 665–7210	www.accucaps.com	X			Validation, development, gelatin, capsules
Akorn	Lake Forest, IL	(800) 932–5676 x6165	www.akorn.com	X			Solutions, sterile fill, injectables, controlled substance
Aptuit	Multiple	(816) 767–3900	www.aptuit.com	X	X		Discovery, analytical
American Radiolabeled Chemicals	St. Louis, MO	(314) 991–4545	www.arc-inc.com		X		
Boehringer Ingelheim	Germany	+49 6132-77-0	www.boehringer-ingelheim.com	X		X	Validation, formulations, Microsystems
Cambrex Bio Science	Charles City, IA	866–286-9133	www.bscp.com	X			Development, QC, QA, validation
Cangene Corp.	Ontario, Canada	(416) 675–8290	www.cangene.com	X			Label & packaging, fermentation, purification, formulation, filling and lyophilization
Chromos Molecular Systems Inc.	Burnaby, BC, Canada	(604) 415–7100	www.chromos.com			X	

Company	Location	Phone	Website				Services
CPL	Ontario, Canada	(905) 821-7600	www.cplltd.com	X			Oral and topical, package, manufacture
Dalton Chemical Laboratories Inc.	Toronto, Canada	(416) 661-2102	www.dalton.com		X`		Peptide synthesis, analytical, formulation development, aseptic filling
Doosan Serdary Research Labs	Ontario, Canada	(416) 742-0774		X			Excipients, manufacture
Dow Chemical	Midland, MI Smithfield, RI	(800) 304-1488	www.dow.com	X	X		Method validation, stability
DSM Pharmaceutical Products	Parsippany, NJ	(973) 257-8011 (973) 257-8220 (Biologics)	www.dsmcatalytica-pharm.com	X	X		Develop, manufacturing
Formatech	Andover, MA	(877) 853-5397	www.formatech.com	X			
Gelda Scientific & Indust. Dev. Corp.	Mississauga, Ontario, Canada	(905) 673-9320	www.gelda.com	X			Manufacture
Genzyme	Cambridge, MA	(617) 252-7500	www.genzyme.com/pharmaceuticals	X			
Girindus	Cincinnati, OH	(513) 679-3000	www.girindus.com	X		X	QA, QA, radiochemistry
Glatt Pharmaceuticals Services	Binzen, Germany Ramsey, NJ	07621-664 319 (201) 825-8700	www.glattpharmaceuticals.com	X			Validation
HyClone	Logan, UT	(800) 492-5663	www.hyclone.com	X			Liquids, package

(continued)

Vendor	Location	Phone #	Website	CGMP synthesis	Synthesis of radiolabeled Compound	Biologic product manufacture	Additional services
Lyne Labs	Brockton, MA	(800) 525–0450	www.lyne.com	X			Manufacture, stability, package
Magellan Labs	RTP, NC	(919) 481–4855	www.magellanlabs.com	X			Stability, validation
Medicago Inc.	Quebec, Canada	(418) 658–9393	www.medicago.com	X		X	Plant growth, manipulation, product recovery and purification
MediChem	Barcelona, Spain	+34 93 477 64 40	www.medichem.com	X			
Microbix Biosystems Inc.	Toronto, Ontario, Canada	(416) 234–1624	www.microbix.com	X		X	Develop, project management
Midwest Research Institute	Kansas City, MO	(816) 753–7600	www.mriresearch.org	X	X		Method validation
National Cancer Institute	Bethesda, MD	(800) 4-CANCER	www.nci.nih.gov		X		
Nucro Technics	Scarborough, Ontario, Canada	(416) 438–6727	www.nucro.com	X			Phase II, III, IV, method validation
OctoPlus	Netherlands	+31 (0)71524 40 44	www.octoplus.nl	X			QC
Norwich Pharmaceuticals	Norwich, NY	(607) 335–3100	www.norwichpharma.com	X			Manufacture, package, QV,QC, validation

Facility	Location	Phone	Website			Services
Pisgah Labs Inc.	Pisgah Forest, NC	(828) 884–2789	www.pisgahlabs.com	X		Validation, manufacture
PPD, Inc.	Austin, TX	(512) 581–9156	www.ppdi.com	X		QA, QC, pharmacokinetics
Quality Chemical Laboratories	Wilmington, NC	(910) 796–3441	www.qualitychemlabs.com	X		Development, validation, stability
RTI International	Research Triangle Park, NC	(919) 485–2666	www.rti.org		X	Radiochemistry, pharmacokinetics/toxicokinetics
Sequani	United Kingdom	+44 (0) 1531 634121	www.sequani.com	X		QA, program management
SGS Group	Switzerland	+41 22 739 91 11	www.pharmardqc.sgs.com	X		
Sigma-Aldrich	St. Louis, MO	(800) 336–9719	www.sigma-aldrich.com/safe	X		Manufacture
Southern Research Institute	Birmingham, AL	(888) 322–1166	www.southernresearch.com	X		Cancer, phase II,III
U. of Iowa Div. Of Pharm. Science	Iowa City, IA	(319) 335–8674	www.pharmacy.uiowa.edu/uip/index.html	X		Method validation
Univ. of Rhode Island	Kingston, RI	(401) 874–5842	www.uri.edu/pharmacy/		X	
Viromed Laboratories	Minnetonka, MN	(952) 563–3300	www.viromed.com	X		QA
Viron Therapeutics Inc.	Ontario, Canada	(519) 858–5109	www.vironinc.com		X	

(continued)

Vendor	Location	Phone #	Website	CGMP synthesis	Synthesis of radiolabeled Compound	Biologic product manufacture	Additional services
Yale Pharmaceutical Research Institute	Bethesda, MD	(301) 571–2388	www.yalepharma.com		X		QA, QC, development
National Cancer Institute	Bethesda, MD	(800) 4-CANCER	www.nci.nih.gov		X		
Neurochem Inc.	Quebec, Canada	(514) 337–4646	www.neurochem.com			X	
NeuroMed Technologies Inc.	Vancouver, Canada	(604) 822–9970	www.neuromedtech.com			X	
New Life Resources	Northvale, NJ	(201) 750–7880	www.newliferecources.net	X			Manufacture, hard-gel caps
Nexia Biotechnologies Inc.	Quebec, Canada	(450) 424–3067	www.nexiabiotech.com			X	
Northview Biosciences	Spartanburg, SC; Northbrook, IL; Berkeley, CA	(864) 574–7728; (847) 564–8181; (510) 548–8440	www.northviewlabs.com	X			Biocompatibility, validation
Nucro Technics	Scarborough, Ontario	(416) 438–6727	www.nucro.com	X			Phase II,III,IV, method validation

					QC
OctoPlus	Netherlands	+31 (71) 524 40 44	www.octoplus.nl	X	
Oncolytics Biotech Inc.	Calgary, Canada	(403) 670–7377	www.onloyticsbiotech.com		X
OSG Norwich	Norwich, NY	(607) 335–3000	www.norwichpharma.com	X	Manufacture, package, QV,QC, validation
Pharm Eco	North Andover, MA	(978) 784–5000	www.pharmeco.com	X	Manufacture, development
Pharmacor Inc.	Quebec, Canada	(450) 973–1710	www.pharmacor.com		X
Pisgah Labs Inc.	Pisgah Forest, NC	(828) 884–2789	www.pisgahlabs.com	X	Validation, manufacture
PPD, Inc.	Austin, TX	(512) 5819156	www.ppdi.com	X	QA, QC, pharmacokinetics
Quality Chemical Laboratories	Wilmington, NC	(910) 796–3441	www.qualitychemlabs.com	X	Development, validation, stability
RTI International	RTP, NC	(919) 485–2666	www.rti.org	X	Radiochemistry, pharmacokinetics/toxicokinetics
RusGen	Moscow, Russia	007-095–253-92-36	www.rusgen.com	X	
Sequani	United Kingdom	+44 (0) 1531 634 121	www.sequani.com	X	QA, program management

(continued)

Vendor	Location	Phone #	Website	CGMP synthesis	Synthesis of radiolabeled Compound	Biologic product manufacture	Additional services
Siegfried Actives	Pennsville, NJ Switzerland	(877) 763–8630 +44 62 746 1212	www.siegfried.ch	X			QC, QA
Siegfried Exclusives	Pennsville, NJ Switzerland	(856) 678–3601 +41 62 746 1221	www.siegfried.ch	X			Storage, QC, QA
Siegfried Ventures	San Diego, CA Pennsville, NJ Switzerland	(858) 546–4346 (856) 678–3809 +41 62 746 1111	www.siegfried.ch	X			QC, QA
Sigma-Aldrich	St. Louis, MO	(800) 336–9719	www.sigma-aldrich.com/safe	X			Manufacture
Southern Research Institute	Birmingham, AL	(888) 322–1166 (205) 322–7472	www.southernresearch.com	X			Cancer, phases II, III
Stiefel Research Institute	Oak Hill, NY	(800) 633–7647	www.stiefelresearch.com	X			Topicals, development, validation
U. of Iowa Div. Of Pharm. Science	Iowa City, IA	(319) 335–8674 (319) 335–4096	www.uiowa.edu/~pharmaser www.uiowa.edu/~cadd	X			Method validation
Univ. of Rhode Island	Kingston, RI	(401) 874–5842	http://www.uri.edu/pharmacy/		X		

							QA
Viromed Laboratories	Minneapolis, MN St. Paul, MN Marietta, GA Camden, NJ	(800) 582–0077 (800) 582–0077 (888) 847–6633 (800) 622–8820	www.viromed.com	X			
Viron Therapeutics Inc.	Ontario, Canada	(519) 858–5109	www.vironinc.com		X		Validation
Vital Pharma Inc.	Riviera Beach, Florida	(561) 844–3221	www.vitalpharma. com	X			
Yale Pharmaceutical Research Institute	New Haven, CT	(301) 571–2388	http://www. yalepharma.com/ ADME.htm			X	QA, QC, development

Appendix F: Formulation

© Springer Nature Switzerland AG 2020
S. C. Gad et al., *Contract Research and Development Organizations-Their History, Selection, and Utilization*, https://doi.org/10.1007/978-3-030-43073-3

Vendor	Location	Phone #	Website	Formulation	Additional services
Alcami	4620 Creekstone Drive, Durham NC 27703	(800) 575–4224 info@alcaminow.com	www.alcaminow.com	X	Method validation, project management, packaging, manufacturing, delivery, phases II, III, and IV
Akorn	1925 West Field Court, Suite 300, Lake Forest, IL 60045	(800) 932–5676	www.akorn.com	X	Solutions, ophthalmic, ointments, delivery, manufacture
Astellas	2-5-1, Nihonbashi-Honcho, Chuo-Ku, Tokyo 103–8411, Japan	+81-3-3244-3000	www.astellas.com	X	Manufacture, validation, stability, solid dose
Avecia Pharma Services	10 Vanderbilt Irvine, CA 92618	(877) 445–6554	www.aveciapharma.com	X	Validation, inhalation, QC, environmental, analytical chemistry, development, biopharmaceuticals, stability, manufacturing
BASi	2701 Kent Ave W. Lafayette, IN47906	(800) 845–4246 (765) 463–4527	www.basinc.com	X	Method validation
Baxter BioPharma Solutions	One Baxter Parkway, DF4-3 W Deerfield, IL 60015	(800) 422–9837 (224) 948–1812	www.baxterbiopharmasolutions.com	X	Stability, packaging, manufacturing, solutions, drug delivery, irrigation products
Boston Analytical Inc.	14 Manor Parkway Salem, NH 03079	(603) 893–3758	www.bostonanalytical.com	X	Method validation, stability
Cardinal Health	7000 Cardinal Place, Dublin, OH 43017	(614) 757–5000	www.cardinalhealth.com	X	Development, publishing, compliance, manufacturing, training, Stable, validation

					QC, QA, validation
Cambrex Corporation	East Rutherford, NJ	(866) 286–9133	www.cambrex.com	X	
Catalent Consumer Health	720 Wright Street Strathroy, Ontario N7G 3H8	(888) 689–9794	www.consumerhealth. catalent.com	X	Validation, OTC, health and nutritionals, Pharma chem., small peptides, GMP manufacturing, stability, preformulation, cytotoxic/ high-potency
Charles River Laboratories	Wilmington, MA	(877) 274–8371	www.criver.com	X	Manufacture, Method validation, stability, safety, efficacy, rapid detection, analytical, microbiological, QA
CMC pharma	7100 Euclid Ave Suite 152 Cleveland OH 44103	216–505-9632	www.cmcpharm.com		
CPL	7600 Danbro Crescent, Mississauga, Ontario, L5N 6 L6, Canada	(905) 821–7600	www.cplltd.com	X	Oral and topical, package, manufacture
CPTC (Consumer Product Testing Company)	70 New Dutch Ln Fairfield, NJ 07004	(973) 828–8137	www.cptclabs.com	X	Method validation, stability, product testing
Dow Chemical	2211 H.H. Dow Way Midland, MI 48674	(989)636–1000	www.dow.com	X	Excipients, manufacture
DPT	318 McCullough San Antonio, TX 78215	(866) 225–5378	www.dptlabs.com	X	Management, production, compounding, package, manufacturing, semi-solids, liquids

(continued)

Vendor	Location	Phone #	Website	Formulation	Additional services
DSM Dyneema	5750 Greenville Blvd. DE Greenville, NC 27834	(252) 707–2547	www.dsm.com	X	Method validation, stability
Elite Pharmaceuticals Inc.	165 Ludlow Ave. Northvale, NJ 07647	(201) 750–2646	www.elitepharma.com	X	Manufacture
Emergent Biosolutions	155 Innovation Drive Winnipeg, MB, CA R3T 5Y3	(204) 275–4200	www.emergentbiosolutions.com	X	Label and packaging, manufacturing, bio defense, donor programs
Ferro	6060 Parkland Boulevard Suite 250 Mayfield Heights, OH 44124	(216) 875–5600	www.ferro.com	X	Manufacture, method validation
Fujifilm (Diosynth Biotechnologies)	101 J Morris Commons Lane, Morrisville, NC 27560	(919) 337–4400	www.fujifilmdiosynth.com	X	Manufacture, method validation, microbial, preformulation studies
GEA	9165 Rumsey Rd. Columbia, MD 21045	(844) 432–2329	https://www.gea.com/en	X	Chemical, evaporator, pharma systems, liquids
GSK	5 Crescent Drive Philadelphia, PA 19112	888–825–5249	www.gsk.com	X	Topicals, development, validation, dermatology
Glatt	20 Spear Road Ramsey, NJ 07446	(201) 825–8700	www.glatt.com	X	Validation, manufacturing

IQVIA	International RTP, NC	(866) 267–447	www.iqvia.com	X	Package, manufacture, phase I-IV, biopharmaceuticals, devices, MBDD, ECG
Irisys	6828 Nancy Ridge Drive, San Diego, CA 92121	(858) 623–1520	www.irisys.com	X	Liquid-filled capsules, peptides, proternal, organics, manufacturing
Laureate Pharma	201 college road East Princeton, NJ 08540	(608) 920–4400	www.laureatepharma.com	X	QC, package, development, aseptic fill, preclinical production
Lubrizol Life Science	3894 Courtney St. Bethlehem, PA 18017–8920	610–861-4701	https://lubrizolcdmo.com/	X	(Formerly particle services)
Lyne Labs	10 Burke Drive Brockton, MA 02301	(800) 525–0450	www.lyne.com	X	Manufacture, stability, package, validation, formulations
MERCK	2000 Galloping Hill Road, Kenilworth, NJ 07033	(908) 740–4000 (908) 423–1000	www.merck.com	X	Stability, scale-up, vaccines, discovery, development
Meridian Medical Technologies	6350 Stevens Forest Rd., Suite 301 Columbia, MD 21046	(443) 259–7800	www.meridianmeds.com	X	Package
Metrics Contract Services	1240 Sugg Parkway, Greenville, NC 27834	(252) 752–3800	www. metricscontractservices. com	X	Validation, storage
Midwest Research Institute	425 Volker Boulevard Kansas City, MO 64110	(816) 753–7600	www.mriglobal.org	X	Method validation, GMP/GLP Bioanalytical services

(continued)

Vendor	Location	Phone #	Website	Formulation	Additional services
MiKart	1750 Chattahoochee Ave. NW, Atlanta, GA 30318	(888) 4MIKART (404) 351–4510	www.mikart.com	X	Validation, stability, package, manufacturing, product development
Millipore Sigma	International	(800)325–3010	www.sigmaaldrich.com	X	Cell and gene bases therapeutics and vaccines, scale-up, supply chain, analytical testing, cell engineering, manufacturing, biopharmaceuticals, diagnostics
Motega Health	Topeka, KS	(785)371–2287	https://motegahealth.com/	X	Solid sustained release, liquid, injectable, nutritional, health and beauty
OctoPlus	B.V. Zermikedreef 12, 2333 CL Leiden. The Netherlands	+31 (0) 71524 40 44	www.octoplus.nl/nl/home	X	QC, delivery, ophthalmic, clinical trials
Pall Corporation	25 Harbor Park Dr. Port Washington, NY	(516) 484–3600	www.pall.com	X	Validation, liquids, biochemistry, capsules, iv, and solutions
Patheon	4815 Emperor Blvd Durham, NC 27703–8580	(919)226–3200	www.patheon.com	X	Manufacture, dosage from development and manufacturing services, pharma and biotech, packaging
Pfizer	New York, NY	(212)733–2323	www.pfizer.com	X	Packaging, liquid and topical, manufacturing
Pharmaceutics International, Inc.	10 819 Gilroy Rd. Hunt Valley, MD	(410) 584–0001	www.pharm-int.com	X	Packaging, project management, stability, CTM, formulation, manufacturing

Proclinical Consulting	Eldon House 2–3 Eldon St. London EC2M 7LS, UK	+44–207–437–6824	www.proclinical.com	X	Packaging, stability, global clinical support
Sanofi Genzyme	Bridgewater, NJ	(800) 981–2491	https://www.sanofi.us/	X	Manufacture, lipids, amino acid derivatives, custom peptides
Southern Research Institute	757 Tom Martin Drive Birmingham, AL 35211	(800) 967–6774	www.southernresearch.org	X	Cancer, phase II, phase III, immunology, ADME, PK, pathology, bioanalytical
SRI International	333 Ravenswood Ave., Menlo Park, CA 94025–3493	(650) 859–2000	www.sri.com	X	Pharmacokinetics, QC, QA
University of Iowa Pharmaceuticals.	115 South Grand Ave, G-20 Iowa City, IA 52242	(319) 335–8674	https://uip.pharmacy.uiowa.edu/	X	Method, validation, formulation, SA
UPM Pharmaceuticals	501 fifth St. Bristol, TN 37620	(423) 989–8000	www.upm-inc.com	X	SUPAC Guidance, Training, formulation, manufacturing

Appendix G: Dosage Forms

Vendor	Location	Phone #	Website	CTM	Label	Additional services
Akorn	Lake Forest, IL	(800) 932–5676	www.akorn.com	X		Solutions, ointments, delivery, manufacture
ARC Biopharmaceutical Research Inc.	St. Louis, MO	(314) 991–4545	www.arc-inc.com		X	
	Vancouver, Canada	(604) 432–9237	www.bripharm.com		X	Stability, QA, QC
Cangene Corp.	Winnipeg, Canada	(204) 275–4200	www.cangene.com		X	
CATO Research	Durham, NC	(919) 361-CATO	www.cato.com		X	Packaging
Chem Syn	Lenexa, KY	(800) 233–6643	www.chemsyn.com	X	X	
Dow Pharma	Petaluma, CA	(707) 793–2600	www.dowpharm.com		X	Process, method validation
DSM Catalytica Pharmaceutical	Parsippany, NJ	(973) 257–8011	www.dsmcatalytica-pharm.com	X		Method validation, stability
Elite Pharma	Northvale, NJ	(201) 750–2646	www.elitepharma.com	X		
EMMCORP	Hempstead, NY	(800) 835–2393	www.easternmarking.com		X	Manufacture
FLEXcon	Spencer, MA	(508) 885–8200	www.flexcon.com			
Formatech	Andover, MA	(877) 853-KEYS	www.formatech.com	X	X	Development, manufacture
Girindus	Cincinnati, OH	(513) 679–3000	www.girindus.com	X		Project management
Glatt Contract Services	Ramsey, NJ	(201) 825–8700	www.glattair.com	X		Validation
Hollister-Stier	Spokane, WA	(509) 489–5656	www.hollister-stier.com	X	X	Package, project management, validation
Irisys	San Diego, CA	(858) 623–1520	www.irisys.com	X		Liquid-filled capsules, peptides, proternal, organics
Lyne Labs	Brockton, MA	(800) 525–0450	www.lyne.com	X		Manufacture, stability, package

Magellan Laboratories	RTP, NC Somerset, NJ San Diego, CA Albuquerque, NM	(919) 481–4855 (732) 302–1400 (858) 547–7800 (815) 338–9500	www.magellanlabs. com	X	X	Stability, validation
Meridian Medical Technologies	Columbia, MD	(410) 309–6830	www.meridianmeds. com	X		Package
Metrics, Inc.	Greenville, NC	(252) 752–3800	www.metricsinc.com	X		Validation, storage
Midwest Research Institute	Kansas City, MO	(816) 753–7600	www.mriresearch.org		X	Method validation
MiKart	Atlanta, GA	(404) 351–4510	www.mikart.com	X		Validation, stability, package, manufacture
Mova	Caguas, Puerto Rico	(800) 468–5201	www.movapharm.com	X		Manufacture, package
OSG Norwich	Norwich, NY	(607) 335–3000	www.norwichpharma. com	X		Manufacture, package, QV, QC, validation
Paragon Data Systems, Inc.	Cleveland, OH	(800) 211–0768	www. paragondatasystem. com		X	
Patheon	Ontario, Canada	(888) PATHEON	www.patheon.com	X		Manufacture, many dosage forms
PCI Services	Philadelphia, PA	(215) 637–8100	www.pciservices.com	X		Manufacture, package, validation
Pharmaceutical Research Company, Inc.	Exton, PA	(484) 875–9000	www. pharmaceuticalrc.com		X	
Pharmatek	San Diego, CA	(858) 350–8789	www.pharmatek.com	X		Pharma chem., small peptides
PPD, Inc.	Austin, TX	(512) 5819156	www.ppdi.com	X		QA, QC, pharmacokinetics

(continued)

Vendor	Location	Phone #	Website	CTM	Label	Additionalservices
Quadrel Labeling Systems	Mentor, OH	(440) 602–4700	www.quadrel.com		X	
Quintiles	Kansas City, MO	(816) 767–3900	www.quintiles.com	X		Package, manufacture
	RTP, NC	(877) 988–2100				
RCC	Switzerland	+41 61 975 11 11	www.rcc.ch	X		
Ricerca	Concord, OH	(888) 742–3722	www.ricerca.com	X		Inhalation, phases II, III
SAFC	San Diego, CA	(858) 523–9544	www.molecularmed.com	X	X	
Schwarz	Seymour, IN	(812) 523–5490	www.schwarzusa.com	X		Cell and gene bases therapeutics and vaccines, scale-up, manufacturing
Siegfried Exclusives	Pennsville, NJ	(856) 678–3601	www.siegfried.ch	X		Manufacture, package, support, method
	Switzerland	+41 62 746 1221				Storage, QC, QA
Southern Research Institute	Birmingham, AL	(800) 967–6774	www.southernresearch.com	X		Cancer, phases II, III
		(205) 581–2000				
SRI International	Menlo Park, CA	(650) 859–2000	www.sri.com	X		Pharmacokinetics, QC, QA
Star Labeling Products	Fairless Hills, PA	(800) 394–6900	www.starlabel.com		X	
Stiefel Research Institute	Oak Hill, NY	(800) 633–7647	www.stiefelresearch.com	X		Topicals, development, validation
Tapecon	Buffalo, NY	(215) 295–3340	www.tapecon.com		X	
		(800) 333–2407				
Taro	Hawthorne, NY	(800) 544–1449	www.tarousa.com		X	
Toxcon	Edmonton, Can.	(780) 435–9028	www.toxcon.com	X		Risk assessment
U. of Iowa Div. Of Pharm. Science	Iowa City, IA	(319) 335–8674	www.uiowa.edu/~cadd	X		Method validation
U. Pharmaceuticals of Maryland, Inc.	St. Baltimore, MD	(410) 843–3700	www.upm-inc.com	X		SUPAC Guidance, training

Appendix H: Clinical Testing

© Springer Nature Switzerland AG 2020
S. C. Gad et al., *Contract Research and Development Organizations-Their History, Selection, and Utilization*, https://doi.org/10.1007/978-3-030-43073-3

Vendor	Location	Phone #	Website	Clinical support	Phase I clinical	Clinical trial management	Clinical Statistics	Additional services
AACT	Camperdown, Australia	+61 2 9993 4523	www.academicalliance.com		X	X	X	Project management, electronic data capture, phases II–III
ABT Associates	Cambridge, MA	(617) 492–7100	www.abtassociates.com		X		X	Project management
ACE Pharmaceuticals	The Netherlands	+31 (0) 365227201	www.acepharmaceuticals.nl		X			Manufacturing, packaging
ACM Medical Lab	Rochester, NY	(800) 525–5227	www.acmgloballab.com	X	X	X		Phases II–IV, data management
Advanced Clinical Research	Salt Lake City, UT	(801) 355–4126	www.acr-research.com			X		
Advanced Clinical Services	Chicago, IL	(847) 267–1176	www.advancedclinical.com	X			X	Validation, programming, data management
Algorithme Pharma	Laval, Quebec	**(450) 973–6077**	www.algopharm.com		X			Phases I–IV, regulatory
Alquest	Minneapolis, MN	(763) 287–3830	www.alquest.com			X	X	Medical devices, data management
Aptuit	Greenwich, CT	(816) 767–3900	www.aptuit.com	X	X			Manufacturing, packaging
Arkios	Virginia Beach, VA	(757) 631–2114	www.arkios.com		X		X	Data management

Company	Location	Phone	Website				Services
ARUP Labs	Salt Lake City, UT	(800) 242–2787	www.arup-lab.com		X		
Barton and Polansky Associates, Inc.	New York, NY	(212) 759–6341	www.bpa-mcs.com	X			
BDH Clinical Research Services	Durham, NC	(919) 477–9542	www.bdhclinical.com		X		QA
Beardsworth Consulting Group, Inc.	Flemington, NJ	(800) 788–6046	www.beardsworth.com		X		QA, phase IV, development
BioClin Health Research, Inc.	British Columbia, Canada	(604) 276–2580	www.bioclin.ca		X	X	Phase II–IV
Biostat International, Inc.	Tampa, FL	(813) 979–1619	www.biostatinc.com	X	X		SAS, validation, data management
Biotechnical Services, Inc.	North Little Rock, AR	(501) 758–6290	www.biotechnicalservices.com	X	X		Validation, data management, QA/QC
CAP Trials	Framingham, MA	(508) 620–2700	www.captrials.com		X		Training, educational materials
Cardinal Systems	Paris, France	+33 1 40 21 19 00	www.cardinal-sys.com	X	X		eCTD
Carolinas Research Associates	Charlotte, NC	(704) 503–3216	www.carolinasresearch.com	X	X		Phase II–IV
CATO	Durham, NC	(919) 361-CATO	www.cato.com	X	X		Phases II–IV, monitoring, regulatory

(continued)

Vendor	Location	Phone #	Website	Clinical support	Phase I clinical	Clinical trial management	Clinical Statistics	Additional services
Cenetron	Austin, TX	(888) 834–6632	www.cenetron.com	X				Trial supplies
Certus International, Inc.	Bedford, NH	(512) 439–2000 (603) 472–8400	www.certusintl.com			X	X	Project management, imaging, monitoring
Chiltern International	Berkshire, United Kingdom	+44 (0)1753 512 000	www.chiltern.com		X	X	X	Phases II–IV, regulatory filings
Cirion	Laval, Quebec	(450) 682–2231	www.cirion.ca	X				Biologics, immunology, microbiology
Clinical R&D Services	Wayne, NJ	(973) 696–0824	www.clinicalrdservices.com		X			Phases II–IV
Clinical Research Consulting, Inc.	Boston, MA	(508) 865–8907	www.eclinicalresearchconsulting.com			X		Project management, monitoring
Clinical Trial Management Services, Inc.	Bristol, TN	(800) 422–3596	www.ctmsinc.com			X	X	QA
ClinSmart	Langhorne, PA	(215) 710–3200	www.clinsmart.com				X	
ClinStat Consulting	Cardiff by the Sea, CA	(760) 207–5260	www.clinstatconsulting.com			X		Project management

Name	Location	Phone	Website					Services
Covance	Princeton, NJ	(888) COVANCE	www.covance.com		X	X	X	Stability, clinical design and management, consulting
CPT Co.	Fairfield, NJ	(973) 808–7111	www.cptclabs.com		X		X	Method validation. Stability, analytical
CRL	Lenexa, KS	(800) 445–6917	www.crlcorp.com	X				Bioanalytical, data management
DATAMAP GmbH	Freiburg, Germany	+49 (761) 4 52 08–0	www.datamap.de	X			X	Programming, data management
DP Clinical	Rockville, MD	(301) 294–6226	www.dpclinical.com			X	X	Data management, regulatory, QA
DPT	San Antonio, TX	(866) CALL DPT	www.dptlabs.com			X	X	Analytical, clinical trial material
Ecron Acunova	Princeton, NJ	(973) 396–2742	www.ecronacunova.com	X	X	X	X	Phases II–IV
Emissary	Austin, TX	(512) 918–1992	www.sendemissary.com			X	X	QA, electronic data capture, regulatory
Emphusion	San Francisco, CA	(415) 776–0660	home.pdd.net		X	X		Statistics
EPS Company, Ltd.	Tokyo, Japan	+81-3-5804–7577	www.eps.co.jp				X	Programming, QA, data management
Esoterix Inc	Cranford, NJ	(877) 788–8861	www.esoterix.com	X			X	Project management
Frontage	Exton, PA	(610) 232–0100	www.frontagelab.com	X			X	Regulatory, pharmacokinetics
Genzyme	Cambridge, MA	(617) 252–7500	www.genzyme.com	X	X	X	X	Phases II–IV
Global Pharma Alliance	Bridgewater, NJ	(908) 672–3686	globalpharmalliance.com	X	X			Project management

(continued)

Vendor	Location	Phone #	Website	Clinical support	Phase I clinical	Clinical trial management	Clinical Statistics	Additional services
GNB Limited	UK	NA	www.gnblimited.co.uk				X	Validation, trial design
Grayline Clinical Drug Trials	Wichita Falls, TX	(800) 782–0895	www.graylinecdt.com		X	X		Phases II–IV
Gulf Coast Research Associates, Inc.	Baton Rouge, LA	(225) 757–1084	www.gulfcoastra.com		X			Phases II–IV
Health Decisions	Durham, NC	(888) 779–3771	www.healthdec.com		X	X	X	Project management, electronic data capture, phases II–IV
Health Research Associates, Inc.	Mountlake Terrace, WA	(425) 775–6565	www.hrainc.net				X	Consulting, project management
Healthcare Project Management (HPM)	Geneva, Switzerland	+41 22 596 44 44	www.hpmgeneva.com			X		
Huntingdon Life Sciences Group Plc	Cambridgeshire, United Kingdom	+44 (0) 1480 892 000	www.huntingdon.com		X			Phases II–III
ICON Clinical Research	Dublin, Ireland	+353 (1) 2912000	www.iconclinical.com	X	X	X	X	Project management, QA, phases II–IV
idv Data Analysis and Study Planning	Munich, Germany	+49 (89) 850 80 01	www.idvgauting.com				X	Programming, data management
Inc Research	Raleigh, NC	(919) 876–9300	www.incresearch.com	X	X		X	Data management, phases II–IV

Name	Location	Phone	Website				Services
Integrated Research, Inc.	Montreal, Canada	(514) 683–1909	www.iricanada.com			X	Regulatory, data management
International Drug Development Institute (IDDI)	Louvain-la-Neuve, Belgium	+32 (0)10 61 44 44	www.iddi.com		X	X	
inVentiv Clinical	Houston, TX	(281) 829–1110 (877) 559–6699	inventivclinical.com/solutions/cro-services/default.aspx		X	X	Software, validation, project management
Kendle Intl. Inc.	Cincinnati, OH	(800) 733–1572	www.kendle.com	X	X		Data management, randomization
Köhler GmbH, Dr. Manfred	Freiburg, Germany	+49 761 50318	www.koehler-freiburg.de		X	X	Phases II–IV
Lovelace Respiratory Research Institute	Albuquerque, NM	(505) 348–9400	www.lrri.org	X			
MAJARO InfoSystems, Inc.	San Jose, CA	(408) 330–9400	www.majaro.com			X	Data management, project management
Medfiles	Helsinki, Finland	+358 20 7446 840	www.medfiles.fi	X	X	X	Phase II-IV, regulatory
MediMentum ApS	Hilleroed, Denmark	+45 48 229 410	N/A			X	Consulting, programming
Medpace LLC	Cincinnati, OH	(513) 579–9911	www.medpace.com		X	X	Project management, regulatory QA/QC
Microbiotest Laboratories	Sterling, VA	(703) 925–0100	www.microbiotest.com	X			

(continued)

Vendor	Location	Phone #	Website	Clinical support	Phase I clinical	Clinical trial management	Clinical Statistics	Additional services
Micromedex	Greenwood Village, CO	(303) 486–6400	www.micromedex.com	X				Electronic data capture
Msource Medical Development	Kraainem, Belgium	+32–2-768.01.66	www.msource-cro.com	X	X	X	X	Project management, phases II–IV, QA/QC
NOCCR	New Orleans, LA	(504) 821-CARE	www.noccr.com		X			Phases II–IV
Northwest Kinetics, L.L.C.	Tacoma, WA	(253) 593–5304	www.nwkinetics.com		X			Phases I, II, pharmacokinetics, QA
Novella Clinical	Durham, NC	(919) 484–1921	www.novellaclinical.com			X		Staffing
Nth Analytics	Princeton, NJ	(908) 672–5649	www.nthanalytics.com				X	Validation, programming
Nucro Technics	Scarborough, Ontario	(416) 438–6727	www.nucro.com	X	X			Phases II–IV, method validation, QA
Omnicare Clinical Research	King of Prussia, PA	(800) 290–5766	www.omnicarecr.com			X	X	Project management, medical devices, Phases II–IV
Operatix Consulting Inc.	Waterdown, Ontario	(905) 690–1200	www.operatrix.com			X		Project management
P3 Research, Ltd.	Tauranga, New Zealand	+64 7 579 0453	www.p3research.co.nz		X			Phases II–IV
Paragon	Irvine, CA	(949) 224–2800	www.parabio.com				X	Programming, project management, QA, regulatory

Company	Location	Phone	Website					Services
PAREXEL Intl. Corp.	Boston, MA	(781) 487–9900	www.parexel.com	X	X	X	X	Phases II–IV, validation
Patheon	Mississauga, Ontario	(888) 728–4366	www.patheon.com	X			X	Packaging
Pierrel Research	Essen, Germany	+49 201 89900	www.pierrel-research.com		X	X	X	Data management, regulatory
Pharma Medica	Ontario, Canada	(905) 624–9115 (877) PHARMA1	www.pharmamedica.com	X	X	X	X	Phases II–IV, development, validation
PharmaNet	Princeton, NJ	(609) 9516800	www.pharmanet.com	X	X	X	X	Phases II–IV, medical devices
Phase Forward	Waltham, MA	(888) 703–1122	www.phaseforward.com	X		X		Data management
PPD, Inc.	Wilmington, NC	(910) 251–0081	www.ppd.com	X	X	X	X	QA, pharmacokinetics, phases II–IV
PRA International	Raleigh, NC	(919) 786–8200	www.prainternational.com		X	X	X	Phases II–IV, QA
PRACS	Fargo, ND	(701) 239–4750	www.pracs.com		X			Phases II–IV, bioanalytical
Premier Research	Philadelphia, PA	(215) 282–5500	www.premier-research.com		X		X	Data management, QA
Prologue Research	Columbus, OH	(614) 324–1500	www.procro.com		X		X	Programming, project management, development
PSI	Zug, Switzerland	+41 41 228 10 00	www.psi-cro.com		X		X	Phases I, II, III, development, consulting

(continued)

Vendor	Location	Phone #	Website	Clinical support	Phase I clinical	Clinical trial management	Clinical Statistics	Additional services
Research Dynamics Consulting Group, Ltd.	Pittsford, NY	(585) 381–1350	www.resdyncg.com			X		Consulting, monitoring
Research Pharmaceutical Services, Inc.	Fort Washington, PA	(215) 540–0700	www.rpsweb.com			X	X	Programming, project management, QA/QC
Rho, Inc.	Chapel Hill, NC	(919) 408–8000	www.rhoworld.com			X	X	Programming, randomization
SciAn Research Services	Toronto, Canada	(416) 231–8008	www.scian.com		X	X	X	Consulting
	King of Prussia, PA	(610) 945–1763						
	Walnut Creek, CA	(925) 407–2069						
Sequani	United Kingdom	+44 (0) 1531 634 121	www.sequani.com		X			QA, management
SGS Biopharma	Wavre, Belgium	(877) 677–2667	www.sgsbiopharma.com		X	X	X	QA/QC
Simbec	United Kingdom	+441 443 690 977	www.simbec.co.uk		X			Phases II, III, QA
SMO-USA, Inc.	Big Timber, MT	(406) 930–1970	www.smo-usa.com		X	X		Phases II–IV
Southern Research Institute	Birmingham, AL	(888) 322–1166	www.southernresearch.com		X			Cancer, phases II, III

Company	Location	Phone	Website				Programming
Statisticians WithOut Borders	Bahama, NC	(919) 477–4007	www.statisticinaswithout borders.com			X	Programming
Statking Consulting Inc.	Fairfield, OH	(513) 858–2989	www. statkingconsulting.com		X	X	Programming, development, randomization
Symbiance, Inc.	Princeton Junction, NJ	(609) 243–9050	www.symbiance.com		X	X	Programming, project management, development
SyMetric Sciences	Lery, Quebec, Canada	(450) 691–0183	www.symetric.ca		X	X	
Symfo	Boston, MA	(617) 577–9484	www.symfo.com	X	X	X	Project management, randomization
Synteract, Inc.	Carlsbad, CA	(760) 268–8200	www.synteract.com	X	X	X	Programming, project management, develop, randomization
Target Health Inc.	New York, NY	(212) 681–2100	www.targethealth.com			X	
Trial Form Support (TFS)	Lund, Switzerland	+46 46 280 18 00	www.trialformsupport. com	X	X	X	Phases II–IV
Trial Management Group, Inc.	Toronto, Canada	(416) 929–7717	www.tmginvestigators. com		X	X	Phases II–IV
U. of Iowa Div. Of Pharm.	Iowa City, IA	(319) 335–8674 (319) 335–4096	www.pharmacy.uiowa. edu/uip				Method validation
United Biosource	Chevy Chase, MD	(866) 458–1096	unitedbiosource.com	X		X	Phases IIIb–IV, health economics, project management

(continued)

Vendor	Location	Phone #	Website	Clinical support	Phase I clinical	Clinical trial management	Clinical Statistics	Additional services
Uppsala Monitoring Centre	Uppsala, Sweden	+46 1865 6060	www.who-umc.org				X	
Virtu Stat, Ltd.	North Wales, PA	(215) 699–2424	www.virtustat.com				X	Validation, programming, randomization, phase I through IV study design
Westat	Sarasota, FL	941–926-2922	www.westat.com					Consulting
West Pharmaceutical Service	Lionville, PA	(610) 594–2900	www.westpharma.com		X		X	Device and package components, drug-package, interactions
Worldwide Clinical Trials	King of Prussia, PA	(610) 964–2000	www.wwctrials.com	X	X	X		Phases II–IV

Appendix I: Genealogy of Contract Research Organizations (CROs)

Legend:

Gray = closed, absorbed , or acquired

White = active at time of publication

CROs displayed alphabetically by most current lab name

Closed Individual CROs

Arthur D Little	Bioresearch (Philadelphia, PA)	Tegaris Labs
Bioresearch (Cambridge, MA; hamsters)	Maccine Pte Ltd (Singapore)	Utah Biomedical
Bioassay Systems	Sitek	U Miami

Closed (or "Extinct") CRO Family Trees

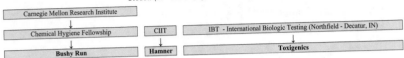

Carnegie Mellon Research Institute
↓
Chemical Hygiene Fellowship
↓
Bushy Run

CIIT
↓
Hamner

IBT - International Biologic Testing (Northfield - Decatur, IN)
↓
Toxigenics

© Springer Nature Switzerland AG 2020
S. C. Gad et al., *Contract Research and Development Organizations-Their History, Selection, and Utilization*, https://doi.org/10.1007/978-3-030-43073-3

Legend:

Gray = closed, absorbed , or acquired

White = active at time of publication

CROs displayed alphabetically by
most current lab name

Active Individual CROs

Absorption Systems (PA + CA)	Korean Institute of Toxicology (KITOX)	Sequani (UK)
American Preclinical Sciences	Lovelace	Sinclair (MO)
Battelle	Luvo Biosciences	Southern Research
Bioneeds (India)	MB Research	SRI International
BoZo Research Center	NAMSA	Stillmeadow
CARE Research	Northern Biomedical	SWRI - South West Research Institute
Comparative Biomedical	Nelson Labs	Toxikon
Experimur	Parsolt	Xenometrics
ILS - Integrated Laboratory Systems	Pharmaron (China)	
ITR Labs - International Toxicology Research Labs (Canada)	RTI	

Legend:

Gray = closed, absorbed , or acquired

White = active at time of publication

CROs displayed alphabetically by
most current lab name

Active (or "Living") CRO Family Trees: BASi, Battelle, and Bioreliance

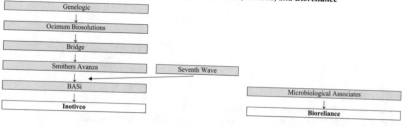

Genelogic
↓
Ocimum Biosolutions
↓
Bridge
↓
Smithers Avanza ← Seventh Wave
↓
BASi
↓
Inotivco

Microbiological Associates
↓
Bioreliance

Legend:

Gray = closed, absorbed , or acquired

White = active at time of publication

CROs displayed alphabetically by
most current lab name

Active (or "Living") CRO Family Trees, continued: Charles River Labs (CRL)

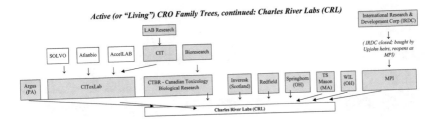

Legend:

Gray = closed, absorbed , or acquired

White = active at time of publication

CROs displayed alphabetically by
most current lab name

Active (or "Living") CRO Family Trees, continued: Covance

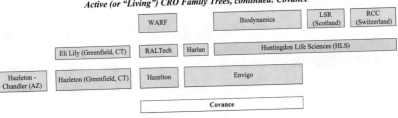

Legend:

Gray = closed, absorbed , or acquired

White = active at time of publication

CROs displayed alphabetically by
most current lab name

Active (or "Living") CRO Families, continued: Calvert, Eurofins, Frontage Labs, and Liberty Labs

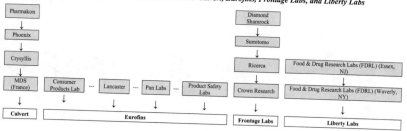

Legend:

Gray = closed, absorbed , or acquired

White = active at time of publication

CROs displayed alphabetically by
most current lab name

Active (or "Living") CRO Families, continued: Mérieux NutriSciences, MRIGlobal, Northview Chicago, Pacific BioLabs, and Smithers

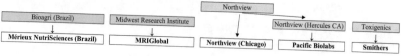

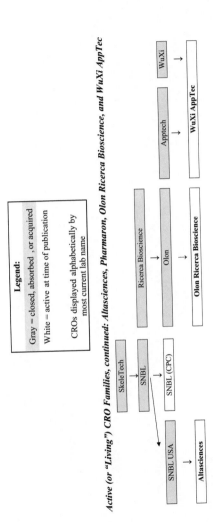

Active (or "Living") CRO Families, continued: Altasciences, Pharmaron, Olon Ricerca Bioscience, and WuXi AppTec

Legend:

Gray = closed, absorbed , or acquired

White = active at time of publication

CROs displayed alphabetically by most current lab name

Appendix J: Contract Manufacturer Audit Check List

Client	Revision:	Title: CONTRACT MANUFACTURER AUDIT CHECKLIST (GMP)	Page 1 of 5

Audit#:_____   Date:_____   Auditor:_____

1.   Project Title:_____

2.   Facility:_____

3.   Address:_____

4.   Date of Audit:_____

5.   Auditor:_____

6.   Date of Last FDA Inspection of Facility:_____

7.   Facility number:_____

8.   Facility Manager:_____

9.   Study Director:_____

10. Quality Assurance Unit:_____

© Springer Nature Switzerland AG 2020
S. C. Gad et al., *Contract Research and Development Organizations-Their History, Selection, and Utilization*, https://doi.org/10.1007/978-3-030-43073-3

		Unaccept	Needs Imp.	Accept	Excellent
11.	**Batch Records:**				
a.	Title and Purpose of Synthesis				
b.	Identification of Drug and Devices Articles				
c.	Name of Sponsor and Name and Address of Facility				
d.	Description of Process				
e.	Rationale for Process				
f.	Procedure for Identification of Process				
g.	Description of Process Design and Equipment				
h.	Description / Specification on Drug				
i.	Initiation of Synthesis				
j.	Type and Frequency of Tests, Analyses, and Measurements				
k.	Records to be Maintained				
l.	Date of Approval and Dated Signature of Manager				
m.	Analytical Methods to be Used				
n.	Changes (with Reasons) Approved and Maintained with Batch Record				

Client	Revision:	Title: CONTRACT MANUFACTURER AUDIT CHECKLIST (GMP)			Page 2 of 5

			Unaccept	Needs Imp.	Accept	Excellent
12.		Current Summary of Training and Experience and Job Description for Each Individual				
13.		Personnel Qualifications				
14.		**Quality Assurance (QA) Unit:**				
	a.	Independent of Personnel Engaged in Study				
	b.	Written Procedure for Operation of QA Unit				
	c.	Maintains copy of Master Schedule Sheet				
	d.	Maintains Copy of All Protocols				
	e.	Inspections at Intervals Adequate to Assure Integrity				
	f.	Written Reports of Periodic Inspections				
	g.	Significant Problems Reported to Study Director and Management				
	h.	Written Status Reports on Each Study				
	i.	Reviews Final Study Report				
	j.	All QA Unit Records are Kept in One Location				
15.		**Written Procedures:**				
	a.	Starting Materials				
	b.	Retology				
	c.	Materials Acceptance Transfer and Identification				
	d.	Characterization of Reagents and Intermediates				
	e.	Handling of Reagents and Intermediates				
	f.	Methods of Synthesis, Fabrication, or Derivation of Intermediate Test and Final Articles				
	g.	Determination of Stability of Process and Final Molecules				
	h.	Determination of Stability of Carrier Mixtures				
	i.	Test System Observations				
	j.	Laboratory Testing				
	k.	Handling of Intermediate				
	l.	Personnel Safety				
	m.	Collection and Identification of Samples				
	n.	Analytical Processes				
	o.	Inspection, Cleaning, Maintenance, Testing, Calibration, and Standardization of Equipment				
	p.	Data Handling and Storage				
16.		Testing Facilities of Suitable Size and Construction				
17.		Spaces for Cleaning, Sterilizing, and Maintaining Equipment and Supplies				
18.		**Equipment:**				
	a.	Adequate Equipment Including Environmental Control Equipment				
	b.	Equipment Cleanliness				
	c.	Adherence to Cleaning, Maintenance, Calibration, and Standardization Schedules				

Client		Revision:	Title: CONTRACT MANUFACTURER AUDIT CHECKLIST (GMP)				Page 3 of 5

			Unaccept	Needs Imp.	Accept	Excellent
	d.	Records of All Inspection, Maintenance, Testing, Calibration, and Standardization Operations				
	e.	Records Include Defects, How and When Defects were Found, and Remedial Action				
19.		Labeling of Reagents and Solutions (Identity, Titer or Concentration, Storage Requirements, and Expiration Date)				
20.		**Test and Control Articles:**				
	a.	Records of Identity, Strength, Purity, and Composition of Each Batch				
	b.	Stability Determined				
	c.	Records of Stability Testing				
	d.	Labeling of Storage Containers				
	e.	Storage				
	f.	Retention of Reserve Samples				
	g.	Handling				
	h.	Testing of Carrier Mixtures				
	i.	Records of Stability Testing of Carrier Mixtures				
	j.	Labeling of Carrier Mixtures				
21.		**Production Facilities:**				
	a.	Sufficient Number of Rooms and Areas:				
		(1) Separation of Materials and Processes				
		(2) Isolation of Individual Projects				
		(3) Isolation of Newly Received Materials				
		(4) Routine and Specialized Housing of Materials				
		(5) Isolation of Projects Using Biohazardous Materials				
	b.	Facilities for Collection and Disposal of Waste and Refuse				
	c.	Storage Areas Before Cleaning				
	d.	Cleaning Procedures				
22.		**Care of Drug Substance/ API:**				
	a.	Isolation of Newly Produced Drug				
	b.	API Tracking				
	c.	Stability Analysis				
	d.	Records of Periodic Analyses				
	e.	Records of Use of Pest Control Materials in Facilities				
	f.	Environmental Records (Humidity and Temperatures)				

Client	Revision:	Title: CONTRACT MANUFACTURER AUDIT CHECKLIST (GMP)				Page 4 of 5
			Unaccept	Needs Imp.	Accept	Excellent
23.	Identification of Specimens (Test System, Study, Nature, and Date of Collection)					
24.	Records of All Deviations from Written Procedures, Including Authorization					
25.	All Records Specified in Batch Record are Maintained					
26.	Data Entries (Manual and Computer)					
27.	Availability of Laboratory Manuals and Written Procedures					
28.	Systems Monitored in Conformity with Protocol					
29.	Personnel Report Adverse Health or Medical Condition					
30.	Final Batch Record Include (as a Minimum) Name and Address of Facility Performing Synthesis, Start and Completion Dates of Project, Objectives and Procedures Stated in the Batch Record, Changes to Protocol, Statistical Methods for Data Analysis, Test and Control Articles Used, Stability of Test and Control Articles, Methods Used, Equipment Used, All Circumstances That Could Have Affected the Data, Names of Key members of Project Team, Operations Performed on the Data, Summary and Analysis of Data, Conclusions Drawn, Signed and Dated Reports of Key Members of Study Team, Data and MAterial Storage Locations, Statement Prepared and Signed by QA Unit, Dated Signature of Project Manager, and Corrections and Additions (in the Form of Amendments) to Final Project Reports, Release Criteria and Documents					
31.	**Data Handling and Storage:**					
a.	Retention of All Raw Data, Documentation, Protocols, Required Specimens, and Final Study Reports					
b.	Archives Orderly and Minimize Deterioration of Documents and Specimens					
c.	An Individual is Responsible for Archives					
d.	Index of Material in Archives					
e.	Historical File of all Obsolete Documents					
f.	Retention Period of at Least 2 Years from Date of Approval by FDA of a Research or Marketing Permit or from Study Termination Date for Studies that are not included in an FDA Submission, Except at Least 5 Years from Date of Submittal to FDA if in Support of an IND or IDE					

Client	Revision:	Title: CONTRACT MANUFACTURER AUDIT CHECKLIST (GMP)	Page 5 of 5

35.   Comments:_____

      _____

      _____

      _____

      _____

      _____

      _____

      _____

36.   Auditors Signature:_____   37.   Date:_____

cc: _____

      _____

      _____

References

Singer, D.C.; Upton, Ronald P.; *Guidelines for Quality Auditing*; ASQC Quality Press, 1993
Robert E. Spinock Consultants; Sample Audit Checklist, 1988

Contract Laboratory Audit Check List (GCP)

Coordinator:		Review Type:	
Sponsor: Visit Type Screen	Protocol #:	Subject Initials: YES/NO	Subject #: If answer is no, then document findings:
Prescreen Report	All Sections Addressed:		
Informed Consent Process	Appropriate # of consents:		
	Appropriate version:		
	All pages initialed:		
	Signed & dated by:		
	Patient:		
	CRC:		
	PI/Sub-I:		
	Process documented:		
	Peer review of consent form:		
Source Checklist	Appropriate procedures completed:		
Cross-reference with applicable source document	Order of procedure evident(if applicable)		
Ratings/Diagnostic Tools	Appropriate, certified rater:		
	Tally(if applicable) meets all inc./no exc.		
	Scales support diagnosis		
PI/Sub-I Progress Note	ICF process documented		
Cross-reference with all	Diagnosis meets all inclusions/no exclusion		
Applicable source documents	History of presenting illness		
	Medical history		
	Concomitant medications		
	Physical examination		

(continued)

Coordinator: _____ Review Type: _____			
Sponsor: Visit Type Screen	Protocol #:	Subject Initials: YES/NO	Subject #: If answer is no, then document findings:
Prescreen Report	All Sections Addressed:		
Medical History Cross-reference with all applicable source documents	Prescreen report		
	PI/Sub-I progress note		
	Medical records (if available)		
	Concomitant medications		
	Medical history meets all inclusion/ no exc.		
Concomitant Medications Cross-reference with all Applicable source documents	Prescreen report		
	PI/Sub-I progress note		
	Previous medication log		
	Con med log		
	Con meds do not meet exclusion		
	If no, was waiver obtained?		
Safety EGG	Vitals (performed per protocol)		
	EGG (performed per protocol)		
	ECG demographics accurate?		
	Timely review of ECG by PI/Sub-I?		
	Any repeats ordered?		
	If so, repeat completed?		
Labs	Labs (performed per protocol)		
	Lab Requisition Demographics Accurate?		
	Timely review of Labs by PI/Sub-I?		

(continued)

Coordinator: _____		Review Type:	
Sponsor: Visit Type Screen	Protocol #:	Subject Initials: YES/NO	Subject #: If answer is no, then document findings:
Prescreen Report	All Sections Addressed:		
	Any repeats ordered?		
	If so, repeat completed?		
Inclusion/Exclusion	Documented and complete through screening		
Protocol Adherence	Any protocol deviation/ violations?		
	Documented?		
	Sponsor/CRO notified?		
	Receipt of approval from sponsor/CRO?		
	Reported to IRB (If applicable)		
Appearance	Source intact and legible?		
	Filing completed?		
	Documented and complete through screening		
	Any protocol deviation/violations?		
	Documented?		
	Sponsor/CRO notified?		
	Receipt of approval from sponsor/CRO?		
	Reported to IRB (if applicable)		
Appearance	Source intact and legible?		
	Filing completed?		
	Headers complete and accurate?		
	CRF completed?		
Reviewed By:	Name:	Date	

(continued)

Coordinator: _____		
Type _____		_____ Review
Sponsor:		
Visit Type: Randomization		
Source Checklist	Appropriate procedures completed:	**YES/NO**
Cross-reference with	Order of procedures evident (if applicable)	
Applicable source documents		
Ratings/Diagnostic Tools	Appropriate, certified rater:	
	Rater changes? If so, explanation provided?	
	Tally (if applicable)meets all inc./no exc.?	
	Scales support diagnosis?	
	Shifts in ratings are explained?	
PI/Sub-I Progress Note	Diagnosis meets all inclusion/ no exclusion	
Cross-reference with all	Confirms subject eligibility	
applicable source documents	Concomitant medications	
	Adverse events	
Concomitant Medications	PI/Sub-I progress note	
Cross-reference with all	Con med log	
applicable source documents	Con meds do not meet exclusion	
	If no, was waiver obtained?	
Adverse Events	PI/Sub-I progress note	
Cross-reference with all	CRC progress note	
applicable source documents	AE log	
	Medical history vs. adverse event	
Drug Accountability	Dispensing recorded	
	Dosing instructions evident (If applicable)	
Safety	Vitals (performed per protocol)	

(continued)

		Review
Coordinator: _____		
Type _____		
Sponsor:		
Visit Type: Randomization		
Source Checklist	Appropriate procedures completed:	**YES/NO**
ECG	Screening ECG available prior to randomization?	
	ECG (performed per protocol) if applicable	
	ECG demographics accurate?	
	Timely review of ECG by PI/Sub-I?	
	Any repeats ordered?	
	If so, repeat completed?	
Labs	Lab Reports available prior to randomization?	
	Labs (performed per protocol) if applicable	
	Lab requisition demographics accurate?	
	Timely review of labs by PI/Sub-I?	
	Any repeats ordered?	
	If so, repeat completed?	
Inclusion/Exclusion	Documented and complete through randomization	
Protocol Adherence	Any protocol deviation/violations?	
	Documented?	
	Sponsor/CRO notified?	
	Receipt of approval from sponsor/CRO?	
	Reported to IRB (if applicable)	
Appearance	Source intact and legible?	
	Filing completed?	
	Headers complete and accurate?	
	CRF completed?	
Reviewed By:		
	Name	Date

(continued)

Coordinator: _____ Review		
Type _____		
Sponsor:		
Visit Type: Interim Visit		
Source Checklist	Appropriate procedures completed:	**YES/NO**
Cross-reference with	Order of procedures evident (if applicable)	
Applicable source documents		
Ratings/Diagnostic Tools	Appropriate, certified rater:	
	Rater changes? If so, explanation provided?	
	Tally (if applicable) meets all inc./no exc.?	
	Scales support diagnosis?	
	Shifts in ratings are explained?	
PI/Sub-I Progress Note	Concomitant medications	
Cross-reference with all	Adverse events	
applicable source documents	Dosage changes documented (if applicable)	
Concomitant Medications	PI/Sub-I progress note	
Cross-reference with all	Con med log	
applicable source documents	Con meds do not meet exclusion	
	If no, was waiver obtained?	
Adverse Events	PI/Sub-I progress note	
Cross-reference with all applicable source documents	AE log	
	Medical history vs. adverse event	
Drug Accountability	Returned drug recorded (if no, reason document?)	
	Dispensing recorded	
	Dosing instructions evident (if applicable)	

(continued)

		Review
Coordinator: _____		
Type _____		
Sponsor:		
Visit Type: Interim Visit		
Source Checklist	Appropriate procedures completed:	**YES/NO**
Safety	Vitals (performed per protocol)	
ECG	Screening ECG available prior to randomization?	
	ECG (performed per protocol) if applicable	
	ECG demographics accurate?	
	Timely review of ECG by PI/Sub-I?	
	Any repeats ordered?	
	If so, repeat completed?	
Safety (continued)	Random. lab reports available prior to current visit?	
Labs	Labs (performed per protocol) if applicable	
	Lab requisition demographics accurate?	
	Timely review of labs by PI/Sub-I?	
	Any repeats ordered?	
Protocol Adherence	Any protocol deviation/violations?	
	Documented?	
	Sponsor/CRO notified?	
	Receipt of approval from sponsor/CRO?	
	Reported to IRB (if applicable)	
Appearance	Source intact and legible?	
	Filing completed?	
	Headers complete and accurate?	
	CRF completed?	
Reviewed By:		
	Name	Date

(continued)

Coordinator: _____ Review		
Type _____		
Sponsor:		
Visit Type: EOS/ET		
Source Checklist	Appropriate procedures completed:	**YES/NO**
Cross-reference with	Order of procedures evident (if applicable)	
Applicable source documents		
Ratings/Diagnostic Tools	Appropriate, certified rater:	
	Rater changes? If so, explanation provided?	
	Tally (if applicable)meets all inc./no exc.?	
	Scales support diagnosis?	
	Shifts in ratings are explained?	
PI/Sub-I Progress Note	Concomitant medications	
Cross-reference with all	Adverse events	
applicable source documents	Dosage changes documented (if applicable)	
	Reason ET (if applicable)	
Concomitant Medications	PI/Sub-I progress note	
Cross-reference with all	Con med log	
applicable source documents	Con meds do not meet exclusion	
	If no, was waiver obtained?	
	Ongoing meds closed out or noted "ongoing"	
Adverse Events	PI/Sub-I progress note	
Cross-reference with all		
applicable source documents	AE log	
	Medical history vs. adverse event	
	Ongoing AEs closed out or noted "ongoing"	
Drug Accountability	Returned drug recorded (if no, reason document?)	
	Dispensing recorded	

(continued)

		Review
Coordinator: _____		
Type _____		
Sponsor:		
Visit Type: EOS/ET		
Source Checklist	Appropriate procedures completed:	**YES/NO**
	Dosing instructions evident (if applicable)	
Safety	Vitals (performed per protocol)	
ECG	Screening ECG available prior to randomization?	
	ECG (performed per protocol) if applicable	
	ECG demographics accurate?	
	Timely review of ECG by PI/Sub-I?	
	Any repeats ordered?	
	If so, repeat completed?	
Safety (continued)	Random. lab reports available prior to current visit?	
Labs	Labs (performed per protocol) if applicable	
	Lab requisition demographics accurate?	
	Timely review of labs by PI/Sub-I?	
	Any repeats ordered?	
Protocol Adherence	Any protocol deviation/violations?	
	Documented?	
	Sponsor/CRO notified?	
	Receipt of approval from sponsor/CRO?	
	Reported to IRB (if applicable)	
Appearance	Source intact and legible?	
	Filing completed?	
	Headers complete and accurate?	
	CRF completed?	
Reviewed By:		
	Name	Date

Vendor/Supplier/Subcontractor Quality Assurance GLP Compliance Assessment Form

Organization Name		
Address:		
Organization Representative(s):	Name	Title

Organization and Personnel

Documentation:	Adequate	Deficient	Not applicable	Comments
Organizational Chart				
Floor Plans				
SOP Index/Listing				
Recent Inspection EIR or Letter				
Management Responsibilities:				
Procedures to Assign and replace a Study Director				
Procedures for control of Study Director work load				
Establishment and support of the Quality Assurance Unit (QAU), including assuring that deficiencies reported by the QAU are communicated to the Study Directors and acted upon.				

(continued)

Appendix J: Contract Manufacturer Audit Check List

Documentation:	Adequate	Deficient	Not applicable	Comments
Procedures to Assure test and control articles are appropriately tested for identity, strength, purity, stability, and uniformity				
Assuring that study personnel are informed of and follow test and control article handling and storage procedures.				
Provide required study personnel, resources, facilities, equipment, and materials.				
Review and approve protocols and standard operating procedures (SOPs).				
Provide GLP or appropriate technical training.				
Personnel:				
Training and position descriptions are maintained and current.				
Personnel are technically and GLP trained				
Practices are in place to ensure that employees take necessary health precautions, wear appropriate clothing and report illnesses that may adversely affect the study.				

(continued)

Documentation: **Validation (if the organization chooses to maintain records electronically and/or use electronic signatures):**	Adequate	Deficient	Not applicable	Comments
Who was involved in the design, development and validation of the computer system?				
Who is responsible for the operation of the computer system (inputs, processing and output of data).				
Corrective action plan for achieving Part 11 compliance				
High Level Systems Document				
Accurate and complete electronic and human readable copies of electronic records.				
Employees are held accountable and responsible for actions taken under their electronic signatures.				
If computer system personnel have training commensurate with their responsibilities (technical and GLP)				

(continued)

Documentation:	Adequate	Deficient	Not applicable	Comments
Determine if some computer system personnel are contractors or on-site employees.				
QAU SOPs for the inspection of computer Validation processes				
Archiving of computerized operations and data under appropriate environmental conditions.				
Validation Study documentation				
Maintenance of equipment, back up procedures.				
Change control procedures				
Evaluation of test data if interfaced with a computer.				
Emergency back up procedures				
Historical file of outdated or modified computer programs is maintained.				
Formal system retirement procedures				
Study Director:				
Assures the Protocol and any amendments have been properly approved and followed.				
Assures all data has been accurately recorded and verified.				

(continued)

Documentation:	Adequate	Deficient	Not applicable	Comments
Assures that all study personnel are familiar with and adhere to the study protocol and SOPs. Data are collected according to the protocol and SOPs.				
Documents unforeseen circumstances that may affect the quality and integrity of the study, implements corrective action.				
Assures that study data are transferred to the archives at the close of the study.				
Quality Assurance Unit SOPs for the following:				
Maintenance of the Master schedule				
Maintenance of copies of all protocols and amendments.				
Scheduling of in-process inspections and audits.				
Inspection of each non-clinical study at adequate intervals to assure the integrity of the study.				
Maintenance of records for each inspection.				

(continued)

Documentation:	Adequate	Deficient	Not applicable	Comments
Immediately notify the Study Director and Management of any problems that are likely to affect the integrity of the study.				
Submit periodic status reports on each study to the Study Director and Management.				
Review of the final study report.				
Preparation of a QA statement (which includes: the type of inspection, the dates inspections were made and the findings reported to Management and the Study Director) to be included in the final report.				
Inspect computer validation processes				
Facilities:				
Security				
Environmental controls and monitoring procedures (temp/humidity, ventilation, lighting, emergency/ backup management).				
SOPs for cleaning critical areas and equipment.				

(continued)

Documentation:	Adequate	Deficient	Not applicable	Comments
Appropriate areas for the receipt, storage, mixing and handling of test and control articles.				
Separation between species and functions requiring separation is maintained.				
Computerized operations and archived computer data are housed under appropriate environmental conditions.				
Equipment:				
Maintenance of Equipment				
SOPs and Manuals				
Maintenance schedule and logs				
Standardization/ calibration procedures, schedules and logs.				
Malfunction reporting/ Corrective action procedures				
Standard Operating Procedures				
Ensure written procedures exist for specified areas (58.81).				
Only current SOPs are available.				
Proper authorization (signatures and dates).				

(continued)

Documentation:	Adequate	Deficient	Not Applicable	Comments
Changes to SOPs are properly authorized and dated. Historical files of SOPs are maintained.				
SOPs to ensure the quality and integrity of data.				
Verify SOPs are periodically reviewed for current applicability.				
Reagents and Solutions:				
Procedures for purchasing, receiving and labeling.				
Reagents and solutions are labeled to indicate identity, concentration (titer), storage and exp. Date.				
Automated analytical: Profile data for each batch of controls is used.				
Animal Care:				
SOPs to cover environment, housing, feeding, handling and care of laboratory animals.				
Appropriate areas for animal supplies (feed, bedding)				
Pest control procedures: list of chemicals used.				
IACUC committee is established.				
Recent IACUC inspection reports/minutes.				

(continued)

Documentation:	Adequate	Deficient	Not applicable	Comments
All animals are isolated and identified and their health status is evaluated.				
Treatment of diseased animals is authorized by the Study Director.				
Animals are appropriately identified.				
Observation procedures for reporting of dead or moribund (gross lesions/masses) animals.				
Separation of species.				
Sanitization procedures for cages, racks and equipment. Appropriate bedding is used.				
Feed and water samples are collected and analyzed, documentation is maintained.				
Test and Control Articles:				
Procedures for acquisition, receipt and storage. Prevention of contamination and deterioration procedures.				
Characterization of each batch are determined and documented.				
Documentation of Stability.				

(continued)

Documentation:	Adequate	Deficient	Not applicable	Comments
Transfer of samples from collection to analysis is documented.				
Storage containers are appropriately labeled.				
Reserve/retention samples are maintained for studies lasting longer than 4 wks.				
Test and Control Article Handling:				
Documentation for receipt and distribution.				
Proper identification and storage.				
Process to avoid contamination, deterioration or damage during distribution.				
Mixtures of Articles with Carriers:				
Uniformity of mixtures is periodically determined.				
Stability determined under study conditions.				
Study Conduct:				
SOPs for protocol approval and preparation.				
Protocol contains required elements.				
Amendments (revisions) to the protocol are authorized, signed and dated by the Study Director.				

(continued)

Documentation:	Adequate	Deficient	Not applicable	Comments
All copies of the approved protocols contain all amendments (changes/revisions).				
Records and Reports:				
Requirements of 21 CFR 58.185 (a) (1-14)				
Dated signature of the Study Director.				
Corrections or additions to the final report are made in compliance with 21 CFR 58.185 (c).				
Storage and retrieval of records and data:				
Verify that raw data, documentation, protocols, final reports and specimens have been retained.				
Individual responsible for the archives. Delegation of duties to other individuals.				
Archived material is indexed to permit expedient retrieval.				
Access to the archives is controlled. Environmental controls to minimize deterioration.				

Documentation:	Adequate	Deficient	Not Applicable	Comments
Controlled procedures for adding or removing material from the archives.				
Storage of computer data and backup data.				

Confidential Disclosure Agreement

This Agreement entered into between Company, with an address of Address Line 1, Address Line 2, City, State Zip (hereinafter "COMPANY") and _____
_____ (hereinafter "Sponsor") confirms the terms and conditions under which Sponsor will disclose to COMPANY, and COMPANY may receive, certain proprietary information or materials or samples (hereinafter, "INFORMATION") for the sole purpose of enabling COMPANY to evaluate the INFORMATION and advise Sponsor on means to further develop the INFORMATION or to establish its utility.

1. COMPANY agrees to hold in confidence and not to disclose to third parties, without Sponsor's prior written consent, for a period of five (5) years from the date hereof, all INFORMATION disclosed by Sponsor whether orally, in writing, or by way of samples.
2. COMPANY shall take all necessary and reasonable steps to assure that INFORMATION is maintained in confidence.
3. COMPANY shall not have any obligation of confidentiality with respect to any INFORMATION that:

   A. Is in the public domain at the time of disclosure or which, after disclosure, becomes part of the public domain by publication or otherwise through no fault of COMPANY, its employees, or its affiliates; or.
   B. Is already in COMPANY 'S possession at the time of disclosure, was not received directly or indirectly from Sponsor, and is identified by COMPANY to Sponsor within twenty (20) days of COMPANY 'S receipt of such INFORMATION from Sponsor; or.
   C. Is properly received by COMPANY from a third party with a valid legal right to disclose such INFORMATION and such third party is not under a confidentiality agreement to Sponsor.

Confidentiality Agreement.
  page 2

4. COMPANY shall not, without the prior written consent of Sponsor, use INFORMATION for any purpose other than to enable it to evaluate and advise Sponsor as set forth herein.

5. It is understood by COMPANY and Sponsor that no patent right or license is hereby granted by this Agreement and that the disclosure of INFORMATION does not result in any obligation to grant COMPANY any right in or to such INFORMATION other than for evaluation as specified herein.

6. At the request of Sponsor, COMPANY shall promptly return to Sponsor all INFORMATION provided in either written or sample form and destroy all copies of documents containing INFORMATION in the possession of COMPANY, except that COMPANY may retain one copy of such INFORMATION in its confidential files, solely for record purposes.

7. At the request of Sponsor, COMPANY shall provide in written form a report in English, of any and all findings from its evaluation of the INFORMATION.

The following individuals who are authorized to do so have hereinafter indicated each party's acceptance of this Agreement.

COMPANY.

By: _____ By: _____

Title: _____ Title: _____

Date: _____ Date: _____

Master Services Agreement

This Master Services Agreement (the "Agreement") is made as of this _____ day of _____, 2018 (the "Effective Date"), by and between Company, Address Line 1, Address Line 2, State (hereinafter referred to as "Company") and _____ (hereinafter referred to as "Client") to govern the testing to be performed by Company for Client during the term of this Agreement.

1. *Services*

    (a) Company will perform, from time to time during the term of this Agreement, a study (each, the "Study") for the Client in accordance with a detailed protocol document (the "Protocol"), which will be (i) supplied by Client or (ii) prepared by Company under Client's direction and approved in writing by Client. The Protocol will specify the Study design, information desired, estimated duration of the Study, and other pertinent matters. Each Protocol will be (i) set forth in writing, (ii) executed by both parties, (iii) specifically reference this Agreement, and (iv) incorporated herein upon execution and delivery by both parties. To the extent that any terms or conditions of a Protocol conflict or are inconsistent with or are in addition to the terms and conditions of this Agreement, the terms and conditions of the Agreement shall control unless the Protocol specifically states otherwise. Each Protocol shall remain effective until the obligations of each party described in it are performed or it is otherwise terminated pursuant to the terms of this Agreement.

(b) If requested by Client, Company will consult with Client or Client's authorized representative to aid Client in developing the Study design and Protocol in a manner consistent with current regulatory guidelines. Company does not warrant that the Study design and/or the Study results will satisfy the requirements of any regulatory agency at the time of, provided, however, that if Company reasonably believes that a Study design will not meet the requirements of any regulatory authority, it shall promptly disclose same to Client.

(c) Company shall provide at its cost (i) all licenses, permits, and other items necessary and appropriate for it to fully and timely perform the Study and (ii) insurance adequate in amounts to fulfill its obligations and liabilities hereunder.

2. *Protocol Revisions.* The Protocol may be revised by agreement between the parties, provided that the party suggesting the revision communicates the same in writing to the other party, and within ten (10) days thereafter, the other party indicates acceptance thereof in writing. In the event that the revision has an impact on the price quoted in the original Protocol, Company shall promptly advise the Client of any cost adjustment related to a proposed amendment to the previously executed Protocol.

3. *Property Ownership.* Client may supply to Company certain materials, information, or other data necessary or desirable for Company to conduct the Study (collectively, "Client Materials"). Company agrees that all (i)

Client Materials and (ii) raw data, laboratory work sheets, reports, analyses, and any other such materials relating to the Study ("Deliverables") are and shall remain the exclusive property of the Client and will be held at Company's archiving facility for the specified period of time set forth in the Protocol or, in the absence of a specified time period, for ten (10) years following the completion of the Study, where they will be available for inspection by the Client or an authorized agent designated by the Client. Company will assist the Client in scheduling these inspections at mutually agreed times during normal business hours. To the extent any Deliverable is copyrightable, it shall be deemed a "Work Made for Hire" or alternatively a "Specially Commissioned Work" under the Copyright Act of 1976 and shall become and remain the sole property of Client. To the extent any Deliverable may not be a Work Made for Hire, Company agrees to assign and does hereby assign or shall cause to have assigned such Deliverable to Client. Company warrants that it has entered into written agreements with its employees and agents sufficient to ensure compliance with the assignment obligations set forth herein.

4. *Confidentiality.*

   (a) To facilitate the Study, certain confidential information and Client Materials may be sent to Company and placed in Company's custody by the Client's personnel or be developed pursuant to the Study and maintained in Company's custody (collectively, "Confidential Information"). Confidential Information includes, but is not limited to, information relating to clinical trials, new drug or device applications, business plans, products, trade secret processes or methodologies, chemical structures, synthetic, analytical or other steps or processes relating to the manufacture of any Client Material, and any intellectual property (including know-how) directly relating to Client Materials. Any Confidential Information related to Client's proprietary material shall be referred to herein as "Agent-Related Information."

   (b) Notwithstanding the foregoing, Confidential Information does not include any information that (a) was in Company's possession before receipt from Client, as evidenced by Company's written records, provided, however, that such Confidential Information is not Agent-Related Information; (b) is or becomes available to the public through no fault of or breach of this Agreement by Company or any of its employees or agents; or (c) is received in good faith by Company without obligations of confidentiality from a third party, which, to the knowledge of Company, is legally entitled to disclose it, provided, however, that such Confidential Information is not Agent-Related Information.

(c) Company agrees that the Confidential Information constitutes the property of the Client and that Company will not use or disclose any such Confidential Information, during or after the term of this Agreement in perpetuity, without the prior written consent of the Client. Company shall use Client's Confidential Information only for the purpose of fulfilling its obligations hereunder. Company shall protect Client's Confidential Information by using the same degree of care, but no less than a reasonable degree of care, as Company uses to protect its own Confidential Information. Notwithstanding the foregoing, Company may disclose Client's Confidential Information to its employees, officers, and agents ("Representatives"), but only to the extent reasonably necessary to fulfill its obligations hereunder, and Company warrants that any and all Representatives receiving access to the Confidential Information of Client are bound by confidentiality and nonuse obligations at least as stringent as those set forth herein. Company shall be solely responsible for informing its Representatives of the terms of this Agreement, and Company shall be liable for any breach of the provisions of this Agreement by any of its Representatives receiving Confidential Information hereunder.

(d) Test articles in Company's custody shall be promptly delivered to the Client upon termination of the Study, except archive samples as set forth in Sect. 12.

(e) When Company is required by law to disclose any Confidential Information to an authorized government agency or any other party, Company shall promptly notify the Client of the request prior to any disclosure so that Client may seek to obtain a protective order. In the event Client is unable to secure a protective order or other remedy to prevent or limit disclosure, Company shall limit its disclosure only to that Confidential Information required pursuant to the compulsory legal process. Company and Client agree that Company will not act as an intermediary in any negotiation between any authorized government agency and the Client. To that end, Company and Client agree that any and all discussions regarding any confidentiality issue between an authorized government agency and the Client will take place between the authorized government agency and the Client. Company will follow the instructions of the Client and attempt to fulfill the requests of the authorized government agency within the legal boundaries established between the authorized government agency and the Client.

(f) Company agrees to either destroy or return all Confidential Information received from Client upon written request, except that Company may retain in its confidential files one copy of written Confidential Information for compliance purposes only.

(g) Company acknowledges, understands, and agrees that a breach of this Sect. 4 may cause irreparable injury to Client and that no adequate or complete remedy at law may be available to Client for such breach. Accordingly, Company agrees that Client shall be entitled to seek enforcement of this Agreement by injunction or any other equitable relief.

5. *Emergency*. Company shall take any reasonable action which it deems necessary to protect the Client's Study in the case of an emergency condition in the laboratory. The Client shall be notified of such action as soon as reasonably possible.

6. *Quality Standards*. Company shall ensure that all Studies and Protocols (and any amendments thereto) are performed in compliance with 21 C.F.R. Part 58, Good Laboratory Practice for Nonclinical Laboratory Studies. If Company, in regard to its activities under this Agreement, commits a technical error which invalidates the Study according to any FDA or USDA rule or regulation, then the parties shall (i) jointly review the invalidation notification and respond to the regulatory agency with Client's input and approval, and (ii) at Client's option, (x) Company shall repeat the exact same Study promptly without additional cost to the Client or (y) provide a credit for a future study(s) up to the amounts paid by Client for this Study, as mutually agreed.

7. *Report*. The format of the final report shall be in accordance with the format set forth in the appropriate regulatory guidelines or in a format agreed to prior to the initiation of the Study. Two (2) copies (1 bound and 1

unbound) of the final report for non-acute studies will be supplied. This number may be changed by mutual written agreement prior to termination of the Study. If additional reports are requested after submission, they will be supplied to Client at Company's out-of-pocket cost. Company represents and warrants that all information and data contained in the final report shall be complete and accurate.

8. *Indemnification: Company to Client.* Company agrees to indemnify and defend Client, its officers, directors, employees, and agents against any loss, claim, suit, liability, or expense (including attorney's fee) stemming from (i) injuries or damages to persons or property which occur on or in the vicinity of Company's premises in the course of services being provided by Company hereunder, (ii) any breach by Company of any representation or warranty contained herein, and (iii) Company's or its employees' or agents' negligence, gross negligence, or willful misconduct in the performance of the Study hereunder, in each case unless such loss, claim, suit, liability, or expense is the result of action or inaction on the part of Client or its employees entitling to Company to be indemnified as set forth in Sect. 9.

9. *Indemnification: Client to Company.* Client agrees to indemnify and defend Company, its officers, directors, employees, and agents against any loss, claim, suit, liability, or expense (including attorney's fees) arising out of the Client's use of any Client Materials tested by Company hereunder, unless such loss, claim, suit, liability, or expense is the result of any action or inaction on the part of Company or its employees entitling Client to be indemnified as set forth in Sect. 8.

10. *Limited Warranty.* The undertaking of Company to perform the Study is a contract for services only. Except as otherwise set forth herein, the sole warranties with respect to its services are that Company will perform the Study with due care in a professional and workmanlike manner in strict accordance with the Protocol and any amendments thereto signed by the Client and adhering to generally prevailing industry standards, and applicable laws, rules, regulations, ordinances, and guidances. Any alleged claim by the Client for a breach of such warranty shall be made in writing to Company on or before the first anniversary of the date that the final report is delivered to the Client. After receipt by Company of such alleged claim of breach by Client, then either the Chief Scientific Officer or the Chief Executive Officer of Company will review such alleged claim with

the Client in person or by teleconference to determine whether Company in fact breached such warranty by not adhering to prevailing industry standards, and applicable laws, rules, regulations, ordinances, and guidance's during the conduct of the Study. The sole remedies of the Client for breach of such warranty shall be at Client's option (a) to require Company to re-perform the exact same Study (or such portions thereof as may reasonably be required to be re-performed) at Company's sole cost and expense, and in such event, Company shall diligently pursue the re-performance of the Study or portions thereof until completion, or (b) to terminate the Agreement and Company will issue a credit to Client equal to the amounts paid to Company for conducting the study for future work. The warranty set forth in this paragraph and the warranties set forth in this Agreement are in lieu of any and all other warranties relating to the services to be performed, expressed, or implied, including, without limitation, any implied warranties of merchantability or fitness for a particular purpose.

11. *Independent Contractor.* It is understood that the status of Company under this Agreement is that of an independent contractor without the capacity to legally bind the Client and Company is not as an agent or employee.

12. *Archiving of Materials.* All experimental data (including all Deliverables such as tissues, slides, records, and other materials generated during the conduct of the Study performed on the Client's behalf) shall be retained by Company unless otherwise indicated by the Client. Company will retain all such experimental data and Deliverables in accordance with regulatory and legal requirements or as otherwise set forth in the Protocol. Two (2) years after completion of the Study, Company shall notify the Client in writing requesting specific determinations as to the disposition of such material and Deliverables. Upon expiration of this two-year period, Company will invoice Client monthly for stored material on a space by storage basis, unless Client instructs that all materials and Deliverables are to be delivered to it at its expense. In no event will Company destroy any materials or Deliverables prior to obtaining Client's consent. All test materials that were furnished to Company by the Client that are not used during the Study or for required samples stored with Study data will be returned to the Client at the Study's conclusion.

13. *Governmental Inspections.* Client is to be notified immediately in the event that Company's facilities or Client's Study is the subject of an inspection by any duly authorized agency of federal, state, or local govern-

ment which may involve the subject matter of this Agreement. Company shall provide Client with the purpose of visit, name of inspector and credential number, and a copy of form(s) issued by the inspector, if any, and, if permitted, shall allow Client or its authorized representative to attend such inspection. Company shall use reasonable efforts to incorporate any Client comments or feedback in any written response to any regulatory authority. In addition, Company shall advise the Client that the Client's Study is involved and will withhold confidential data from the applicable regulatory authority until further instructions are received from the Client, or until the Client and the inspecting agency have reached an appropriate agreement. At no time are any copies of the Client's specifications to be given to the inspector; any request for such documents is to be redirected to the Client. If the Client does not comply in a timely manner with any request by the applicable regulatory authority and such delay by Client results in the issuance of a Form 483 to Company, then the Client will provide a letter to the applicable regulatory authority (with a copy sent to Company) within 10 business days of the issuance of such Form 483 to Company exonerating Company of any culpability related to the violation(s) listed on the Form 483 only if the issuance of the Form 483 to Company was based upon the lack of responsiveness or lack of cooperation by the Client.

14. *Inspection by Client.* Client or its authorized representatives shall have the right to inspect the facilities on the premises of the laboratory during normal working hours during the course of the Study to ensure compliance with the Agreement, and Company shall reasonably cooperate with any such inspection. Client may review, or request copies of, data derived from the Study at any time.

15. *Access to Study.* Neither Client nor Company will unreasonably withhold access by the other to Study material, wherever located, if such access is required for validation of laboratory results or procedures pursuant to government regulatory agency requests or applicable law.

16. *Publication.* Company agrees not to publish the results of any of its work hereunder without the prior written approval of the Client. Both parties agree that they will not use the name of the other party or any of its personnel for promotional literature or advertising without the prior written approval of the other party. This paragraph is in addition to those require-

ments set forth in the paragraph delineating the confidentiality requirements of this Agreement.

17. *Patents.* If, in the reasonable judgment of Company, a patentable situation arises during the course of the Study, Company will promptly notify Client of, and cause to be assigned to Client the rights to, any and all inventions, whether patentable or not, discovered directly as a result of performing Client's Study. If Client requests and at Client's expense, Company will provide Client with reasonable assistance to obtain these patents.

18. *Term and Termination.* This Agreement shall commence as of the Effective Date and shall expire on the three (3) year anniversary of the Effective Date, unless earlier terminated as set forth herein. Either party shall have the right at any time to terminate this Agreement upon sixty (60) days written notice to the other party, provided, however, that this Agreement will remain in full force and effect until any then-effective Studies are completed. Either party may terminate this Agreement for a material breach by the other party that is not cured within thirty (30) days of that party's receipt of written notice of the breach. Client shall have the right to earlier terminate a Study prior to completion upon the giving of written notice. In the event that such notice is given, Company shall immediately use its best efforts to reduce loss and cost to Client as the result of such termination. Client's obligations will be to reimburse Company for costs incurred plus pro rata fees as of the date of termination, including any uncancellable legal obligations to third parties relating to this Agreement, such as purchase orders, which were entered into prior to receiving the notice of termination with Client's approval.

19. *Termination Obligations.* The termination of the Agreement shall not relieve either party of its obligations to the other in respect of (a) maintaining the confidentiality of information, (b) assignment of rights to patentable inventions and Deliverables, (c) reporting rights of previously ongoing studies, (d) obtaining consents for advertising purposes and publications, and (e) indemnification.

20. *Force Majeure.* If any event occurs which is not reasonably foreseen by either Company or the Client at the date of the Protocol and which may result in gross inequity to either Company or the Client, then at the request of the party on whom the inequity shall fall, the Client and Company shall meet and renegotiate the terms of this Agreement. Examples of such an event leading to impossibility or impracticability of performance would

include, but are not limited to, fire, strike, governmental action, acts of God, explosion, hostility of war, or riot. In the event such force majeure event delays the Study by more than thirty (30) days, Client may terminate this Agreement with notice and without liability hereunder.

21. *Delays.* If, during the course of the term of the Agreement, delays are experienced owing to the Client's inability to make available to Company necessary materials or data required to perform the work detailed in the Protocol, Company reserves the right to reschedule resources reserved to complete performance on this contract and to adjust the original pricing of the Protocol where appropriate. Should a Study be canceled by the Client after costs have been incurred by Company, such costs will be billed to the Client at the time of cancellation.

22. *Assignment: Subcontracting.* This Agreement shall not be assigned by Company without the prior written consent of the Client; however, Company's services shall inure to the benefit of any assigns, successors in business, or subsidiaries or affiliates of the Client. Company shall not assign, delegate, or subcontract any of the services to be provided hereunder without the prior written approval of Client.

23. *Notice.* All notices required or permitted to be given under this Agreement shall be in writing and shall be delivered personally, by overnight courier, or mailed by certified mail, postage prepaid, return receipt requested to the person named and addresses set forth below.

If to Client

If to Company:

    Company
    Address Line 1
    City, State Zip

24. *Amendment.* Any amendments, changes, or revisions to this Agreement must be in writing and duly executed by both parties.

25. *Waiver.* No waiver of any term, provisions, or conditions of this Agreement, whether by conduct or otherwise, in any one or more instances shall be deemed to be or construed as a further or continuing waiver of any such term, provision, or condition or of any other term, provision, or condition of this Agreement.

26. *Price and Terms.* In consideration of the performance of the Study, Client shall pay Company the total sum agreed upon in each Letter of Acceptance for a particular Study/Protocol, or amendment thereto. Any subsequent changes to the Protocol or work to be performed as referred to in paragraph 2 shall require a written amendment to this price through agreement between the parties, and execution of a corresponding Letter of Acceptance for such amendment. Payment shall be made according to invoices submitted by Company to Client for tests performed and in accordance with the schedule outlined in the Letter of Acceptance. Delinquent accounts may at the discretion of Company be subject to late payment fees at 1.5% per month of the outstanding delinquent balance.

27. *Choice of Law.* The validity, interpretation, performance, rights, and duties with respect to this Agreement, and all actions arising hereunder, by the terms of this Agreement, shall be determined by the laws of the applicable state.

28. *Severability.* If any provision of this Agreement is declared void or unenforceable, such provision shall be deemed modified to the extent necessary to allow enforcement, and all other portions of this Agreement shall remain in full force and effect.

29. *Entire Agreement.* This Agreement is the entire agreement between the Client and Company regarding the subject matter hereof, and it is agreed that no modifications of this Agreement shall be effective unless agreed to in writing by authorized representatives of both parties. This Agreement becomes effective and binding on both parties only when signed by each party below and delivered to Company.

30. *Execution.* This Agreement and all Protocols related hereto may be executed in one or more counterparts, each of which shall be deemed an original but all of which together shall constitute one and the same document. This Agreement and all Protocols related hereto may be executed and delivered by facsimile or electronically (including PDF). The parties agree that facsimile and electronic copies of signatures have the same effect as original signatures.

Signature Page

Client

Company

By:_____

By:_____

Title:_____

Title:_____

Date:_____

Date:_____

Draft Protocol

TITLE:	**A DOSE-RANGE-FINDING AND 7-DAY REPEAT-DOSE ORAL TOXICITY STUDY OF _____ IN S PRAGUE-DAWLEY RATS**
STUDY NO.:	_____
TESTING FACILITY:	_____
STUDY SPONSOR:	_____

Introduction

Title
A Dose-Range-Finding and 7-Day Repeat-Dose Oral Toxicity Study with
_____ in Sprague Dawley Rats

Objective
The purpose of this study is to determine the maximum tolerated dose (MTD) of
_____ when administered via oral gavage once daily to Sprague Dawley Rats
using an ascending/descending dose design (phase I), and to characterize the
repeat-dose toxicity and toxicokinetics of _____ when administered via oral
gavage once daily to Sprague Dawley Rats for a minimum of 7 days (Phase II).

Regulatory Compliance
This is a non-regulated study. However, it will be run according to the Standard
Operating Procedures (SOPs) of _____. There will be no formal involvement
of the Quality Assurance Unit.

Study Number

_____

Testing Facility

_____

Sponsor

_____

Study Director

_____

Study Monitor

_____

Principal Investigator – Bioanalytical Evaluation

_____

Principal Investigator – Toxicokinetics

_____

Key Study Dates

Proposed Experimental Start Date:
Proposed First Day of Dosing (Phase I):
Proposed First Day of Dosing (Phase II):
Proposed Necropsy (Phase II):
Proposed Experimental Completion Date:

Materials and Methods

Test Article

1. **Test Article**

Identification:	
Lot/Batch No.:	To be documented in study data
Physical Description:	To be documented in study data
Storage Conditions:	

2. **Vehicle**
   5% DMSO in water.

Lot/Batch No.:	To be documented in the study data
Physical Description:	
Storage Conditions:	

3. **Dose Preparation**
   Please add preparation instructions and frequency Daily – to be provided.
   Is dose formulation analysis needed?

4. **Reserve Archive Samples**

5. **Accountability and Disposition**
   Unused test article will be disposed of, returned to the Sponsor or designee at the completion of this study or retained for use on related future studies. The Sponsor will be notified in advance of shipping and a transmittal letter will accompany the shipment. The material will be packed in a suitable container to maintain the conditions specified by the Sponsor during transit plus an adequate margin of safety to account for any possible transit delays.

Test System (Animals and Animal Care)

1. Description

Species:	Rat
Stock:	Sprague Dawley – Hsd:SD
Total Number:	136
Gender:	68 males and 68 females
Age Range:	Approximately 7–9 weeks at start of dosing; records of dates of birth for animals used in this study will be retained in the _____ archives.
Body Weight Range:	170–325 grams for the males and females at the outset (Day 1) of the study.
Animal Source:	_____
Experimental History:	Purpose-bred and experimentally naïve at the outset of the study
Identification:	Ear tag and cage card

2. Rationale for Choice of Species and Number of Animals

The rat is a species that is commonly used for nonclinical toxicity studies with human drugs and satisfies the regulatory requirement for using a rodent species for such studies. The number of animals used in this study is considered the minimum required to achieve the objectives of the study for assessment of toxicity/tolerance of the test article, account for variability among animals, and provide an assessment of the toxicokinetic profile of the test article (1, 2).

Successful experience with predecessor (structurally similar) compound. Animal number required to validly assess dose levels for GLP study.

Husbandry.

Housing:	Animals will be group housed by sex upon receipt and individually housed upon assignment to study in compliance with National Research Council "Guide for the Care and Use of Laboratory Animals." The room in which the animals will be kept will be documented in the study records. No other species will be kept in the same room.
Lighting:	12 hours light/12 hours dark, except when room lights will be turned on during the dark cycle to accommodate blood sampling or other study procedures.
Room Temperature:	20–26 °C

Relative Humidity:	30–70%
Food:	All animals will have access to Teklad Rodent Diet (certified) or equivalent ad libitum, unless otherwise specified. The lot number(s) and specifications of each lot used are archived at _____. No contaminants are known to be present in the certified diet at levels that would be expected to interfere with the results of this study. Analysis of the diet was limited to that performed by the manufacturer, records of which will be maintained in the _____ archives.
Water:	Water will be available ad libitum, to each animal via an automatic watering device. The water is routinely analyzed for contaminants as per _____ SOPs. No contaminants are known to be present in the water at levels that would be expected to interfere with the results of this study. Results of the water analysis will be maintained in the _____ archives.
Acclimation:	Study animals will be acclimated to their housing for a minimum of 5 days prior to their first day of dosing.

3. **Pre-study Health Screen and Selection Criteria**

All animals received for this study will be assessed as to their general health by a member of the technical staff or other authorized personnel. During the acclimation period, each animal will be observed at least once daily for any abnormalities or for the development of infectious disease. Only animals that are determined to be suitable for use will be assigned to this study. Any animals considered unacceptable for use in this study will be replaced with animals of similar age and weight from the same vendor.

4. **Assignment to Study Groups**

Animals will be assigned to study groups using Pristima version 6.3.2. Animals will be randomly assigned to groups using selection designed to achieve similar group mean body weights.

5. **Humane Care of Animals**

Treatment of animals will be in accordance with the study protocol and also in accordance with _____ SOPs which adhere to the regulations outlined in the USDA Animal Welfare Act (9 CFR Parts 1, 2, and 3) and the conditions specified in the Guide for the Care and Use of Laboratory Animals (ILAR publication, NRC, 2011, The National Academies Press). The ___ Institutional Animal Care and Use Committee (IACUC) will approve the study protocol prior to finalization to insure compliance with acceptable standard animal welfare and humane care.

No alternative test systems exist which have been adequately validated to permit replacement of the use of live animals in this study. Every effort has been made to obtain the maximum amount of information while reducing to a minimum the number of animals required for this study. The assessment of pain and distress in study animals and the use or nonuse of pain alleviating medications will be in accordance with Standard Operating Procedure VET-19, Criteria for Assessing Pain and Distress in Laboratory Animals. The study will be terminated in part or whole for humane reasons if unnecessary pain occurs. To the best of our knowledge, this study is not unnecessary or duplicative.

6. **Study Endpoints**

The maximum tolerated dose (MTD) is the highest dose that does not cause mortality or overt clinical signs of toxicity. In order to determine the MTD, the dose level will be increased incrementally until toxicity is observed. Any signs of pain or distress will be reported to and addressed by DLAM and any treatments or interventions determined by the Study Director in consultation with DLAM and the Sponsor Representative/Study Monitor. Decisions to not treat or euthanize animals displaying signs of pain or distress will require justification in an IACUC-approved protocol amendment.

Test Article Administration

1. Group Assignments and Dose Levels

Phase I

Group	Treatment	Dose Level[a] (mg/kg)	Concentration (mg/ml)	Dose volume (ml/kg)	Number of animals	
					Male	Female
1	Dose 1	500	XXX	10	3	3
2	Dose 2		TBD	10	3	3
3	Dose 3	TBD	TBD	10	3	3
4	Dose 4	TBD	TBD	10	3	3

TBD To be determined

[a]The first group of rats will be dosed at 500 mg/kg. For subsequent doses, the dose level will be increased or decreased until the MTD, maximum feasible dose is established, or the dose limit of XX is reached. Females to be dosed only at highest tolerated dose

Phase II
Toxicology Groups

Group	Treatment	Dose level[a] (mg/kg)	Concentration (mg/ml)	Dose volume (ml/kg)	Number of animals	
					Male	Female
5	Vehicle control	0	0	10	5	5
6	Low dose	TBD	TBD	10	5	5
7	Mid dose	TBD	TBD	10	5	5
8	High dose	TBD	TBD	10	5	5

Toxicokinetic Groups

Group	Treatment	Dose level[a] (mg/kg)	Concentration (mg/ml)	Dose volume (ml/kg)	Number of animals	
					Male	Female
9	Low dose	TBD	TBD	10	12	12
10	Mid dose	TBD	TBD	10	12	12
11	High dose	TBD	TBD	10	12	12

TBD To be determined.
[a]Dose levels in phase II will be based on phase I results.

(a) *Phase I*

_____ will be administered to three naïve male rats (/Group) at 500 mg/kg via oral gavage once. The rats will be observed at intervals post-dose for clinical signs of effect or toxicity.

After a period of at least 2 days (minimum of 44 hours) following the previous dose of _____, an additional dose level (either increased or decreased depending on clinical observation assessment of the previous dose level) will be administered to an additional six naïve rats (3/sex). The rats will again be observed at intervals post-dose for clinical signs of effect or toxicity.

This dosing scheme (dose escalation or de-escalation) will continue until a maximum tolerated dosage (MTD), maximum feasible dose, or the dose limit of 1000 mg/kg is reached.

(b) *Phase II*

Phase II will proceed following completion of dosing in Phase I. The doses selected for Phase II will be based on the results of Phase I.

_____ will be administered to 112 naïve rats (5/sex/group for toxicology and 12/sex/group for toxicokinetic evaluation) once daily for 7 days (Groups 5–11) via oral gavage.

1. Dosing

Route:	Oral gavage
Frequency:	Phase I – Once at each dose level. Minimum of at least 2 days (minimum 44 hours) between dosing, until the MTD or dose limit is reached.
	Phase II – Once daily for 7 days.
Procedure:	Each animal will receive a dosing volume based upon the most recent body weight.

2. Justification for Route, Dose Levels, and Dosing Schedule

The oral route was chosen as it is the intended route of administration in humans. Drug is an NSAID and intended for daily oral clinical use.

In-Life Observations and Measurements (Phase I, Groups 1–4)

1. Mortality/Morbidity

Frequency:	Twice daily (a.m. and p.m.). Once prior to scheduled sacrifice on Day 3.
	Each animal observed for evidence of death or impending death (as per _____ SOP VET-14).

2. Clinical Observations

Frequency:	On the day of dosing, prior to each dose administration, approximately 1–3 hours post-dose. On non-dosing days, once daily. Once prior to scheduled sacrifice.

3. Body Weight

Frequency:	Body weights will be recorded for all animals prior to randomization/selection, prior to each dose level administration on Day 1 and prior to scheduled sacrifice on Day 3 (non-fasted).

1. Food Consumption

Frequency: Full feeder weights and/or feeder weigh backs will be recorded on Days 1 and 3 for determination of food consumption.

In-Life Observations and Measurements (Phase II, Groups 5–8)

1. Mortality/Morbidity

Frequency: Twice daily (a.m. and p.m.). Once prior to scheduled sacrifice on Day 8.
Each animal observed for evidence of death or impending death (as per _____ SOP VET-14).

2. Clinical Observations

Frequency: Prior to each dose administration, and approximately 1–3 hours post-dose, and additionally as needed. Once prior to scheduled sacrifice on Day 8.

3. Body Weight

Frequency: Body weights will be recorded for all animals prior to randomization/selection and prior to dose administration on Days 1 and 7.

4. Food Consumption

Frequency: Full feeder weights and/or feeder weigh backs will be recorded on Days 1 and 7 for determination of food consumption.

Clinical Pathology Evaluation (Phase II, Groups 5–8)

1. Sample Collection

Blood samples for evaluation of serum chemistry, hematology, and coagulation parameters and urine for urinalysis will be collected from all surviving animals (targeted 5/sex/group) prior to terminal sacrifice on Day 8. Animals will be anesthetized by CO_2 inhalation prior to blood collection. Immediately following exsanguination by cardiocentesis for terminal blood collection, rats will be returned to the CO_2 chamber to ensure euthanasia. Animals will be fasted overnight (approximately 12–24 hours) prior to blood collection for clinical pathology evaluation and during urine collection. If an animal is euthanized due to moribund condition prior to scheduled sacrifice, an attempt will be made to collect blood samples (non-fasted) as described above.

2. **Collection Procedures, Processing, and Analysis**
   (a) *Hematology*

Method of Collection:	Cardiocentesis
Anticoagulant:	K_2-EDTA

   Parameters analyzed:

Hematology parameters	
Red blood cell (RBC) count and morphology	Platelet count (PLT)
White blood cell (WBC) count[a]	Hematocrit (HCT)
Mean corpuscular hemoglobin (MCH)	Hemoglobin (HGB)
Mean corpuscular hemoglobin concentration (MCHC)	Reticulocyte count (Retic)
Mean corpuscular volume (MCV)	

   [a]Total and differential white blood cell counts, including neutrophils, basophils, eosinophils, monocytes, lymphocytes, and large unstained cells

   (b) *Coagulation*

Method of collection:	Cardiocentesis
Anticoagulant:	Sodium citrate

   Parameters analyzed:

Coagulation parameters	
Activated partial thromboplastin time (APTT)	Prothrombin time (PT)

   (c) *Serum Clinical Chemistry*

Method of collection:	Cardiocentesis
Anticoagulant:	None

Parameters analyzed:

Clinical chemistry parameters	
Alanine aminotransferase (ALT)	Globulin (calculated) (GLOB)
Albumin (ALB)	Glucose (GLU)
Albumin/globulin ratio (calculated)(A/G)	Phosphorus (PHOS)
Alkaline phosphatase (ALP)	Potassium (K)
Aspartate aminotransferase (AST)	Sodium (NA)
Calcium (CA)	Total bilirubin (T-BIL)
Chloride (CL)	Total protein (TP)
Cholesterol (CHOL)	Triglycerides (TRIG)
Creatinine (CREAT)	Urea nitrogen (BUN)

(d) *Urinalysis*

Method of collection:	Collection in metabolism cages

Parameters analyzed:

Urinalysis parameters	
Specific gravity	Nitrite
pH	Appearance/color
Protein	Bilirubin
Glucose	Blood
Ketone	Leukocytes
Urobilinogen	Microscopic examination of formed elements

Terminal Procedures and Anatomic Pathology (Phase I, Groups 1–4, and Phase II, Groups 5–8)

1. Termination

(a) *Scheduled Sacrifice*

Phase I – All surviving animals of each dose level will be euthanized on Day 3 by CO_2 asphyxiation, and a gross necropsy will be performed.

Phase II – All surviving animals will be euthanized by CO_2 asphyxiation and necropsied on Day 8 of Phase II.

(b) *Unscheduled Sacrifice*

Any animal judged to be in moribund condition or undergoing excessive pain will be euthanized by CO_2 asphyxiation, and a necropsy will be performed. A final body weight (non-fasted) will be recorded for such animals.

(c) *Final Body Weight*

A fasted terminal body weight will be recorded prior to sacrifice on Day 8 for phase II Groups 5–8 animals. This body weight will be used to calculate organ to body weight ratios.

2. Gross Necropsy (Phase I, Groups 1–4, and Phase II, Groups 5–8)

A complete gross necropsy will be performed by ____ personnel on all animals that are sacrificed or found dead during the study. The necropsy will include examination of:

- The external body surface.
- All orifices.
- The cranial, thoracic, and abdominal cavities and their contents.

All abnormalities will be described completely and recorded.

At the completion of phase I necropsy, tissues will not be retained and carcasses will be appropriately discarded.

3. Organ Weights (Phase II, Groups 5–8)

At scheduled sacrifice on Day 8, the following organs (when present) will be weighed before fixation, after dissection of excess fat and other excess tissues. Organ weights will not be recorded for animals found dead or sacrificed moribund. Paired organs will be weighed together unless gross abnormalities are present, in which case they will be weighed separately. The thyroids/parathyroids will be weighed fixed.

Organs weighed	
Adrenals	Testes
Brain	Ovaries
Heart	Spleen
Kidneys	Thyroid/parathyroid
Liver	

Organ to body weight ratios will be calculated (using the final body weight obtained prior to necropsy), as well as organ to brain weight ratios.

3. **Tissue Collection and Preservation (Phase II, Groups 5–8)**

For all animals in Groups 5–8 in the repeat-dose phase, the tissues listed in the table below will be preserved in 10% neutral buffered formalin (except for the eyes, which will be preserved in Davidson's fixative and the testes that will be preserved in Modified Davidson's fixative for optimum fixation).

Tissues collected	
Cardiovascular	*Urogenital*
Aorta	Kidneys
Heart	Urinary bladder
Digestive	Ovaries
Salivary gland(s)	Uterus
Tongue	Cervix
Esophagus	Vagina
Stomach	Testes
Small intestine	Epididymides
Duodenum	Prostate
Jejunum	Seminal vesicles
Ileum	*Endocrine*
Large intestine	Adrenals
Cecum	Pituitary
Colon	Thyroid/parathyroid
Rectum	*Skin/musculoskeletal*
Pancreas	Skin
Liver	Mammary gland

Respiratory	Skeletal muscle (thigh)
Trachea	Femur with articular surface
Larynx	*Nervous/special sense*
Lung with mainstem bronchus	Eyes with optic nerve
Lymphoid/hematopoietic	Sciatic nerve
Sternum with bone marrow	Brain
Thymus	Spinal cord – cervical
Spleen	Spinal cord – midthoracic
Lymph nodes	Spinal cord – lumbar
Mandibular	Lacrimal glands
Mesenteric	*Others*
	Gross findings
	Unique animal identifier (not for evaluation)

There is no histopathologic assessment intended for the preserved tissues on this study. If histopathologic assessment is considered required (at additional cost to the Sponsor), the appropriate information will be added to the protocol via amendment.

In-Life Observations and Measurements (Phase II Toxicokinetics, Groups 9–11)

1. Mortality/Morbidity

Frequency: Twice daily (a.m. and p.m.). Once prior to scheduled sacrifice. Each animal observed for evidence of death or impending death (as per _____SOP VET-14).

2. Clinical Observations

Frequency: Observations will be recorded as needed, but not reported.

3. Body Weight

Frequency: Body weights will be recorded for all animals prior to randomization/ selection, prior to each dose administration on Day 1 and Day 7.

4. Food Consumption

Frequency: Will not be recorded.

Toxicokinetics (Phase II, Groups 9–11)

1. **Blood Sampling**
   On Day 1 and Day 7, whole blood samples (approximately 0.5–1.0 mL/sample) will be collected from 3 animals/sex/group/timepoint in Groups 9–11 at the following timepoints:

PRE-DOSE	4 hours post-dose
1 hour post-dose	8 hours post-dose
2 hours post-dose	24 hours post-dose

The total volume collected, in consideration with other parameters that require blood collection, is not to exceed 1% of body weight for the animals during a 2-week period. Each animal will be bled no more than four times with the fourth bleed only occurring after anesthetization, immediately prior to euthanasia. Animals will be anesthetized by CO_2 inhalation immediately prior to each blood collection. Following the last scheduled blood collection, each animal will be euthanized by CO_2 asphyxiation. Blood samples will be collected by retro-orbital puncture into tubes containing K_2 EDTA. Following collection, blood samples will be chilled on ice. Blood samples will be spun in a refrigerated (2–8 °C) centrifuge (approximately 3000 rpm for approximately 10 minutes) to separate the plasma. Plasma samples will then be collected and stored frozen at −70 °C or lower.

2. **Bioanalytical Evaluation**
   Plasma samples will be shipped to and bioanalytical evaluation will be done under the direction of:

TBD targeted total

Number of samples:	216

Sample storage.

Conditions:	−70 °C or lower

Testing requirements:
Analytical methods:
Automated data.
Collection systems:

If any samples need to be reanalyzed, the Study Director will be notified, and details will be included in the bioanalytical report. If samples need to be evaluated for incurred sample reproducibility (ISR), the Principal Investigator will determine which samples will be tested and results will be noted in the bioanalytical report.

The bioanalytical report will be provided to the Study Director for inclusion as an appendix in the ____study report.

3. **Toxicokinetic Evaluation**
   Data from the bioanalytical evaluation will be provided to, and toxicokinetic evaluation will be done under the direction of:

   _____.

   Parameters examined: At least the following areas will be examined if feasible, AUC_{0-inf}, AUC_{0-last}, C_{max}, C_{last}, T_{last}, T_{max}, $T_{1/2,e}$
   Data evaluation.

   Software:

   The toxicokinetic report will be provided to the Study Director for inclusion as an appendix in the ____ study report.

Terminal Sacrifice (Phase II, Groups 9–11)

(a) *Scheduled Sacrifice*
   All animals will be euthanized by CO_2 asphyxiation on their scheduled day of blood collection and discarded properly without examination. Euthanasia will be ensured as outlined in SOP VET-16.

(b) *Unscheduled Sacrifice*
   Any animals sacrificed for humane reasons will be euthanized by CO_2 asphyxiation and discarded without examination. Euthanasia will be ensured as outlined in SOP VET-16.

Records and Reports

Data Collection and Analysis

In-life data (clinical observations, body weights, feeder weights, dose administration, and/or other related data) will be collected using Pristima version

6.3.2 or on paper when necessary. Hematology data will be collected using the Advia 120 Hematology analyzer. Coagulation data will be collected using the Diagnostica STA Compact Coagulation Analyzer. Clinical chemistry data will be collected using the AU480 Chemistry analyzer. Once collected on their respective instruments, hematology, coagulation, and clinical chemistry data will be transferred to Pristima version 6.3.2 via a validated interface. In the event of hardware or software maintenance, testing or malfunction or network connection issues, data will be collected on paper or on the appropriate clinical pathology instrument and then entered into Pristima version 6.3.2 at a later date. Necropsy data will be collected on paper and then entered into Pristima version 6.3.2. Any other data not collected online will be manually tabulated for inclusion in the report.

In-life data, clinical pathology data, and necropsy data will be tabulated and/or statistically evaluated using Pristima version 6.3.2.

Statistical evaluation will be performed on in-life, clinical pathology, and organ weight numerical data. The software will determine statistical significance by following a decision tree. First, the homogeneity of the data will be determined by Bartlett's test. If the data is homogeneous, a one-way analysis of variance will be performed to assess statistical significance. If statistically significant differences between the means are found, Dunnett's test will be used to determine the degree of significance from the control means ($p < 0.05$, $p < 0.01$ and $p < 0.001$). If the data is nonhomogeneous, the Kruskal-Wallis nonparametric analysis will be performed to assess statistical significance. If statistically significant differences between the means are found ($p < 0.05$, $p < 0.01$, and $p < 0.001$), the Mann-Whitney U-Test will be used to determine the degree of significance from the control means ($p < 0.05$, $p < 0.01$, and $p < 0.001$).

Storage of Records

Test article preparation, test article tracking, in-life data, clinical pathology data, necropsy data, protocol, protocol amendments (if applicable), slides, draft report(s), and the original final report generated as a result of this study will be archived at _____. After 2 years, the Sponsor will be contacted to determine final disposition of all study materials.

All bioanalytical and toxicokinetic data will be archived at.... _____ for 1 year.

Ninety days following the submission of the draft report, if there are no client comments generated by the Sponsor and/or Study Monitor, the Sponsor/Study Monitor will be notified, and the report may be finalized and archived according to the terms stated in the protocol.

Miscellaneous

Confidentiality Statement
The information contained herein is for the personal use of the intended recipient(s).

References
Gad, S. C. (Ed.). (2014). *Drug safety evaluation* (3rd ed.). Hoboken, NJ: Wiley.
Speid, L.H., Lumley, C.E., & Walker, S.R. (1990). Harmonization of guidelines for toxicity testing of pharmaceuticals by 1992. *Regulatory Toxicology and Pharmacology, 12,* 179–211.

Protocol Approval Signature

Study Director	Date
_____Laboratories, Inc.	
Scientific Management	Date
_____ Laboratories, Inc.	
IACUC	Date
_____ Laboratories, Inc.	
Study Monitor	Date

Appendix K: Regulatory Services

© Springer Nature Switzerland AG 2020
S. C. Gad et al., *Contract Research and Development Organizations-Their History, Selection, and Utilization*, https://doi.org/10.1007/978-3-030-43073-3

Vendor	Location	Phone #	Website	IND Preparation	NDA Preparation	Annual update preparation	Regulatory advisors	Additional services
Advanced Clinical Services	10 Parkway North Suite 350 Deerfield, IL 60015	(847) 267–1176	www. advancedclinical.com	X		X	X	QA, SAS
Agalloco and Associates	P.O. Box 899 Belle Mead, NJ 08502	(908) 874–7558	www.Agalloco.com		X			Validation, manufacturing
Alta Sciences	575 boul. Armand-Frappier Laval, Quebec, H7V 4B3 Canada	(450) 973–6077	www.altasciences. com				X	QA/QC, development
Allied Clinical Research	2485 Sunrise Boulevard Gold River, CA 95670	(916) 281–2262	www.alliedclinical. org	X				Phases II and III, method development
AON	200 East Randolph St. 12th floor Chicago, IL60601	(312) 381–1000	https://www.aon.com/ risk-services/ professional-services/ global-regulatory-compliance.jsp				X	
ArisGlobal, LLC	3119 Ponce de Leon Blvd. Coral Gables, FL 33134	(609) 360-4042	www.arisglobal.com				X	
Brand Institute, Inc.	200 SE first St. 12th floor Miami, FL 33131	(305) 374-2500	www.brandinstitute. com		X	X	X	Consulting, validation

Company	Address	Phone	Website				Notes
Cambridge Regulatory Services	2 Cabot House, Compass point Business Park St. Ives, PE27 5JL Cambridgeshire, United Kingdom	+44 (0) 1480 465 755	www.cambreg.co.uk			X	
Cardinal Health	7000 Cardinal Place Dublin, OH 43017	(614) 757–5000	www.cardinalhealth.com	X	X	X	Development (acquired Magellan Labs), stability, validation
CCS Associates	2001 Gateway Place Suite 350 W San Jose, CA 95110	(650) 691–4400	www.ccsainc.com	X		X	QA
Cerner	2800 Rock Creek Pkwy Kansas City, MO 64117	(866) 221–8877	www.cerner.com		X	X	Acquired Galt Associates LLC.
Certus International, Inc.	1422 Elbridge Payne Rd. Suite 200 Chesterfield MO 63017	(636) 519–1699	www.certusintl.com	X		X	Development, project management
Charles River	Morrisville, NC	(877) 274–8371	www.criver.com			X	(Inveresk was acquired by Charles River) Project management

(continued)

Vendor	Location	Phone #	Website	IND Preparation	NDA Preparation	Annual update preparation	Regulatory advisors	Additional services
Clinipace Clinical Research	3800 Paramount Pkwy, Suite 100 Morrisville, NC 27560	(919) 224–8800	www.clinipace.com				X	Programming, project management, QA/QC (acquired Paragon Biomedical)
Covance Inc.	210 Carnegie Center Princeton, NJ 08540	(888) 268–2623 (609) 452–4440	www.covance.com			X	X	Consulting
DrugLogic	934 Douglass Drive McLean, VA 22101	(800) 393–1313	www.druglogic.com		X			(Acquired RCN Associates, Inc.)
DXC Technology	1775 Tysons Blvd Tysons, VA 22102	(703) 245–9700	www.dxc.technology.com	X	X			BLA prep, consulting
EAS Consulting Group	1700 Diagonal Road Suite 750, Alexandria, VA 22314	(877) 327–9808	www.easconsultinggroup.com	X	X		X	Validation (acquired Phoenix Regulatory Associates, Ltd.)
EMMES Corporation	401 N.Washington St. Suite 700 Rockville, MD 20850	(301) 251–1161	www.emmes.com	X				QC, project management

Company	Address	Phone	Website				Specialty
eResearch Technology	1818 Market St. Suite 1000 Philadelphia, PA 19103	(215) 972–0420	www.ert.com	X			Development
EZ Associates	37 Falcon Way Washington, NJ 07882	(908) 531–8148	www.ezassociates.com	X		X	Development
Gad Consulting Services	4008 Barrett Dr. Raleigh, NC 27608	(919) 233–2926	www.gadconsulting.com	X	X	X	Development, IB
General Dynamics	3150 Fairview Park Dr. Falls Church, VA 22042	(703) 995–8700	www.gdit.com	X		X	
Health Decisions	2510 Meridian Parkway Suite 100 Durham, NC 27713	(919) 967–1111	www.healthdec.com			X	Project management
Icagen, Inc.	4222 Emperor Blvd. Suite 350 Durham, NC 27703	(919) 941–5206	www.icagen.com	X		X	Development
ICON Clinical Research	2100 Pennbrook Pkwy North Wales, PA 19454	(215) 616–3000	https://iconplc.com/		X		QA/QC, project management
IMIC	18 320 Franjo Rd. Palmetto Bay, FL 33157	(786) 310–7477	www.imicinc.com			X	QA/QC

(continued)

Vendor	Location	Phone #	Website	IND Preparation	NDA Preparation	Annual update preparation	Regulatory advisors	Additional services
JSS Medical Research	9400 Henri-Bourassa Blvd. West St. Laurent (Montreal) Quebec H45 1 N8	(514) 934–6116	www.jssresearch.com				X	Development
MAJARO InfoSystems, Inc.	2350 Mission College Blvd., Suite 700 Santa Clara, CA 95054	(408) 330–9400	www.majaro.com		X			Validation, project management
McCarthy Consultant Services, Inc.	14–320 Harry Walker pkwy., Newmarket, Ontario Canada L3Y 7B4	(905) 836–0033	www. mccarthyconsultant. com	X	X	X	X	Consulting, QA/QC
MEIRx RS	100 N. Brand Blvd. Suite 306 Glendale, CA 91203	(818) 552–2503	www.meirxrs.com				X	QA/QC
Medichem	Fructuós Gelabert, 6–8. 08970 Sant Joan Despí, Barcelona, Spain	+34 93 477 64 40	www.medichem.es	X				Develop, scale up
MEDISCRIBE, INC.	315 N. Academy St. Cary, NC 27513	(919) 467–2632	www.mediscribe.com	X	X		X	IB, development
Medpace LLC	5375 Medpace Way Cincinnati, OH 45227	(513) 579–9911	www.medpace.com		X		X	Project management, programming

Company	Address	Phone	Website				Services
MedSource Consulting, Inc.	16 902 El Camino Real, Suite 1A Houston, TX 77058	(281) 286–2003	www.medsource.com	X		X	Project management
MORIAH Consultants	21 380 Abigail Lane Huntington Beach, CA 92646	(714) 970–0790	www. moriahconsultants. com	X	X	X	BLA prep, consulting
Navitas Data Sciences	215 West Philadelphia Ave., Boyertown, PA 19512	(610) 970–2333	www.dataceutics.com		X	X	Validation, consulting, project management (acquired DataCeutics)
Nautic Partners, LLC	50 Kennedy Plaza 12th Floor Providence, RI 02903	(401) 278–5678	www.nautic.com	X			Project management
Nucro-Technics Inc.	2000 Ellesmere Rd. Unit #16 Scarborough, Ontario M1H 2 W4 Canada	(416) 438–6727	www.nucro-technics. com	X		X	QA/QC, stability
ORA Inc.	300 Brickstone Sq. Andover, MA 01810	(978) 685–8900	www.oraclinical.com	X			Project management
Parexel International	2520 Meridian Parkway Suite 200 Durham, NC 27713	(919) 544–3170	https://www.parexel. com/	X	X	X	Validation (acquired Liquent Inc.) BLA prep, consulting

(continued)

Vendor	Location	Phone #	Website	IND Preparation	NDA Preparation	Annual update preparation	Regulatory advisors	Additional services
PharmaLex	One Presidential Way Suite 109, Woburn, MA 01801	(617) 475–3470	www.pharmalex.com			X	X	Consulting, CTX prep, (acquired Wainwright Associates Ltd.)
PPD	929 North Front St. Wilmington, NC 28401	(910) 251–0081	www.ppdi.com	X			X	Project management
PRA Health Sciences	4130 Park Lake Ave. Suite 400 Raleigh, NC 27612	(919) 786–8200	www.prahs.com	X	X		X	Project management (acquired RPS), Programming, project management, QA/QC
PRS Inc. (Pharmaceutical Regulatory Services, Inc.	103 Carnegie Center Suite 103 Princeton, NJ 08540	(609) 799–0021	www. pharmregservices. com	X		X	X	Consulting
PSI International, Inc.	11 200 Waples Mill Road, Suite 200 Fairfax, VA 22030	(703) 352–8700	www.psiint.com			X	X	Consulting
Recruitech International	Now a staffing agency, delete this						X	Project management, QA/QC

Company	Address	Phone	Website					Services
Regulatory Affairs, North America, Inc.	Durham, NC 27717	(919) 949-4617	www.ranainc.com	X		X	X	Consulting, CTX prep, IB
Simbec Research Ltd.	Merthyr Tydfil Industrial Park, Merthyr Rd. Pentrebach, Merthyr Tydfil CF48 4DR, UK	+44-1685-700 870	www.researchuk.co.uk				X	Project management, phase 1
Smith Hanley Associates LLC	107 John St. second Floor Southport, CT 06890	(203) 319-4300	www.smithhanley.com		X			Programming, project management
SRI	333 Ravenswood Ave. Menlo Park, CA 94025	(650) 859-2000	www.sri.com	X				QA, pharmacokinetics
Syneos health	1030 Sync Street Morrisville, NC 27560	(919) 876-9300	www.syneoshealth.com	X	X		X	Project management, development (Kendle International and Pharmanet were acquired by Syneos Health) Phases II, III, IV
Target Health Inc.	261 Madison Ave. 24th Floor New York, NY 10016	(212) 681-2100	www.targethealth.com	X	X		X	Data management

(continued)

Vendor	Location	Phone #	Website	IND Preparation	NDA Preparation	Annual update preparation	Regulatory advisors	Additional services
TFS	212 Carnegie Center Suite 208 Princeton, NJ 08540	(609) 775–9500	www.tfscro.com	X	X			PLA prep, project management
TPIreg	3470 Superior Court Oakville, ON L6L0C4 Canada	(888) 420–5457	www.tpireg.com	X	X	X	X	Consulting, PLA prep
TRI (Technical Resources International, Inc.)	6500 Rock Spring Dr. Suite 650 Bethesda, MD 20817	(301) 564–6400	www.tech-res.com	X				
Waters	34 Maple St. Milford, MA 01757	(800) 252–4752	www.waters.com				X	Validation, project management, QA/QC

Appendix: Representative Contract Manufacturing Organizations (CMOs) for Small Molecule Active Pharmaceutical Ingredients (APIs)

Contract manufacturing organizations that are capable synthesizing small molecule drug candidates are numerous and subject to frequent mergers, reorganizations, and name changes. The following list is meant to be representative, but by no means comprehensive. No endorsement or value judgment is intended by the inclusion or exclusion of any CMO below. Additional CMOs can be found, for example, among the exhibitors at trade shows such as INFORMEX and ChemOutsourcing.

© Springer Nature Switzerland AG 2020
S. C. Gad et al., *Contract Research and Development Organizations-Their History, Selection, and Utilization*, https://doi.org/10.1007/978-3-030-43073-3

Company	Website	nonGMP	GMP			Location(s)			
			P1	P2	P3-C	US	Canada	Europe	Asia
A&C Your Global GMP Partner	www.acgpp.com				X		X	X	
Abbvie	www.abbviecontractmfg.com				X	X		X	
Acebright Pharmaceuticals Group	www.acebright.com								X
Adesis	adesisinc.com	X							
Affinity Research Chemicals, Inc.	www.affinitychem.com	X				X			
Agno Pharma	www.agnopharma.com	X	X	X					
Alcami	www.alcaminow.com	X	X	X	X	X			X
Almac Group ltd	www.almacgroup.com		X	X	X			X	
Ajinomoto Bio-Pharma	ajibio-pharma.com		X	X	X			X	X
AMRI	www.amriglobal.com	X	X	X	X	X			
Asymchem	www.asymchem.com	X	X	X	X				X
BCN Peptides	www.bcnpeptides.com		X	X	X				X
BioDuro	bioduro.com	X						X	
Cambrex Corporation	www.cambrex.com	X	X	X	X	X			
ChemCon	www.chemcon.com	X	X	X	X			X	
Chemic Laboratories, Inc	chemiclabs.com	X	X	X		X		X	
Chempacific Corporation	www.chempacific.com	X	X	X		X			X
Chemspec-API	www.chemspec-api.com	X	X	X		X			X

Company	Website							
Civentichem	www.civentichem.com	X						X
CM-Tec	www.cmtec-inc.com	X					X	
Corden Pharma	www.cordenpharma.com	X	X	X	X		X	X
DavosPharma	www.davos.com	X	X	X	X		X	X
Eurofins CDMO	www.eurofins.com/cdmo	X	X	X	X	X	X	X
Evotec	www.evotec.com	X	X	X	X			X
Fareva	www.fareva.com	X	X	X			X	X
Formosa Laboratories	www.formosalab.com	X	X	X	X	X	X	X
Hovione	www.hovione.com		X	X	X		X	
PharmaScience Ltd. Johnson Matthey	matthey.com	X	X	X	X		X	
J-Star Research Inc	www.jstar-research.com	X	X		X			
Kalexsyn	www.kalexsyn.com	X			X			X
Laurus Synthesis Inc.	www.laurussynthesis.com	X	X	X	X		X	X
Medicilon	www.medicilon.com	X	X		X			X
Neuland Laboratories Limited	www.neulandlabs.com	X	X	X				X
Novick Biosciences	novickbio.com	X					X	
Obiter Research	www.obires.com	X			X		X	
Olon Ricerca Biosciences	www.ricerca.com	X	X					
Patheon	patheon.com	X	X	X	X		X	
PCI Synthesis	www.pcisynthesis.com	X	X	X	X		X	X
Pfizer CentreOne	www.pfizercentreone.com	X	X	X				
PharmaBlock Inc.	www.pharmablock.com	X	X	X		X		X
Piramal Pharma Solutions	www.piramalpharmasolutions.com	X	X	X	X	X	X	X
PolyPeptide Group	www.polypeptide.com	X	X					

(continued)

Company	Website	nonGMP	GMP			Location(s)			
			P1	P2	P3-C	US	Canada	Europe	Asia
Regis Technologies Inc.	www.registech.com	X	X	X	X	X			
SAI Advantium	www.sailife.com	X	X	X					X
Sanofi Active Ingredient Solutions	www.activeingredientsolutions-sanofi.com		X	X	X			X	
ScinoPharm Taiwan, Ltd.	www.scinopharm.com		X	X	X				X
Siegfried	www.siegfried.ch	X	X	X	X	X			X
Solvias AG	www.solvias.com	X	X	X	X	X		X	X
STA Pharmaceutical Co., Ltd.	www.stapharma.com	X	X	X	X	X		X	X
Sterling Pharma Solutions	www.sterlingpharmasolutions.com	X	X	X	X	X		X	
Sundia MediTech	www.sundia.com	X							X
Syngene International Ltd	www.syngeneintl.com	X	X	X	X				X
Vagdevi InnoScience Private Limited (VISPL)	www.vispl.net	X							X
WuXi AppTec Lab Testing Division	www.wuxiapptec.com	X							X

nonGMP = Quality suitable for nonclinical/research purposes
P1 = Quality/capacity suitable for Phase 1
P2 = Quality/capacity suitable for Phase 2
P3-C = Quality/capacity suitable for Phase 3 to commercial
Websites accessed December 2019

Index

© Springer Nature Switzerland AG 2020
S. C. Gad et al., *Contract Research and Development Organizations-Their History, Selection, and Utilization*, https://doi.org/10.1007/978-3-030-43073-3

Printed in the United States
by Baker & Taylor Publisher Services